PREPECTORAL BREAST RECONSTRUCTION:
CURRENT TRENDS AND TECHNIQUES

胸肌前
乳房重建

主编 [英]拉格万·维迪亚（Raghavan Vidya）
　　 [美]希尔顿·贝克（Hilton Becker）
主译　丁志勇　赵海东　唐军

山东科学技术出版社
·济南·

First published in English under the title
Prepectoral Breast Reconstruction: Current Trends and Techniques
edited by Raghavan Vidya and Hilton Becker, edition: 1
Copyright © The Editor(s) (if applicable) and The Author(s), under exclusive license to Springer
Nature Switzerland AG, 2023
This edition has been translated and published under licence from
Springer Nature Switzerland AG.
Springer Nature Switzerland AG takes no responsibility and shall not be made liable for the accuracy
of the translation.
Simplified Chinese translation edition © 2025 by Shandong Science and Technology Press Co., Ltd.
版权登记号：图字 15-2023-156

图书在版编目（CIP）数据

胸肌前乳房重建 /（英）拉格万·维迪亚
(Raghavan Vidya),（美）希尔顿·贝克
(Hilton Becker) 主编；于志勇，赵海东，唐军主译.
济南：山东科学技术出版社, 2025.6. -- ISBN 978-7
-5723-2710-0

Ⅰ. R655.8

中国国家版本馆 CIP 数据核字第 2025D9T873 号

胸肌前乳房重建
XIONGJIQIAN RUFANG CHONGJIAN

责任编辑：李志坚
装帧设计：李晨溪

主管单位：	山东出版传媒股份有限公司
出 版 者：	山东科学技术出版社
	地址：济南市市中区舜耕路517号
	邮编：250003　电话：（0531）82098088
	网址：www.lkj.com.cn
	电子邮件：sdkj@sdcbcm.com
发 行 者：	山东科学技术出版社
	地址：济南市市中区舜耕路517号
	邮编：250003　电话：（0531）82098067
印 刷 者：	日照蓝图仕印务有限公司
	地址：山东省日照市莒县招贤镇罗庄二路西路3号
	邮编：276500　电话：（0633）7770369

规格：16开（184mm×260 mm）
印张：19.5　字数：410千
版次：2025年6月第1版　印次：2025年6月第1次印刷
定价：190.00元

主编

Raghavan Vidya
Birmingham University
The Royal Wolverhampton NHS Trust
Wolverhampton, UK

Hilton Becker
Charles E. Schmidt College of Medicine
Florida Atlantic University
Boca Raton, FL, USA

主　译：于志勇　赵海东　唐　军

副主译：刘兆芸　刘宪强　张　梅　李　彤

译　者：王　磊　王新昭　王福凯　卞晓丽　尹永硕
　　　　孔令禹　龙厚隆　田西朋　田照坤　冯志浩
　　　　刘　琪　刘文涛　刘在波　刘兆芸　刘岩青
　　　　刘宪强　刘晓宇　孙　政　孙芦浩　孙德峰
　　　　李　彤　李　栋　李　超　李小磊　宋　翔
　　　　宋书彬　张　良　张　梅　张思浩　陈晓洁
　　　　范杰后　赵海东　徐娜娜　唐　军　曹晓珊
　　　　霍志军

前言

胸肌前乳房重建是近年来整形外科领域最重要的发展趋势之一，为了进一步推动该领域的发展，Raghavan Vidya 和 Hilton Becker 编写了本书。

自 Cronin 和 Gerow 于 1962[1] 年首次实施假体置入术后，锐意进取的整形外科医师随即将这项美容技术拓展至乳腺癌治疗领域，并自然衍化出胸肌前内置物直接重建术。随着手术医师对血管分布问题的担忧，以及外形不规则及美学效果相关问题的凸显，乳房假体重建逐渐转向胸肌后假体重建及Ⅱ期重建，并在随后数十年里成了假体乳房重建的主流术式。

近年来，与功能及美学效果相关的争议再度激发了学界对胸肌前乳房重建术的热情。胸肌后重建可能加剧运动性畸形及软组织轮廓不规则问题。与此同时，保留乳头手术与预防性乳房切除术的广泛开展，对假体乳房重建术的形态与功能的平衡提出了更高要求。对兼具美学效果与功能协调性的乳房重建术的期待，促使学界再次关注将假体从有违解剖生理的肌下位置调整至更接近原始解剖结构的位置，即在胸肌前置入假体。乳房切除技术的演进（伴随更可靠的皮瓣技术的应用），也为此术式重焕生机奠定了基础。以 Vidya 及 Becker 为代表的先驱者在此术式的临床运用中发挥了引领作用，他们共同编写的本书汇集了目前关于胸肌前乳房重建术的最新研究成果与临床经验，具有非凡意义。

在本书一开始，Becker 阐明了胸肌前乳房重建的意义，深入分析了这一技术再获重视的深层逻辑。早在胸肌前假体置入乳房重建术成为潮流之前，Becker 便敏锐地意识到这一趋势并努力研发核心技术平台及配套术式（如美国圣巴巴拉 Mentor 公司生产的 Spectrum 假体、Becker 假体），为该技术成为主流奠定了坚实的基础。

本书的编写遵从严格的逻辑顺序，首先详尽阐释肿瘤学与胸肌前术式适应证的交叉领域，继而围绕核心技术（包括不同类型真皮基质与合成补片）论述该技术的合理性与先进性。后续章节系统剖析了多种可行的手术入路。值得注意的是，在胸肌前假体乳房重建再次成为主流技术前，已衍生了包括脂肪移植、直接假体置入、无补片/补片应用等多种改良技术。著者融合既往术式与胸肌前入路的创新成果，对近期技术走向进行了研判。尤为值得关注的是，在放疗背景下，此术式被视为规避胸肌后假体重建中传统畸形及组织移位问题的有效策略。Vidya及Becker也在本书中对该创新术式的手术规划、术式原理及异质性预后进行了全面阐述。

本书共25章，从多个角度详细介绍了胸肌前术式的要点。著者皆系深耕该领域研究且著作等身的著名学者，本书是他们丰富经验的系统总结，有助读者快速突破学习曲线。作为整形外科医师，我们必须不断创新与突破；欲达此目标，我们又必须以鉴往知来与学术共进为基石。Raghavan Vidya与Hilton Becker编写的《胸肌前乳房重建》对两者皆进行了全面诠释，为提高业者技术水平提供了有力的学术支撑。

John Kim MD, FACS
Professor, Division of Plastic and Reconstructive Surgery
Department of Surgery
Northwestern University Feinberg School of Medicine
Northwestern Medicine
Chicago, IL, USA
December 2022

序

在全球范围内，乳腺癌是女性最常见恶性肿瘤，治疗仍以手术为主，但生物学机制认识的深入不断推动治疗方式的革新。乳腺外科手术已由Halsted术式毁损性治疗发展为肿瘤整形与肿瘤美学手术，核心在于肿瘤外科原则与形体重建理念的统合。

乳房重建技术历经了复杂自体组织重建向简易假体重建的演变。胸肌前假体乳房重建术作为最新术式，以保留正常解剖结构为特征。之前的传统皮下假体重建术美学弊端显著，如假体皱褶外露、轮廓形态显露等。因此，假体置入位置逐渐转为胸肌后。近年来，随着运动性畸形、术后迁延性疼痛等问题频现，以及新型补片与假体材料的研发进展，胸肌前假体重建术再度引发学界关注。随着技术日臻成熟，对构建完整胸肌前假体乳房重建术的简明学术体系具有迫切需求。

本书旨在系统阐述胸肌前假体乳房重建术，重点解析当代技术发展动态。为此，对该领域权威先驱学者及既往研究者的卓著贡献表示诚挚感谢。本书编纂逾两载，承蒙所有撰稿者勠力同心，辅以出版团队及编审委员会鼎力相助，终得付梓，在此谨致谢忱。

Wolverhampton, UK	Raghavan Vidya
Boca Raton, FL, USA	Hilton Becker

致谢

在南非接受整形外科住院医师培训期间，笔者观察到非洲原住民采用连续性耳环悬挂实现耳郭组织渐进性扩张的独创方法并深受启发，由此对组织扩张理论尤其是Radovan式扩张器应用于乳房重建的理念产生了浓厚兴趣。

笔者联系Radovan医生后获赠其研发的扩张器并成功应用于临床，初期于改良根治术后将Radovan扩张器置入胸肌前间隙。学界曾推荐假体胸肌后置入方案以降低包膜挛缩发生率并增强假体覆盖效果。实践发现，Radovan扩张器于全肌层覆盖场景中尤具价值，可实现假体低张力置入及术后渐进式扩张。

部分病例因对扩张效果满意拒绝撤除Radovan扩张器的注射阀，促使笔者着手研发配置可拆卸注射阀的盐水扩张器，并进一步开发具备硅胶外壳的双腔室结构假体（Becker 50/50）。肌下重建术式实施数年后，笔者注意到患者群体普遍存在运动性畸形、不适及疼痛主诉。时值Loren Eskenazi医生采用Becker 50/50假体行肌上置入术，笔者视此改良为重要突破，并承袭其理念。然顾虑假体表面切口风险，遂以真皮瓣及脱细胞真皮基质（ADM）构建保护层，继而开启假体胸肌前置入及胸肌后置换实践，术后上述症状消失，整体美学效果获显著改善。

后于美国弗吉尼亚医学院完成第二次住院医师规范化培训期间，有幸师从Robert Diegelman教授研修创面愈合，聚焦组织再生理论与实践，并探索生物合成支架材料研发应用。

谨此向合著者Raghavan Vidya医生致以双重感谢：其一是诚邀笔者参加2017年6月英国伍尔弗汉普顿大学举办的"乳房外科创新与进展"学术会议，在会上双方就胸肌前乳房重建经验进行深入交流并产生编写此书的想法；其二是为该书付梓所贡献的学术智慧与不懈努力。

笔者衷心感谢转诊外科同仁及所有撰稿者贡献的精彩章节，其内容将对读者产生深远影响。

感恩父母谆谆教诲激励我投身医学事业，感谢家人鼎力支持，尤其是我的妻子 Janet——身兼手术第一助手，术中襄助对本项目推进功不可没。

谨向 Springer Verlag 编辑团队致以诚挚谢意。

Hilton Becker

笔者早年在印度一所具有 300 年历史的学术殿堂——Stanley 医学院接受外科培训，师从 CMK Reddy 与 Venkataswami 等著名学者，初涉整形外科领域即醉心于其融合功能复建与形体重塑的学术精要。普外硕士研读期间，Nityanand 与 Palanivel 言传身教，令笔者矢志追求外科技术的至臻之境。后于英国爱丁堡大学乳腺中心研修，幸得 Udi Chetty 医生激发乳腺外科从业志趣，又受 Mike Dixon 教授"少即是多"的理念影响，坚定了学术追求。后于 F. Fatah 与 G. Sterne 先生指导下接受肿瘤整形专科培训，从而深悟肿瘤安全保障与整形技术融合理念，两位先生创立的技术标准至今仍是职业典范。

胸肌后假体重建术式曾盛行一时，但笔者观察到术中对肌肉组织的破坏会导致患者术后运动性畸形及疼痛频发。同时，传统的皮下假体重建术存在较高的并发症发生率及明显的美学缺陷。随着预塑形基质材料的创新推广，以及与 Giorgio Berna 医生、Simon Cawthorn 先生、J. Masia 教授等欧洲同仁的通力合作，我们最终得以证实胸肌前乳房重建术的先进性。该术式因符合解剖保全理念，减少了对胸壁肌肉结构的破坏，获术后患者满意度高、并发症发生率低的积极反馈。经欧洲多中心临床论证后，该术式逐渐成为主流。

本团队通过解剖示教与临床实操培训课程面向业界同人及青年医师传道授业。虽然胸肌前假体乳房重建术已获临床成功证验且技术持续精进，但目前尚少系统阐述理论体系的专著。鉴于此，笔者携手 Becker 等编写了本书，以分享临床实践经验。

书稿付梓之际，谨向我的父亲（已故）Raghavan、母亲 Annapoorani、胞妹 Chitra 及妹夫 Vaidyanthan 致谢，感念家人殷切勉励；同时，感谢我的丈夫 S. Venkatachalam 与爱子 Abhinav 的鼎力支持，本书方得成稿。

感谢本书全体撰稿者无私分享经验，同时感谢 Holy Angels Convent 学校及 Adarsh Vidyalaya 学校诸位老师启蒙教诲。最后，谨以赤忱之心致敬广大病患及本书共同撰稿者，双方的参与乃学术成果成形之基。另外，特此鸣谢 Springer 出版社鼎力支持。

Raghavan Vidya

目 录

1 胸肌前乳房重建术的演变 …………………………………………… 1

2 乳房解剖学 ………………………………………………………… 11

3 乳腺癌肿瘤学分析：乳房切除与腋窝分期的必要性 ……………… 22

4 保留性乳房切除术的肿瘤学安全性及技术进展 …………………… 40

5 胸肌前乳房重建：选择标准与患者考量 …………………………… 53

6 保留皮肤和乳头乳房切除胸肌前重建中的腋窝分期 ……………… 59

7 组织灌注的重要性与乳房切除皮瓣的评估 ………………………… 75

8 胸肌前乳房重建术的补片与内置物选择 …………………………… 84

9 胸肌前假体乳房重建：预成型补片全覆盖 ………………………… 100

10 胸肌前内置物联合补片乳房重建术 ……………………………… 109

11 胸肌前覆盖乳房重建术 …………………………………………… 119

12 使用扩张器的胸肌前重建术 ……………………………………… 128

13 合成补片在胸肌前乳房重建中的应用 …………………………… 139

14 复合式胸肌前乳房重建：联合皮瓣与假体 ……………………… 152

15 无补片胸肌前乳房重建术 ………………………………………… 160

16 胸肌前皮肤缩减术式 ……………………………………………… 176

17 并发症：降低与管理 ……………………………………………… 186

18	Ⅰ期胸肌前乳房重建术后临床、组织学及超声随访观察	201
19	胸肌前假体与放疗	215
20	预期放疗时的胸肌前重建方案	230
21	胸肌前假体重建术中的脂肪移植增容	246
22	LOTUS 胸肌前乳房重建术	254
23	内镜辅助保留乳头和皮肤乳房切除术	262
24	胸肌前乳房重建：功能优势与成本－效益分析	276
25	生物合成支架在胸肌前重建中的应用	293

1 胸肌前乳房重建术的演变

编者：Hilton Becker, Raghavan Vidya, Simon Cawthorn
译者：王新昭

1.1 引言

在过去的几十年里，假体乳房重建技术得到了不断发展和创新。随着假体与生物补片技术的进步，目前已能够成功实施胸肌前或肌肉保护性乳房重建手术。通过回顾从胸肌前重建到胸肌后重建，再到基于假体的胸肌前重建这一演变历程，可深入理解推动生物医学创新与外科技术发展的关键并发症与临床问题，在实现最佳美容效果的同时将并发症风险降至最低。本章将对胸肌前乳房重建技术的发展历程进行了系统性回顾。

1.2 乳房假体

乳房假体的历史可追溯至1951年，Grindlay 与 Clagett 首次通过体内实验研究了聚乙烯醇合成海绵（Ivalon 海绵，Beverly Hills 外科器械公司生产）的应用[1]。随后，Pangman 对该材料进行改良，研制出复合型聚乙烯醇–聚乙烯假体。但无论采用何种改良方案，此类海绵材料均有相似的并发症，包括明显的包膜挛缩、乳房硬化及体积减小，并且多在置入后1年内发生[2]。直至1963年 Cronin 与 Gerow 推出硅凝胶假体，乳房增大手术才重新获得临床关注[3]。1965年，Arion Laboratories 公司进一步推出了盐水充注式假体[4]。随着假体技术的突破，乳房重建手术得以实现。早期术式将假体置于肌肉上方、乳房切除术后形成的皮瓣下方，即皮下或"胸肌前间隙"，但因并发症发生率较高，临床应用受限[5]。

H. Becker
Department of Surgery, Charles E. Schmidt College of Medicine, Boca Raton, FL, USA

Atlantic University, Boca Raton, FL, USA
e-mail: Hilton@beckermd.com

R. Vidya
Breast Department, The Royal Wolverhampton NHS Trust, Wolverhampton, UK
e-mail: Raghavan.Vidya@nhs.net

S. Cawthorn (✉)
Breast Care Centre, Southmead Hospital, Bristol, UK

© The Author(s), under exclusive license to Springer Nature Switzerland AG 2023
R. Vidya, H. Becker (eds.), *Prepectoral Breast Reconstruction*,
https://doi.org/10.1007/978-3-031-15590-1_1

1982年，Radovan首次报道应用组织扩张器（Radovan扩张器）进行乳房重建[6]。随后，Becker于1984年在Radovan技术上开发了可调节式乳房假体，其注射端口可拆卸设计使该装置兼具组织扩张与盐水假体的双重功能[7]。第二代此类假体改进为硅胶外腔结构[8]。随着内置注射端口式组织扩张器的问世，通过渐进性皮肤扩张弥补乳房切除术后的组织缺损，推动了组织扩张器在乳房重建中的应用。此后，学者们相继报道了不同质地、尺寸与形态的组织扩张器的应用经验。早期采用组织扩张器的乳房重建术多将扩张器置于皮下囊袋内（乳房切除术后皮瓣下方，胸大肌表面），该皮下入路操作简便且能保持胸大肌完整性，但存在假体移位、皱褶形成、皮肤破损后继发假体外露及包膜挛缩等并发症，以包膜挛缩多见[6]。

20世纪70年代，胸肌前间隙重建术因术后感染率高、瘢痕组织增生及偶发假体外露等问题逐渐被弃用。1981年，文献首次报道采用胸大肌全层覆盖联合前锯肌部分抬升的全肌下覆盖假体重建技术[9]。随着改良根治性乳房切除术中胸大肌保留技术的普及，学界提出了胸肌后重建可通过加强组织覆盖层为假体提供保护的理论。目前，选择肌下置入假体的原因包括乳房切除术后软组织覆盖不足（尤其大切口病例）、降低假体暴露风险等[10]。

脱细胞真皮基质（Acellular Dermal Matrix，ADM）的问世极大促进了胸肌后平面的应用，使之成为乳房重建的主流方式[11]。全肌层覆盖会导致假体发生压迫性变形和脂肪化，同时限制了假体尺寸选择。部分病例因无法完整分离下筋膜与肌瓣连续结构，需要离断肌肉后重新缝合固定，但该缝合稳定性欠佳，促使外科医生尝试采用各类补片加固肌瓣。

随着临床对胸肌后置入相关并发症（尤其是动态畸形）认识的深入，目前开始重新审视胸肌前术式，以避免形成动态畸形，减轻术后疼痛及缓解胸部紧缩感和肌肉痉挛[12,13]。Eskenazi等率先报道了在胸肌浅层可调节式假体的临床应用[14]。由于当时该术式尚未成为标准治疗方案，术者多持谨慎态度。值得注意的是，美国曾有外科医生因采用胸肌前术式遭起诉（指控其违反诊疗规范）但最终胜诉，激发了学界对该技术的关注。

1.3 脱细胞真皮基质（ADM）技术

生物力学工程的进步催生了ADM技术，该材料可通过在胸肌后构建更大的囊袋空间，实现更大体积的即刻假体重建，对称性与下极饱满度的改善显著提升了美学效果。研究证实，ADM在皮下平面可有效抑制假体下极包膜挛缩的发生，为此术式提供了理论依据。技术要点包括：离断胸大肌下缘附着点，将矩形ADM补片（最大20cm×10cm）缝合于离断肌缘下界，随后在肌下置入适配假体，并将ADM固定于乳房下皱襞上方的胸壁，从而完成I期假体重建。

ADM强化的胸肌后假体重建术可与乳房切除术同期实施，在保证良好的对称性、适度的下垂度及更优凸度的同时，因需广泛剥离胸大肌及部分前锯肌的肋骨附着点，会导致肌功能丧失；同时，损伤肋间神经外侧皮支，会引发急慢性疼痛[15]。此外，当胸肌收缩时，假体上方的乳房组织易出现形态扭曲，进而引发乳房动态畸形[16]。

意大利 Decomed 医疗公司在组织移植物领域取得突破性进展，其创新性外科重建方案提出在保留胸大肌的基础上，采用脱细胞真皮基质（ADM）完整包裹假体并置入皮下层。该术式的理论基础在于 ADM 材料与胸大肌下假体下极周围皮下组织整合过程中未观察到包膜挛缩现象。通过将硅胶假体置于肌肉表面而非深层，并以 ADM 网片完全包裹，不仅可优化乳房形态美学效果和患者舒适度，更能有效规避远期包膜挛缩风险。该创新术式配套的定型 ADM 网片被命名为 Braxon，为英文文胸（B.R.A.）与 ADM 包裹（X）及肌肉表面置入（ON）等关键要素的缩写组合。

Berna 等率先报道了应用 Braxon 脱细胞真皮基质（ADM）辅助胸肌前即刻假体置入乳房重建术的临床研究[17]，通过 25 例手术（平均随访 14 个月）对比了两种 ADM 材料：一种为预成型的猪源 ADM（厚 0.9 mm），需在术前行化学防腐剂冲洗处理；另一种为更薄（厚 0.6 mm）的无化学防腐剂 ADM，仅需生理盐水水化复温即可使用。研究最终选用后者（即 Braxon ADM）。结果显示，0.9 mm 厚 ADM 组的假体取出率为 12%，而 0.6 mm 无化学防腐剂 ADM 组未发生假体取出事件。

2017 年，Vidya 等研究证实，胸肌前乳房重建术具有良好的安全性、可行性及短期预后[18]。一项多中心回顾性分析针对 Braxon ADM 应用于胸肌前乳房重建进行研究，收集了 2014 年以来 6 年间 30 家欧洲中心开展的 1 450 例手术的数据[19]。结果显示，约 6.5% 病例因并发症需要取出假体，糖尿病、吸烟史、假体重量及免疫抑制状态是并发症的影响因素。包膜挛缩与术后放疗相关，但发生率较低（2.1%）。随着首个完全 ADM 包裹假体的创新应用，乳房切除术后即刻胸肌前重建术因为避免

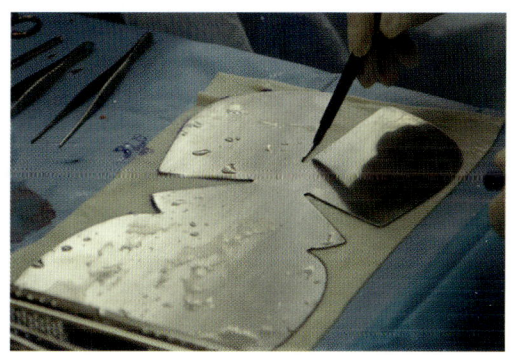

首款预成型 Braxon 网片（厚 0.9 mm）

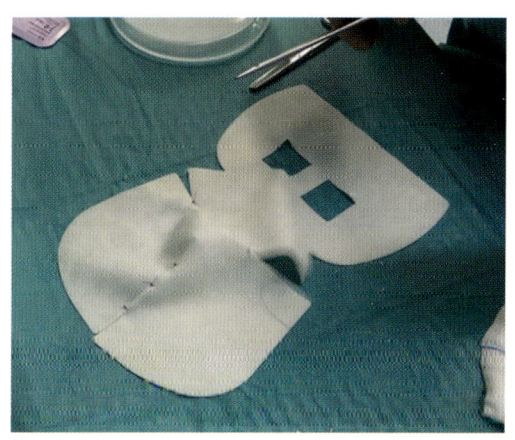

第二款预成型 Braxon 网片（厚 0.6 mm）

了术后疼痛及包膜挛缩等相关并发症而重新变得流行。随着在全球范围内乳房切除后的重建术从胸肌后转向胸肌前，诸多预防包膜挛缩的创新技术仍有待深入评估。

1.4 网片（ADM）与假体联合应用

由于胸肌筋膜可为假体提供充分支撑，胸肌前隆乳术逐渐普及。该术式消除了肌肉运动对假体的牵拉效应，进一步推动了胸肌前平面的临床应用。然而，乳房重建患者因筋膜缺失，需使用脱细胞真皮基质（ADM）替代筋膜进行前方覆盖，使胸肌前重建术成为可行方案[20]。随着保留皮肤及乳头、乳晕的乳房切除术（NSM/SSM）的推广，外科医师多采用乳房下皱襞切口或垂直切口进行手术。针对直接位于 ADM 上方的垂直切口的潜在风险，可将外侧皮瓣部分去表皮处理后内折覆盖于内侧皮瓣下方，从而在 ADM 表面形成额外组织层。

在胸肌前重建术中，ADM 可为软组织提供一定的支撑作用。应用方法主要包括两种：前包裹法，将 ADM 缝合固定于乳房囊袋上缘，随后固定内侧及外侧边缘，最后将假体与 ADM 下缘缝合以确保其在囊袋内稳定贴合[21]；全包裹法，按假体/扩张器尺寸裁剪 ADM 并固定于乳房下皱襞（IMF），随后将假体/扩张器置于胸肌表面并完全包裹 ADM。该技术由 Sbitany 等[22]首次描述，但研究显示其假体取出率、皮瓣坏死率、包膜挛缩率、波纹征及血清肿发生率较高[23]。Vidya 等（2017）对 100 例乳房的研究证实，胸肌前重建术安全可行，短期预后良好，在美学效果及患者满意度方面表现优异[18]。

2015 年，Becker 提出采用垂直切口联合网片/基质支撑的单阶段胸肌前即刻乳房重建术，采用光面可调节生理盐水假体，取得了良好美学效果且并发症发生率低。由于在胸肌前置入假体时切口直接位于假体上方，外科医师常采用去表皮皮瓣或网状 ADM 覆盖来保护假体[24]。乳房切除术的垂直切口设计可使外侧皮瓣部分去表皮化，从而实现更安全的水密性闭合。需要注意的是，该术式可能增加网片相关血清肿、感染风险及手术成本，并延长手术时间[25]。

为减少血清肿的发生，对 ADM 常进行网格化或开窗处理，以促进快速整合并改善液体引流[24]。与非网状 ADM 相比，网状 ADM 可减少术后引流量并缩短引流管留置时间[26]。Vidya 等于 2019 年提出，理想网片应具备低炎症反应、快速整合、易塑形、高强度和成本效益等特性[27]。ADM 可通过开窗或网格化处理来提升其顺应性[28]。

鉴于 ADM 成本较高且存在发生血清肿及感染的风险，外科医师开始探索使用合成网片。2014 年，Casella 等研究表明，钛涂层聚丙烯合成网片用于皮下两阶段重建术安全可行，末次假体置入后中位随访 14 个月显示患者满意度极佳[28]。其他可应用网片包括可吸收网片（薇乔）及长效可吸收网片（T.I.G.R. Phasix）[12, 29]。近期研究的新型单丝 P.D.S. 网片（Durasorb）

初步结果良好[30]。

1.5 胸肌前假体直接置入乳房重建

两阶段假体重建是目前最常用的乳房重建方式，即初期置入组织扩张器或可调节假体，Ⅱ期更换为定容假体。传统乳房切除术常因皮肤覆盖不足需要组织扩张，而现代保皮技术可保留充足的皮肤[31]。2019 年，Jones 证实了单阶段胸肌前直接假体重建术的先进性、安全性及可重复性[32]。

胸肌前重建初期需通过 SPY 荧光成像来评估皮瓣血供，确认条件理想后即刻置入硅胶假体。聚氨酯泡沫涂层硅凝胶假体于 20 世纪 70 年代问世，但在 1991 年因对潜在毒性的担忧而不再在美国应用，在其他地区仍广泛应用。2006 年，Handel 等研究证明，此类假体可降低包膜挛缩风险，安全性与其他硅凝胶假体相当[33]。2015 年，Castel 等研究发现，假体聚氨酯涂层量与包膜挛缩发生率呈负相关[34]。Roy de Vita 率先将聚氨酯涂层假体应用于胸肌前重建[35]。

1.6 脂肪移植

脂肪移植之前用于改善假体与胸壁交界处的阶梯状畸形[36]，亦常用于组织扩张后假体置入阶段，优势在于可将脂肪延迟移植至假体包膜浅层的皮下平面。现有证据表明脂肪移植可促进胸壁愈合，并可能在组织扩张期通过稳定来逆转软组织损伤[37]。

对于存在放疗史、皮瓣菲薄脆弱、乳房明显下垂及超重等非理想条件患者，胸肌前单阶段即刻重建可替代胸肌后假体置入或延期手术，在初期置入扩张器可避免血管损伤[38]。具体操作中，使可调节假体部分充气来发挥占位作用，防止皮瓣与深层肌肉粘连，并避免对皮肤皮瓣（尤其生理盐水积聚的下极）形成压迫。假体充气促使皮瓣增厚上提，从而无须切除皮肤并减少脱细胞真皮基质（ADM）的使用。随访期间通过逐步注气调整乳房形态，待达到预期体积后以生理盐水替换气体[31]。

2020 年的一项研究发现，对于乳房肥大伴下垂患者，保留乳头、乳晕的乳房切除术联合胸肌前重建与即刻乳房悬吊术可获得良好效果，但须完善术前规划、术中皮瓣评估，以降低并发症风险[39]。

1.7 胸肌前间隙乳房重建发展历程年表

主题	作者	时间
胸肌前生理盐水填充组织扩张器[6]	Radovan	1982
胸肌前即刻乳房重建术（应用 Becker 50 假体）[14]	Eskenazi	2007
胸肌前即刻乳房重建术（应用预成型 Braxon 网片）[17]	Berna	2014
胸肌前与皮下重建对比研究（应用钛环 Bra 网片）[29]	Casella	2014
垂直切口胸肌前即刻重建术（联合真皮皮瓣）[25]	Becker	2015

（续表）

主题	作者	时间
胸肌前重建术（联合 ADM 与减容真皮皮瓣）[52]	Caputo	2016
胸肌前假体重建术：理论基础与适应证[40]	Sigalove	2017
Braxon 网片全包裹技术[27]	Vidya	2017
胸肌前即刻乳房重建术：一种安全替代方案[22]	Sbitany	2017
胸肌前重建术（应用充气式组织扩张器）[38]	Becker	2017
胸肌前乳房重建术综述[21]	Ter Louw	2017
胸肌前直接假体重建术（联合吲哚菁绿血管造影）[41]	Jones	2017
胸肌前重建术（应用牛源 ADM）[24]	Schefan	2018
胸肌前可吸收薇乔网片囊袋重建术[12]	Gfrerer	2018
胸肌前重建术与欠充填扩张器组织收缩效应[31]	Becker	2018
胸肌前直接假体重建术[32]	Jones	2019
胸肌前聚氨酯涂层假体直接置入术[35]	de Vita	2019
胸肌前重建术并发症综述[13]	Wagner	2019
非理想患者胸肌前重建（应用间隔物）[42]	Becker	2019
胸肌前直接假体重建术风险分析[43]	Nealon	2020

1.8 放疗

乳房切除术后行放疗放疗是假体重建术的重要风险因素，可导致包膜挛缩、重建失败[44, 45]。研究显示，放疗后胸肌后组的包膜挛缩发生率显著高于胸肌前组（52.2% : 16.1%）[45]。在 Ⅱ 期重建中，接受放疗后胸肌后组的双平面扩张器移位率高于胸肌前组，其机制与放疗诱导的胸大肌纤维化挛缩有关。胸肌前重建术可避免此类移位。

1.9 胸肌前乳房重建的优势

胸肌前重建的主要优势在于显著减轻术后疼痛，减少静脉及口服阿片类镇痛药物使用[28, 40]。多项早期回顾性研究证实了该优势，可能与术式无须行胸肌后分离及软组织重塑、操作创伤更小有关。在当前阿片类药物滥用危机背景下，该术式对提升患者安全性与改善社会医疗环境具有积极意义[46]。

研究显示，该术式可缩短平均住院时间（从 2~3 天降至 1~2 天）[40, 47]，并且不同术式均能明显缩短实际手术时间。此优势源于术中可在乳房切除同时于后台预置 ADM 包裹的扩张器/假体，同时无须制备胸肌后囊袋也进一步节省了手术时间。长期获益包括消除假体动态畸形，减轻胸壁不适与疼痛，改善肩关节活动度及降低相关并发症发生率[48]。

1.10 胸肌前乳房重建术的特异性并发症

包膜挛缩是该术式最常见的并发症，近期综述显示其发生率约为9%[13]。使用脱细胞真皮基质（ADM）可使包膜挛缩率降至2%，显著低于非ADM组的12%。ADM应用与红乳房综合征相关，后者的特征为ADM表面区域红斑，被认为继发于淋巴水肿及淋巴管阻塞，发生率为6%~7%。研究显示，ADM的使用与较高的假体取出率、感染发生率及乳房切除术后皮瓣坏死风险相关[13]。红乳房综合征通常可随时间缓解，多行保守治疗即可，若持续存在则应取出ADM及假体[49]。

皮瓣或乳头坏死是胸肌前重建术的潜在并发症，多因菲薄受损的皮瓣直接受压导致灌注障碍引发[43]。术中采用吲哚菁绿组织灌注评估等皮瓣活性检测技术可有效预防。

感染是假体重建术的常见问题，可能导致假体取出，可通过抗生素、限制手术室人员流动及对腔隙进行冲洗来处理。重建前遗留的较大皮下囊袋可能增加术后血肿/血清肿风险，充分止血和放置引流管有助于降低此类风险[13]。

与胸肌后重建相比，胸肌前重建因乳房上极软组织覆盖较薄更易出现假体皱褶，但新型全壳高填充假体的使用可使该现象的出现率明显降低[22]。在Ⅱ期重建中，组织扩张器或可调节假体应欠充填至预期终末假体体积，以减少皱褶。在乳房切除的皮瓣上极处行脂肪移植，和/或使用ADM、合成网片，可有效改善皱褶[47]。术前应告知接受胸肌前直接假体重建的患者，可能需Ⅱ期脂肪移植以覆盖假体来处理皱褶和假体显形问题。

1.11 小结

乳房重建已从传统胸肌后技术发展为新的胸肌前假体重建术及保留肌肉的重建术。随着对胸肌后假体置入相关并发症认知的深化，胸肌前重建术在经历多次改良后效果显著改善。乳房假体的技术革新为隆乳与乳房重建提供了重要支撑，而精准的软组织评估技术（如吲哚菁绿血管造影）与脱细胞真皮基质（ADM）的应用进一步提升了胸肌前重建的安全性及美学效果。未来研究应聚焦于优化材料性能，降低并发症风险，同时探索个体化重建策略以满足不同患者需求。

参考文献

1. Grindlay JH, Waugh JM. Plastic sponge which acts as a framework for living tissue. Arch Surg. 1951,63:288–97. https://doi.org/10.1001/archsurg.1951.01250040294003.
2. Pangman WJ, Wallace RM, Hills B. The use of plastic prosthesis in breast plastic and other soft tissue surgery. West J Surg Obstet Gynecol. 1955,63:503–12.
3. Cronin T, Gerow FG. Augmentation mammaplasty: a new natural feel prosthesis. Transact III Internat Congr Plast Surg. 1964,51(2):41–9. https://doi.org/10.1016/S0039–6109(16)39388–4.
4. Arion HG. Retromammary prosthesis. C R Soc Fr Gynecol. 1965,5

5. Peters W. The evolution of breast implants. Can J Plast Surg. 2002,10(5):223–36.
6. Radovan C. Breast reconstruction after mastectomy using the temporary expander. Plast Reconstr Surg. 1982,69(2):195–208. https://doi.org/10.1097/00006534-198202000-00001.
7. Becker H. Breast reconstruction using an inflatable breast implant with detachable reservoir. Plast Reconstr Surg. 1984,73(4):678–83. https://doi.org/10.1097/00006534-198404000-00031. PMID: 6709750
8. Becker H. The expandable mammary implant. Plast Reconstr Surg. 1987,79(4):631–7.
9. Apfelberg DB, Laub DR, Maser MR, Lash H. Submuscular breast reconstruction—indications and techniques. Ann Plast Surg. 1981,7(3):213–21.
10. Glasberg SB, Light D. AlloDerm and Strattice in breast reconstruction: a comparison and techniques for optimising outcomes. Plast Reconstr Surg. 2012,129:1223–33. https://doi.org/10.1097/PRS.0b013e31824ec429.
11. Bloom JA, Patel K, Cohen S, Chatterjee A, Homsy C. Prepectoral breast reconstruction: an overview of the history, technique, and reported complications. Open Access Surg. 2020,13:1–9. https://doi.org/10.2147/OAS.S201298.
12. Gfrerer L, Liao EC. Technique refinement in prepectoral implant breast reconstruction with vicryl mesh pocket and acellular dermal matrix support. Plast Reconstr Surg Glob Open. 2018,6(4):e1749. https://doi.org/10.1097/GOX.0000000000001749. Published 2018 Apr 9
13. Wagner RD, Braun TL, Huirong Z, Winocour S. A systematic review of complications in prepectoral breast reconstruction. J Plast Reconstr Aesthet Surg. 2019,72(7):1051–9. https://doi.org/10.1016/j.bjps.2019.04.005.
14. Eskenazi LB. New options for immediate reconstruction: achieving optimal results with adjustable implants in a single stage. Plast Reconstr Surg. 2007,119:28–37.
15. Ducic I, Seiboth LA, Iorio ML. Chronic postoperative breast pain: danger zones for nerve injuries. Plast Reconstr Surg. 2011,127:41–6.
16. Spear SL, Schwartz J, Dayan JH, Clemens MW. Outcome assessment of breast distortion following submuscular breast augmentation. Aesthet Plast Surg. 2009,33:44–8.
17. Berna G, Cawthorn SJ, Papaccio G, Balestrieri N. Evaluation of a novel breast reconstruction technique using the Braxon® acellular dermal matrix: a new muscle-sparing breast reconstruction. ANZ J Surg. 2014,87(6):493–8. https://doi.org/10.1111/ans.12849. Epub 2014 Sep 29
18. Vidya R, Masia J, Cawthorn S, et al. Evaluation of the effectiveness of the prepectoral breast reconstruction with Braxon dermal matrix: first multicenter European report on 100 cases. Breast J. 2017,23(6):670–6. https://doi.org/10.1111/tbj.12810.
19. Masià J, iBAG Working Group. The largest multicentre data collection on prepectoral breast reconstruction: The iBAG study. J Surg Oncol. 2020,122(5):848–60.
20. Antony AK, Poirier J, Madrigano A, Kopkash KA, Robinson EC. Evolution of the surgical technique for "breast in a day" direct-to-implant breast reconstruction: transitioning from dual-plane to prepectoral implant placement. Plast Reconstr Surg. 2019,143(6):1547–56. https://doi.org/10.1097/PRS.0000000000005627.
21. Ter Louw RP, Nahabedian MY. Prepectoral breast reconstruction. Plast Reconstr Surg. 2017,140:51S–9S. https://doi.org/10.1097/PRS.0000000000003942.
22. Sbitany H, Piper M, Lentz R. Prepectoral breast reconstruction: a safe alternative to submuscular prosthetic reconstruction following nipple-sparing mastectomy. Plast Reconstr Surg. 2017,140(3):432–43. https://doi.org/10.1097/PRS.0000000000003627.
23. Nadeem R. Prepectoral implant-based breast reconstruction complete acellular dermal matrix wrap or anterior circumferential cover. Breast J. 2018,24(2):223–4. https://doi.org/10.1111/

tbj.12881. Epub 2017 Aug 1. PMID: 28763153

24. Scheflan M, Grinberg-Rashi H, Hod K. Bovine acellular dermal matrix in immediate breast reconstruction: a retrospective, observational study with SurgiMend. Plast Reconstr Surg. 2018,141:1e–10e.

25. Becker H, Lind JG 2nd, Hopkins EG. Immediate implant-based prepectoral breast reconstruction using a vertical incision. Plast Reconstr Surg Glob Open. 2015,3(6):e412. https://doi.org/10.1097/GOX.0000000000000384. Published 2015 Jul 8

26. Fabrizio T, Serio S, Massariello D, Vestita M, Simeon V. The meshed biological matrix in immediate, definitive breast reconstruction. J Plast Reconstr Aesthet Surg. 2019,72(1):137–71. https://doi.org/10.1016/j.bjps.2018.09.004. Epub 2018 Sep 23. PMID: 30291046

27. Vidya R, Iqbal FM. A guide to prepectoral breast reconstruction: a new dimension to implant-based breast reconstruction. Clin Breast Cancer. 2017,17(4):266–71. https://doi.org/10.1016/j.clbc.2016.11.009. Epub 2017 Jan 9. P.M.I.D.: 28190760

28. Vidya R, Berna G, Sbitany H, et al. Prepectoral implant-based breast reconstruction: a joint consensus guide from U.K., European and U.S.A. breast and plastic reconstructive surgeons. Ecancermedicalscience. 2019, 13:927. Published 2019 May 7. https://doi.org/10.3332/ecancer.2019.927.

29. Casella D, Bernini M, Bencini L, et al. Ti-Loop® bra mesh used for immediate breast reconstruction: comparison of retro pectoral and subcutaneous implant placement in a prospective single-institution series. Eur J Plast Surg. 2014,37(11):599–604. https://doi.org/10.1007/s00238-014-1001-1.

30. Becker H, Lind JG. The use of synthetic mesh in reconstructive, revision, and cosmetic breast surgery. Aesthetic Plast Surg. 2013,37:914–21. https://doi.org/10.1007/s00266-013-0171-8.

31. Becker H, Zhadan O. Tissue contraction-a new paradigm in breast reconstruction. Plast Reconstr Surg Glob Open. 2018,6(7):e1865. Published 2018 Jul 13. https://doi.org/10.1097/GOX.0000000000001865.

32. Jones G, Antony AK. Single-stage, direct-to-implant prepectoral breast reconstruction. Gland Surg. 2019,8(1):53–60. https://doi.org/10.21037/gs.2018.10.08.

33. Handel N, Gutierrez J. Long-term safety and efficacy of polyurethane foam-covered breast implants. Aesthet Surg J. 2006,26(3):265–74. https://doi.org/10.1016/j.asj.2006.04.001. P.M.I.D.: 19338905

34. Castel N, Soon-Sutton T, Deptula P, Flaherty A, Parsa FD. Polyurethane-coated breast implants revisited: a 30-year follow-up. Arch Plast Surg. 2015,42(2):186–93. https://doi.org/10.5999/aps.2015.42.2.186. Epub 2015 Mar 16. PMID: 25798390; PMCID: PMC4366700

35. De Vita R, Buccheri EM, Villanucci A, Pozzi M. Breast reconstruction actualized in nipple-sparing mastectomy and direct-to-implant, prepectoral polyurethane positioning: early experience and preliminary results. Clin Breast Cancer. 2019,19(2):e358–63. https://doi.org/10.1016/j.clbc.2018.12.015. Epub 2018 Dec 27. P.M.I.D.: 30691930

36. Kanchwala SK, Glatt BS, Conant EF, Bucky LP. Autologous fat grafting to the reconstructed breast: the management of acquired contour deformities. Plast Reconstr Surg. 2009,124(2):409–18. https://doi.org/10.1097/PRS.0b013e3181aeeadd. P.M.I.D.: 19644255

37. Hammond DC, O'Connor EA, Scheer JR. Total envelope fat grafting: a novel approach in breast reconstruction. Plast Reconstr Surg. 2015,135(3):691–4. https://doi.org/10.1097/PRS.0000000000000968.

38. Becker H, Zhadan O. Filling the spectrum expander with air-a new alternative. Plast Reconstr Surg Glob Open. 2017,5(10):e1541. Published 2017 Oct 25. https://doi.org/10.1097/GOX.0000000000001541.

39. Manrique OJ, Arif C, Banuelos J, Abu-Ghname A, Martinez-Jorge J, Tran NV. Prepectoral breast reconstruction in nipple-sparing mastectomy with immediate mastopexy. Ann Plast Surg. 2020,85(1):18–23. https://doi.org/10.1097/SAP.0000000000002136. P.M.I.D.: 31855861

40. Sigalove S, Maxwell GP, Sigalove NM, Storm-Dickerson TL, Pope N, Rice J, Gabriel A. Prepectoral implant-based breast reconstruction: rationale, indications, and preliminary results. Plast Reconstr Surg. 2017,139(2):287–94. https://doi.org/10.1097/PRS.0000000000002950. P.M.I.D.: 28121858

41. Jones G, Yoo A, King V, et al. Prepectoral immediate direct-to-implant breast reconstruction with anterior AlloDerm coverage. Plast Reconstr Surg. 2017,140(6S):31S–8S. https://doi.org/10.1097/PRS.0000000000004048.

42. Becker H, Mathew PJ. Immediate prepectoral breast reconstruction in suboptimal patients using an air-filled spacer. Plast Reconstr Surg Glob Open. 2019,7(10):e2470. https://doi.org/10.1097/GOX.0000000000002470. PMID: 31772895; PMCID: PMC6846304

43. Nealon KP, Weitzman RE, Sobti N, Gadd M, Specht M, Jimenez RB, Ehrlichman R, Faulkner HR, Austen WG Jr, Liao EC. Prepectoral direct-to-implant breast reconstruction: safety outcome endpoints and delineation of risk factors. Plast Reconstr Surg. 2020,145(5):898e–908e. https://doi.org/10.1097/PRS.0000000000006721. PMID: 32332523

44. Elswick SM, Harless CA, Bishop SN, Schleck CD, Mandrekar J, Reusche RD, Mutter RW, Boughey JC, Jacobson SR, Lemaine V. Prepectoral implant-based breast reconstruction with postmastectomy radiation therapy. Plast Reconstr Surg. 2018,142(1):1–12. https://doi.org/10.1097/PRS.0000000000004453. P.M.I.D.: 29878988

45. Sinnott CJ, Persing SM, Pronovost M, Hodyl C, McConnell D, Young AO. Impact of postmastectomy radiation therapy in prepectoral versus subpectoral implant-based breast reconstruction. Ann Surg Oncol. 2018,25(10):2899–908. https://doi.org/10.1245/s10434-018-6602-7.

46. Glasberg SB. The economics of Prepectoral breast reconstruction. Plast Reconstr Surg. 2017,140:49S–52S. https://doi.org/10.1097/PRS.0000000000004051.

47. Salibian AA, Frey JD, Choi M, Karp NS. Subcutaneous implant-based breast reconstruction with acellular dermal matrix/mesh: a systematic review. Plast Reconstr Surg Glob Open. 2016,4(11):e1139.

48. Kim SE. Prepectoral breast reconstruction. Yeungnam Univ J Med. 2019,36(3):201–7. https://doi.org/10.12701/yujm.2019.00283.

49. Nahabedian MY. Prosthetic breast reconstruction and red breast syndrome: demystification and a review of the literature. Plast Reconstr Surg. 2019,7(5):e2108. https://doi.org/10.1097/GOX.0000000000002108.

2 乳房解剖学

编者：Robert D. Rehnke
译者：王福凯

2.1 引言

智慧和知识的来源不同。文艺复兴时期前，以希波克拉底、盖伦等先贤的典籍为代表的权威性知识主导医学体系，其真理性鲜受质疑。安德烈亚斯·维萨里被誉为现代医学之父，通过解剖研究人体结构，并于1543年出版了《人体构造》(《De Humani Corporis Fabrica Libri Septem》，下卷)[1]，这种基于观察与实践的实证知识奠定了现代医学的科学基础。

外科医师的知识体系兼具双重属性：通过学习获得的权威性知识，和通过临床观察积累的实证经验。面对人体解剖这一复杂领域，二者缺一不可。借助上述二者，医学生才有可能理解人体庞杂的原始数据。本章融合经典文献与笔者二十余年手术经验，以"乳房浅筋膜系统"重新诠释乳房解剖结构。

通过文字来描述解剖学知识很困难。为此，本文引入类比来阐释乳房解剖层级结构：乳房组织犹如置于"床垫"(被深筋膜被覆的胸肌)上的"羽绒枕"，"枕芯"(外胚层来源的细胞群)包裹于"拉链式枕套"(含包膜的乳腺本体)内，整体再嵌套于"浅筋膜枕套"中。该"枕套–床垫"系统由"床架"(胸廓)支撑的。这一模型为后续精细解剖描述提供框架支撑。

2.2 乳房浅筋膜系统

2.2.1 基础体节

胚胎发育第3周初，囊胚期形成的胚盘已具备外胚层、中胚层与内胚层三重结构[2]。至第3周末，胚盘逐渐演化为管状结构，具备头、尾两端及背、腹两面：背侧形成神经管，腹侧形成原始前肠、中

Supplementary Information The online version contains supplementary material available at https://doi.org/10.1007/978-3-031-15590-1_2. The videos can be accessed individually by clicking the DOI link in the accompanying figure caption or by scanning this link with the SN More Media App.

R. D. Rehnke (✉)
Private Practice Plastic Surgery, The Center for Surgical Excellence, St. Petersburg, FL, USA

© The Author(s), under exclusive license to Springer Nature Switzerland AG 2023
R. Vidya, H. Becker (eds.), *Prepectoral Breast Reconstruction*,
https://doi.org/10.1007/978-3-031-15590-1_2

肠与后肠。此时，中胚层于胚胎纵轴两侧，形成成对的板层结构，随后从头端至尾端分节形成中胚层体节（体节）。若非脑与心脏快速发育，胚胎外形近似蠕虫。这种抽象化的基础管状结构衍生出"基础体节"概念，对理解解剖结构排布具有重要价值。随着分化的进展，四肢与器官依其沿管状体节的定位发育。例如，乳房源于基础体节头端腹侧面细胞群。宏观视角下，胸廓呈管状；若聚焦局部，前胸壁与乳房初为脂肪平面。胚胎组织发育的知识可揭示成体器官排布规律，而成体乳房的实证观察亦可反证胚胎发育认知。值得注意的是，胸腹结构具有同源基础体节模式，故胸部诸多结构可视为腹部结构的同源衍生物（腹部可视为简化版胸部）。例如，胸壁结构可视为腹壁的衍生形态，其腹侧中线以骨性胸骨替代腹白线，腹中线两侧成对的腹直肌在胸部演化为胸肌（其止点延伸至上肢），腹部斜肌的同源结构在胸部分化为肋间肌与肋骨复合体。

腹胸部皮肤与深部肌筋膜间的软组织呈水平层状排列，由垂直走行的皮肤支持带（又称皮肤悬韧带或浅筋膜支持带）维持结构抗剪切稳定性。乳房区域的此类支持带即著名的Cooper韧带[3]。腹部浅筋膜的经典分层（Camper筋膜与Scarpa筋膜）为人所熟知，而胸部前、后层浅筋膜实为其同源结构[4]。鲜为人知的是，浅筋膜系统实为多层水平层叠结构，其排布具有分形特征——相同组织与细胞排列模式可在不同尺度呈现自相似性。因功能需求差异，身体特定区域筋膜层增厚并被命名，而其他区域则隐匿难辨[5]。这种水平筋膜层与细胞层通过垂直支持带（纤维与水平面呈90°交联）相连的架构形似绗缝织物结构。浅筋膜系统概念最早由维萨里提出，他将其描述为"肉膜"，认为该膜贯穿全身皮肤与肌肉，于胸部包裹乳腺组织。维萨里在论及乳房时写道："此刻我们可展示乳房的构造……"[1]

文艺复兴时期的解剖学家将人体结构视为连续交织的膜系结构，这与19世纪盛行的还原论观点截然不同。直至1842年，Astley Cooper爵士的乳房解剖学专著方对浅筋膜系统做出了更详尽的描述："皮肤被毛发覆盖；其下为脂肪及悬韧带；前、后筋膜间夹裹腺体……"其所述的"悬韧带"即垂直支持带，后被命名为Cooper韧带。其解剖图谱至今仍是乳房结构最精准的图示之一[6]，但未明确描述乳房筋膜边界的周缘附着点及其与深筋膜、胸壁的具体连接方式。

[乳房浅筋膜系统实为一种生物张力（biotensegrity）完整性结构。骨科医师Stephen Levin率先提出生物张力完整性理论，以解释肌肉骨骼系统的自然原理。该理论历经近40余年方获学界认可，其不仅精准模拟乳房构造，亦能阐释自组织生物系统的物理与几何特性（参见构造定律：https://www.youtube.com/watch?v=tgEBTPee9ZM）。

20世纪50年代，网格球顶发明者巴克敏斯特·富勒提出"张力完整性"（tensegrity）概念，其核心特征为连续性张力网络作用于非连续性可压缩单元。该理论看似复杂，实则广泛存在于自然界：如气泡膜即由连续张力性塑料网络包裹非连续性可压缩气泡构成。莱文于20世纪80年代提出，张力完整性模型较经典力学更能诠释肌肉骨骼系统。乳房浅筋膜系统——由张力性水平筋膜层与垂直支持带作用于非连续性脂肪小叶——恰似气泡膜结构。其不仅具有类似保护功能，更兼具热调节、代谢、旁分泌及再生等生理作用。21世纪，斯卡尔将张力完整性模型拓展至生物结构物理学领域[7]，该理念最早可追溯至达西·汤普森1917年的研究[8]。（吉姆贝尔托提出疏松结缔组织层面的张力完整性模型，称为"多微泡胶原动态系统"，详见：https://www.youtube.com/watch?v=eW0lvOVKDxE）。]

2.2.2 乳腺体层板

乳房浅筋膜系统的核心层之一是乳腺体层板（图2.1），是介于Cooper前、后层之间的水平浅筋膜层，乳腺本体（corpus mammae）即发育于此。在胚胎乳腺脂肪垫中，外胚层细胞向内迁移并定植于该层。女性乳房发育时，此二维筋膜层扩展为三维宏观结构，而男性乳房未发育，仍保持二维平面状态。在乳房切除或乳房缩小术

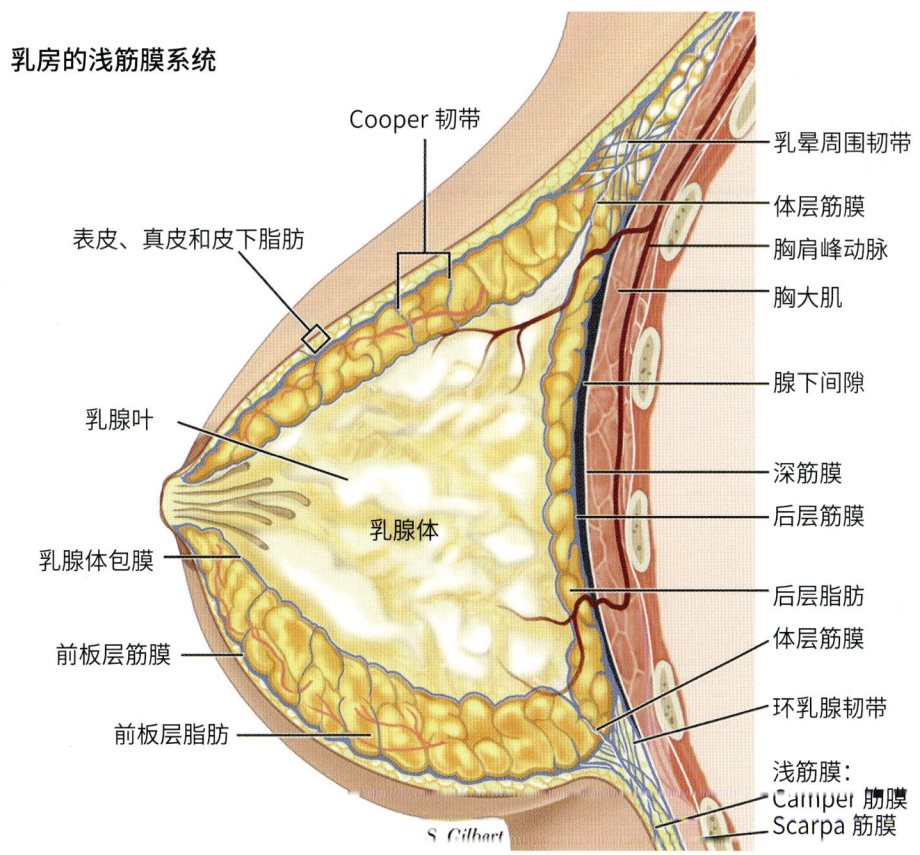

图2.1　乳房浅筋膜示意图，展示重要层次结构：前层、后层及乳腺体层板（Susan Gilbert供图，2020）

中，移除三维乳腺本体后，乳腺体层板仍以二维筋膜层形式存在。

基于基础体节理论，腹部亦存在此类中间层浅筋膜，但需精细解剖方可辨识。Cooper 在《乳房解剖学》中清晰展示了女性乳房从早期胚胎乳芽向成熟乳腺本体的形态演变[6]：未成熟乳腺形似倒置香菇，"菌柄"指向乳晕区；成熟后因导管 – 小叶系统分支生长（类似植物花序结构），扩展为典型圆锥形三维结构。覆盖其上的浅筋膜系统（SFS）与皮肤共同塑造青年女性乳房的半球形凸起轮廓。经多次妊娠及退行性变后，乳腺本体突出度降低，SFS 与皮肤松弛，导致成熟期乳房下垂。

2.2.3 前层与后层结构

浅筋膜系统（SFS）由前层筋膜与后层筋膜构成，两者之间为乳腺体层板。前层脂肪层与后层脂肪层分别位于乳腺本体两侧（图 2.2，图 2.3）。浅筋膜支持带系统由后层筋膜发出的纤维束组成，垂直贯穿多层水平浅筋膜。解剖后层脂肪时可见其纤维纤细；当纤维穿过乳腺本体并延伸至其前表面时，形成三维杯状结构（蛋托状），前层脂肪小叶如蛋体般嵌于该支持带（即 Cooper 韧带）中。这些纤维以 90° 角穿过菲薄的前层筋膜，止于真皮层。部分 Cooper 韧带发育显著，其致密基底

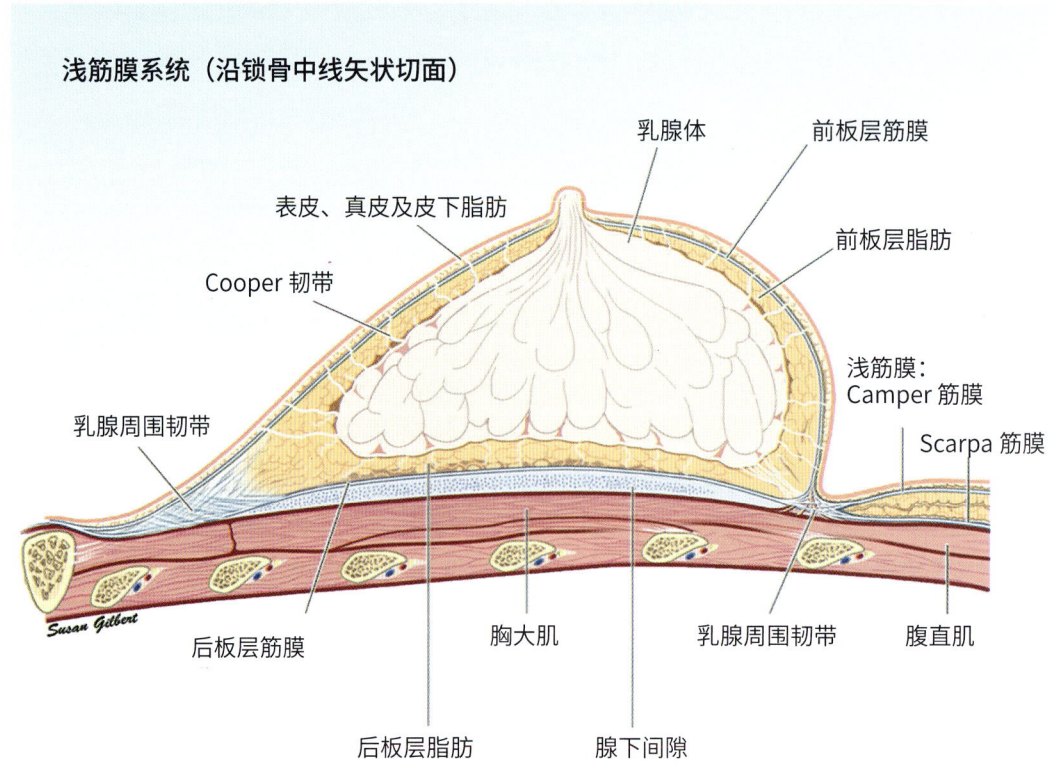

图 2.2　前、后浅筋膜及脂肪层的矢状面视图（Susan Gilbert 供图，2020）

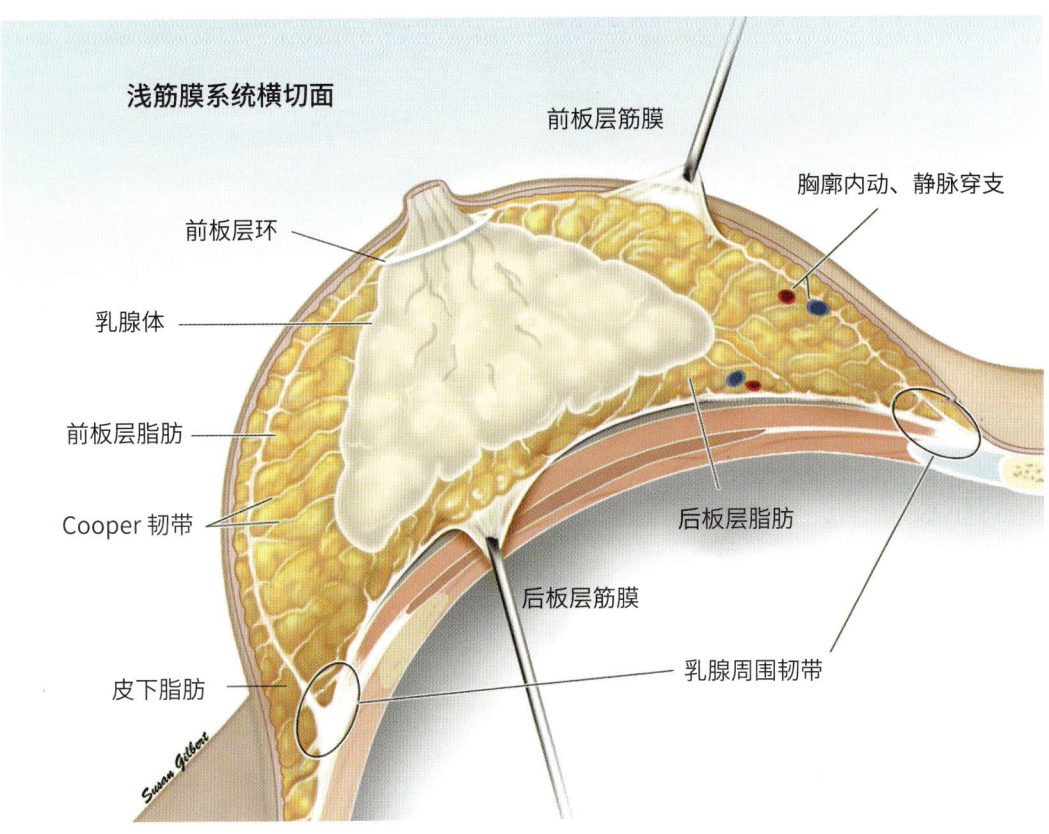

图2.3 前、后浅筋膜及脂肪层的轴向视图（Susan Gilbert 供图，2020）

与乳腺本体前包膜延伸结构（称外周锥状突）融合[9]。基底内包含乳腺实质最外围的终末导管小叶单元。前层筋膜与皮肤间为均匀皮下脂肪层（厚2~3mm）。前层脂肪厚度因个体体脂率的不同而异，但均呈现基底部厚、乳晕缘渐薄的分布特征。乳晕下无脂肪层，此处乳腺本体突破前层脂肪环（称前层环状区）穿入乳头。15~20条输乳管于此致密结缔组织内汇聚，先膨大为集合窦再缩窄穿出乳头皮肤。行保留皮肤及乳头、乳晕的乳房切除术时，可沿乳腺本体与乳晕真皮深面平滑肌纤维间进行锐性分离，但需在集合窦远端切断输乳管以游离乳腺本体（图2.4）。乳腺本体致密白色包膜（表面具锥状突与库珀韧带）与周围黄色前/后层脂肪对比显著（图2.5）。

与前表面相比，乳腺本体包膜的深面更平滑，若不细致观察，其深面穿入的浅筋膜支持带易被忽视。在老年女性体积增大且发生退变的乳房中，包膜结构不明显，切开后难以区分前/后层脂肪与乳腺本体内的间质脂肪。此时，乳房易被误判为无解剖分区的脂肪团块，实则各结构仍存在，仅边界很模糊。通常包膜深面较厚，周缘可见由外周锥状突形成的"活性边缘"，质地粗糙可辨。后层脂肪层（较前层脂肪显著菲薄）深面为后层筋膜，其厚度与强

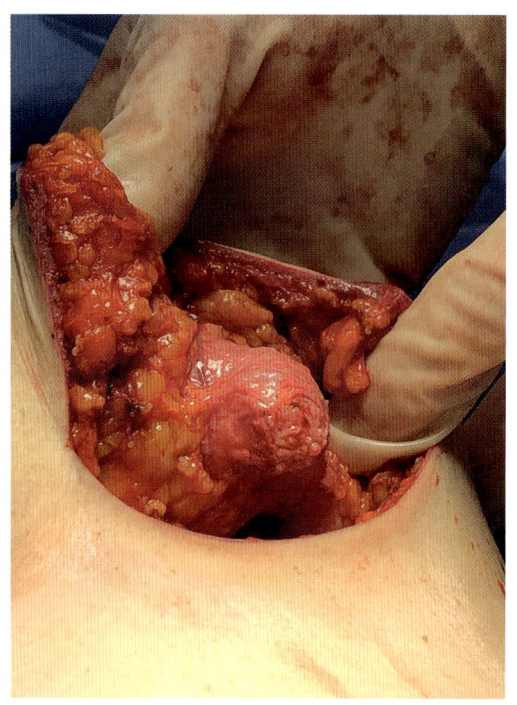

图 2.4 经倒"T"形切口切除乳腺本体后，前层环状区视图。注意皮下脂肪缺失及乳晕真皮深面平滑肌暴露，中央可见输乳管残端穿入外翻的乳头（Robert Rehnke 供图，2020）

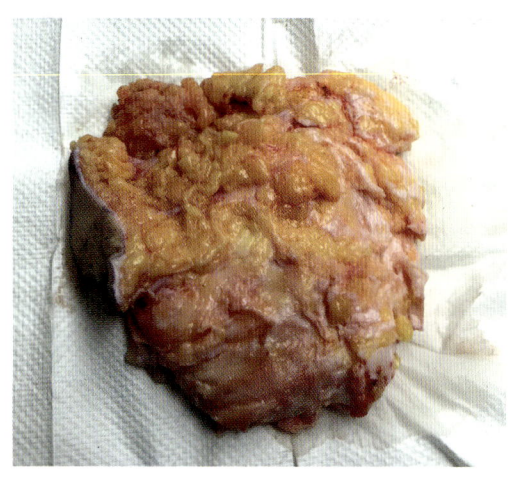

图 2.5 右乳外上象限肿瘤区域行皮肤、前层筋膜及脂肪椭圆形切除后获取的全乳腺本体标本。因 Cooper 韧带存在，前表面呈不规则形态，外周边缘可见粗糙自然分界（Robert Rehnke 供图，2020）

度远超前层筋膜，类似腹部 Camper 筋膜与 Scarpa 筋膜的厚度差异。后层筋膜与胸大肌深筋膜之间存在乳后间隙（或称滑囊），该潜在性筋膜裂隙允许乳房在胸壁上产生剪切运动。除极度肥胖者外，此层疏松结缔组织内无脂肪沉积（不同于 Scarpa 筋膜下的腹部脂肪储区）。通过牵引–反牵引技术在后层脂肪中进行分离，可进入浅筋膜水平面，实现洁净剥离，完整暴露乳腺本体深面包膜。这一操作凸显了后层筋膜与胸肌深筋膜的明确分界，乳后间隙作为无血管平面的解剖优势，以及浅筋膜系统层级结构的可分离性。

2.2.4 环乳韧带

浅筋膜系统通过特定黏附区与深层筋膜室融合[10]。这一解剖现象由 Lockwood 提出，他认为黏附区"决定了体表形态特征——局部脂肪堆积形成隆起，而紧密的薄层粘连则形成软组织皱褶与沟壑"[11, 12]。例如，无论肥胖程度如何，腹股沟皱襞均分隔躯干与下肢；半月线、腹中线及腹直肌腱划仅见于极瘦且肌肉发达者。胸部精细解剖显示，腹部半月线沿乳房外缘延伸，腹中线延续为乳房间沟；乳房下皱襞作为腱划样结构分隔腹直肌与胸大肌；乳房上方的微弱黏附线标示胸大肌胸肋头与锁骨头分界。乳房发育成熟时，浅、深筋膜间的菱形黏附区逐渐演变为泪滴状结构，尖端指向腋窝（图 2.6）。

我们称此环形黏附区为环乳韧带[4]。Gaskin、Peoples 与 McGhee 的尸体研究已证实该结构特征[13]。其厚薄并非如呼啦

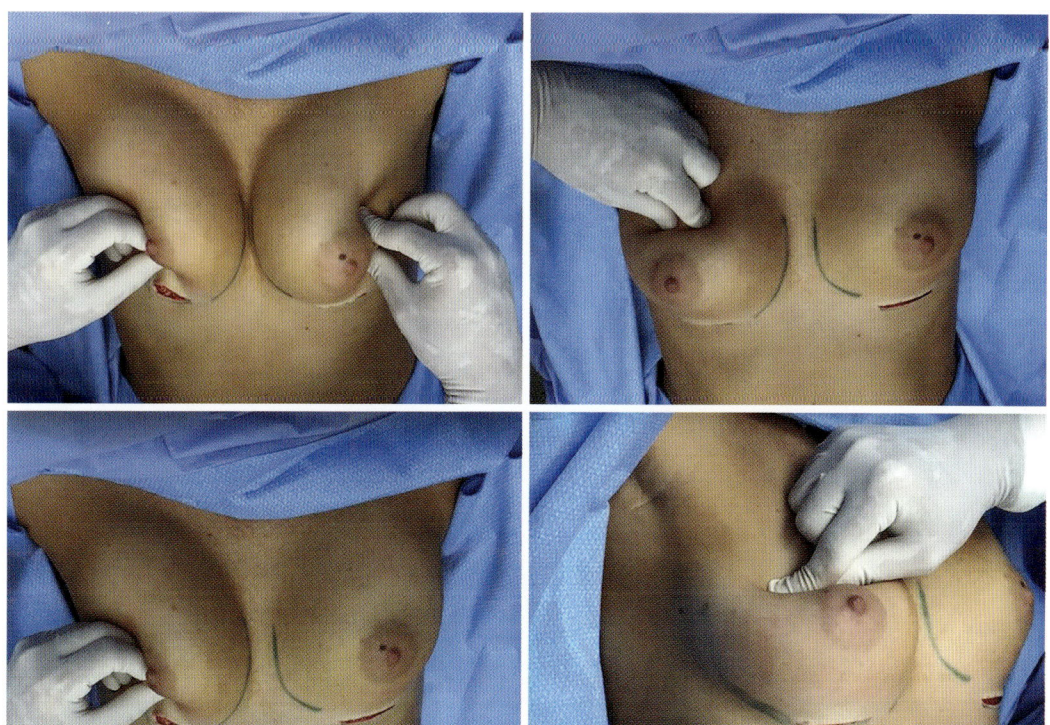

图 2.6 环乳韧带在皮肤与胸壁间形成泪滴形黏附区域（Robert Rehnke 供图，2020）

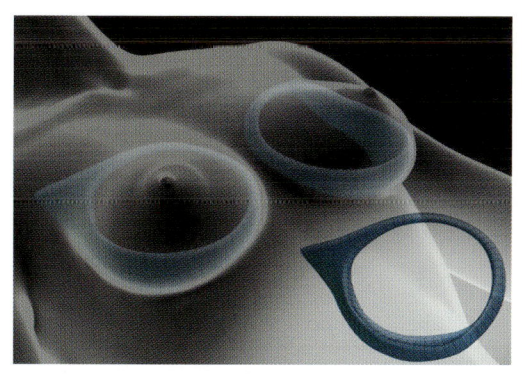

图 2.7 环乳韧带相对厚度示意图（David Killpack 供图，2015）

圈般均匀，而似旧卡车轮胎内胎一样存在直径差异（图 2.7）。该结构作为乳腺本体的环形边界，存在一定的厚度和深度，类似美式橄榄球场端区，而非单纯线性平面。通过施加牵引 - 反牵引力可区分：乳腺本体包膜与环乳韧带纤维，前者为白色纤维致密且不透明，后者呈弯曲环状排列，与脂肪组织交织。Astley Cooper 将其描述为"韧带样或筋膜样环状结构，将乳房连接至胸大肌腱膜"[6]。整体观之，环乳韧带围绕乳腺本体形成致密皮肤支持带区域，其纤维因乳腺发育扩张形成环状弯曲，其间夹杂脂肪组织。神经血管束与淋巴管于此黏附区穿行，分布于乳腺周围软组织被膜（图 2.8b）。

2.2.5 乳房的血液循环系统

乳房的血供来源多样，各血管在乳头-乳晕周边形成的丰富侧支供血循环并相互吻合（图 2.9）。乳房血供可分为浅层与深层两个系统（图 2.9）。浅层系统的主要来源有三个：胸廓内动脉（乳内动脉）

胸肌前乳房重建

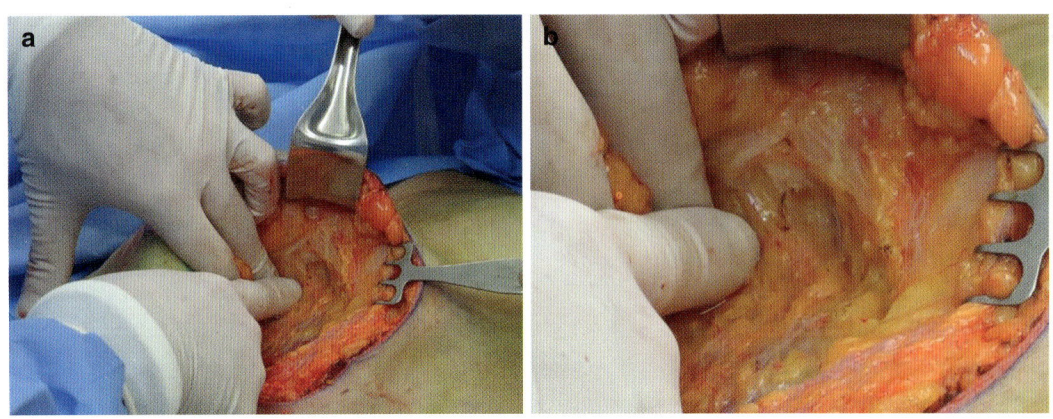

图 2.8 （a）内侧环乳韧带胸骨旁附着部观察。（b）内侧环乳韧带特写，自上而下可见肋间动脉、静脉、神经及淋巴管（Robert Rehnke 供图，2020）

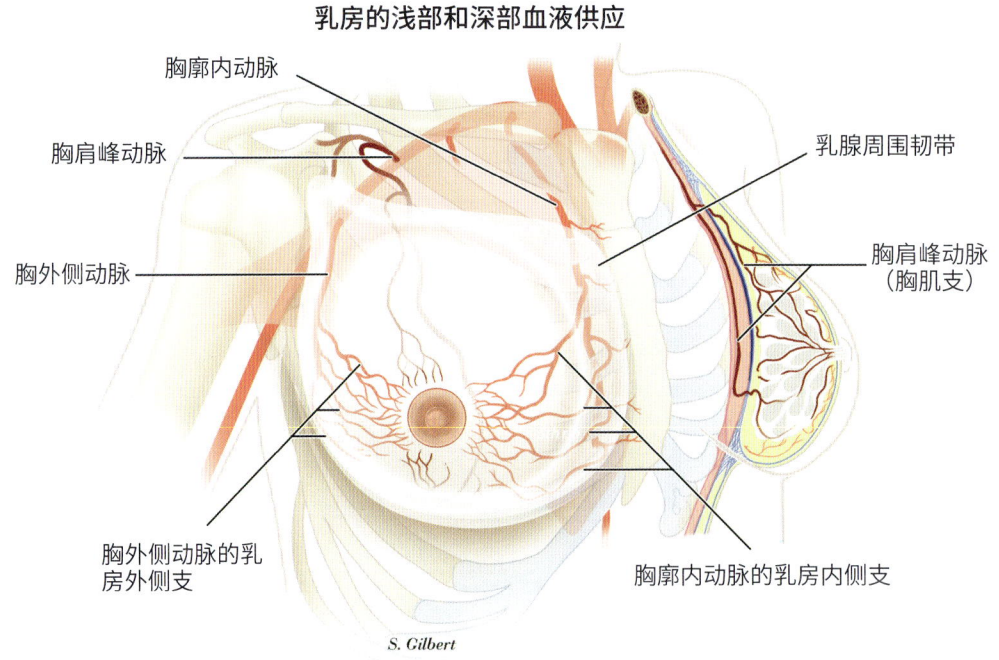

图 2.9 乳房与乳头血供示意图（Susan Gilbert 供图，2020）

及其肋间穿支（第 2、第 3 及偶见第 4 肋间动脉），胸外侧动脉（分支支配乳房区域外下部），肋间动脉前支（尤其支配乳房内下部）。深层系统由第 5 肋间动脉前支及胸肩峰动脉分支（视频 2.10）组成，在胸大肌深部走行并发出穿支（垂直胸壁平面 90° 上行），穿透后层脂肪进入乳腺体深部（第 2~5 肋）。这些血管继续向腺体小叶供血，最终抵达乳头 - 乳晕吻合环（前层筋膜下方）。在此乳晕周区域，浅层与深层系统相连接。浅层血管走行于前层脂肪（即前层筋膜与乳腺体之间），形

18

成乳头。乳晕的节段性血供[14]。

乳房静脉同样存在浅、深两个系统：浅层静脉位于前层浅筋膜下方，有横、纵两种走行模式。横静脉向胸骨缘汇聚，与乳内穿支静脉汇合后注入乳内静脉；纵静脉引流乳房上部及胸部（含下颈部），至胸骨上切迹区汇入颈前静脉。深层静脉与腋动脉分支伴行，汇入腋静脉及无名静脉[15]。

2.2.6 乳房的淋巴系统

传统外科学教材对乳房淋巴系统论述存在过度关注，源于早期"渗透理论"的癌症发展模型。该理论认为肿瘤呈渐进式浸润性生长，逐渐侵犯周围结构，通过淋巴管道播散至腋窝、胸廓及颈部淋巴结区域，而血行转移仅见于疾病终末期。此学说为"根治性"乳房切除术（整块切除腺体、皮肤、胸肌及腋窝内容物）提供了理论依据——术者须详尽掌握乳房的淋巴系统解剖，以避免在乳腺癌手术中残留淋巴通道或淋巴结，即Halstead提出的"完整术式"。随着解剖学进步（如20世纪40年代Grey证实深部乳腺淋巴与胸肌关联甚微），改良根治术成为20世纪后半叶的标准术式。

渗透理论后被Bernard Fisher的癌症生物学理论所颠覆：20世纪60年代实验室研究及70年代多中心随机试验证实——"乳腺癌是宿主-肿瘤复杂交互作用的系统性疾病，血流播散具重要意义，淋巴结转移更似远处转移的预测因子而非始动因素"[16]。这一认知推动了保乳治疗及微创手术的发展。有关乳房淋巴解剖的经典论述可参考Haagensen的著作[15]，Morris在《人体解剖学》中则进行了精辟总结："乳房淋巴管高度密集，形成广泛吻合的网状结构。"乳头-乳晕区皮下淋巴丛汇入乳晕下丛，腺泡间隙深部淋巴管与浅丛自由吻合后多数汇入乳晕下丛，由此发出的主淋巴管联通胸肌、肩胛下、腋窝及中央群淋巴结，故乳腺癌或感染最常转移至腋窝淋巴结。

乳房淋巴引流另有三条次级路径：

1. Grozman路径——直接穿胸大肌至Rotter淋巴结（胸大肌下群）。

2. 内乳动脉穿支伴行淋巴管——汇入纵隔及胸膜淋巴结。

3. Gerota乳房旁路径——可能介导肝转移及上腹壁皮肤转移。胸部皮肤淋巴管网亦可跨中线相互吻合[2]。

乳腺体（乳腺癌起源部位）的淋巴引流最终汇入乳晕下丛[15]。Sappey于19世纪末描述了乳晕下丛，并证实中线外侧胸部及上腹部皮肤淋巴回流至同侧腋窝淋巴结，而乳腺体因源于皮肤，其淋巴先汇入Sappey丛再经皮肤淋巴引流至腋窝。次级淋巴管道主要引流中胚层成分，但因两系统广泛吻合，偶可成为乳腺癌的转移通路。

目前，临床实践已由腋窝淋巴结清扫转向前哨淋巴结活检：通过定位乳房淋巴引流的首个淋巴结检测转移情况，为预后评估及辅助治疗决策提供依据。

2.2.7 乳腺的神经支配

乳房由胸段肋间神经的外侧皮支和前

皮支共同支配。外侧皮支走行于腋前线区域的环乳韧带内层，内侧皮支则与胸骨旁区域的胸廓内动脉穿支伴行于胸骨旁环乳韧带（图 2.8）。此外，乳房上部皮肤接受颈丛锁骨上神经支配，乳头 – 乳晕区主要由第 4、5 肋间神经外侧支支配。

2.3 小结

乳房浅筋膜系统由多层筋膜构成，垂直韧带从最深层贯穿至真皮层，通过锚定作用防止剪切力破坏软组织形态。环乳韧带环绕乳房周缘，呈泪滴状，当乳腺体部在浅筋膜中间层（即体部板层）扩张时形成。乳腺体部夹裹于脂肪层之间：深层为较薄的后板层脂肪，体部前表面与皮肤之间为较厚的前板层脂肪。乳房内垂直支持带高度发育，结构呈蛋托状，其间的垂直韧带即 Cooper 韧带，分隔前板层脂肪小叶。整个系统包裹于由前板层筋膜与后板层筋膜构成的筋膜容器内。此系统在乳头 – 乳晕下方存在特殊开口区域（即前板层环状区，图 2.10），此处无皮下脂肪及前板层脂肪。该软组织系统整体覆盖于骨肌系统基础之上（图 2.11，图 2.12）。底层骨性结构的大小、形态及轮廓特征，既是导致乳房外形个体差异的重要因素，也能解释为何某些乳房具有更好的支撑性，可随年

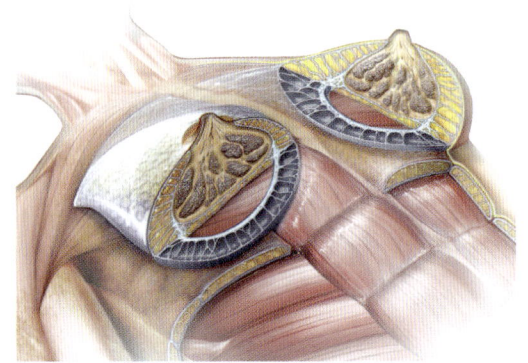

图 2.10　乳房浅筋膜系统示意图（David Killpack 供图，2015）

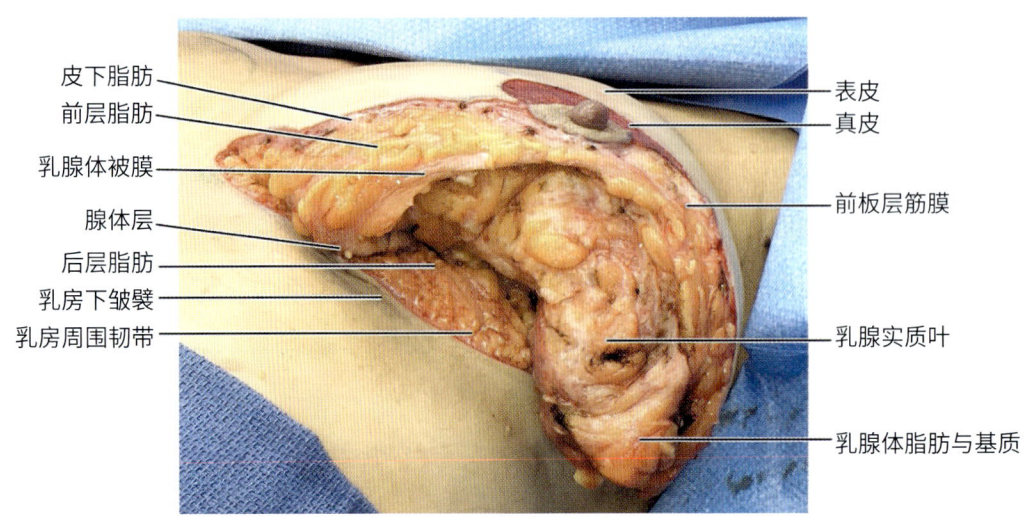

图 2.11　上蒂法乳房缩小术（Susan Gilbert 供图，2020）

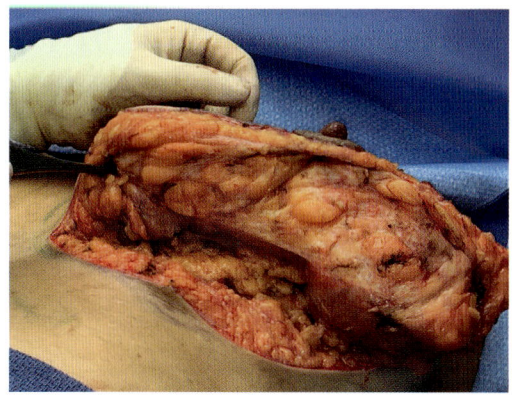

图 2.12 同图 2.11 所示乳房，牵拉显露乳腺体包膜（Susan Gilbert 供图，2020）

龄增长避免下垂（乳房松垂）。浅筋膜中胶原纤维与弹性纤维的固有质量与强度差异，则阐释了相同体积与质量的乳房为何下垂程度各异。充分理解浅筋膜系统是开展各类乳腺手术的重要基础。

参考文献

1. Andreas Vesalius, On the fabric of the human body. In Book V: The organs of nutrition and generation, transl. William Frank Richardson in collaboration with John Burd Carman, Novato, CA, Norman Publishing, 2007, pp. xix, 257, illus (hardback 978–0–930405–88–5). Medical History. 2009,53(1):153.
2. Schaeffer JP, Arey LB. Morris' human anatomy: a complete systematic treatise. JAMA. 1942,120(11):869.
3. Bland KI, Klimberg VS, Copeland EM, Gradishar WJ. The breast: comprehensive management of benign and malignant diseases. 5th ed. Philadelphia, PA: Elsevier; 2018.
4. Rehnke RD, Groening RM, Buskirk ERV, Clarke JM. Anatomy of the superficial fascia system of the breast. Plast Reconstr Surg. 2018,142(5):1135–44.
5. Abu-Hijleh MF, Roshier AL, Al-Shboul Q, Dharap AS, Harris PF. The membranous layer of superficial fascia: evidence for its widespread distribution in the body. Surg Radiol Anat. 2006,28(6):606–19.
6. Cooper A. On the anatomy of the breast. Longman, Orme, Green, Brown, and Longmans: London; 1840.
7. Scarr G. Biotensegrity: the structural basis of life. 2nd ed. Pencaitland: Handspring Publishing; 2018.
8. Thompson DAW. On growth and form. D'Arcy Wentworth Thompson. Am Nat. 1942, 76(767):614–6.
9. Stiles HJ. The surgical anatomy of the breast and axillary lymphatic gland. Edinburgh: Oliver and Boyd; 1892.
10. Rohrich RJ, Smith PD, Marcantonio DR, Kenkel JM. The zones of adherence: role in minimizing and preventing contour deformities in liposuction. Plast Reconstr Surg. 2001,107(6):1562–9.
11. Lockwood TE. Superficial fascial system (SFS) of the trunk and extremities. Plast Reconstr Surg. 1991,87(6):1009–18.
12. Lockwood T. Reduction mammaplasty and mastopexy with superficial fascial system suspension. Plast Reconstr Surg. 1999,103(5):1411–20.
13. Gaskin KM, Peoples GE, Mcghee DE. The attachments of the breast to the chest wall: a dissection study. Plastic Reconstr Surg. 2020, 146(1):11e–22e.
14. Deventer PVV. The blood supply to the nipple-areola complex of the human mammary gland. Aesthet Plast Surg. 2004,28(6):393–8.
15. Haagensen CD. Diseases of the breast.... 2nd ed. Philadelphia, PA: Saunders; 1971.
16. Fisher B, Anderson SJ. The breast cancer alternative hypothesis: is there evidence to justify replacing it? J Clin Oncol. 2010,28(3):366–74.

3 乳腺癌肿瘤学分析：乳房切除与腋窝分期的必要性

编者：Kate R. Pawloski, Audree B. Tadros

译者：王 磊 卞晓丽

3.1 引言

在乳腺癌多学科综合治疗时代，与20世纪早中期高侵袭性手术相比，创伤更小的局限性手术不仅可行，而且符合肿瘤学安全原则。早期乳腺癌患者多可选择保乳手术联合全乳放疗（BCT）或乳房切除术，两种治疗方式的生存预后均较理想。新辅助系统治疗的广泛应用，使得按既往标准被判定为"不可手术"的局部进展期乳腺癌患者得以成功接受根治性手术。近30年来，腋窝处理策略亦发生了重大改革，前哨淋巴结活检已成为临床腋窝淋巴结阴性患者的标准分期手段。本章将系统阐述乳腺癌外科治疗策略及其演进历程，着重探讨乳房切除术患者的多学科管理。

3.2 乳腺癌外科治疗的历史沿革

20世纪中期之前，Halsted根治性乳房切除术，即整块切除乳腺组织、覆盖皮肤、胸肌及腋窝内容物是乳腺癌的主要治疗方式[1]。20世纪后半叶，辅助化疗与放疗被常规纳入乳腺癌治疗体系，有效降低了局部复发和全身性转移的风险。随着影像技术的进步及乳腺癌筛查的常规化，局限于乳腺的早期肿瘤检出率显著提高，此类病例现已成为目前最常见的乳腺癌患者[2, 3]。筛查与早期诊断技术的进步，推动了缩小乳腺癌手术范围的可行性及肿瘤学安全性的研究。

限制性手术（即全乳切除术）对总体生存率的影响，通过具有里程碑式意义的NSABP B-04随机临床试验（美国国家乳腺与肠道外科辅助治疗项目，National Surgical Adjuvant Breast and Bowel Project）首次获得验证[4]。1971~1974年，1 665例患者被随机分配接受根治性乳房

K. R. Pawloski · A. B. Tadros (✉)
Breast Service, Department of Surgery, Memorial Sloan Kettering Cancer Center, New York, NY, USA
e-mail: tadrosa@mskcc.org

© The Author(s), under exclusive license to Springer Nature Switzerland AG 2023
R. Vidya, H. Becker (eds.), *Prepectoral Breast Reconstruction*,
https://doi.org/10.1007/978-3-031-15590-1_3

切除术或全乳切除术（联合/不联合腋窝放疗）。根治术实现乳腺组织、覆盖皮肤、胸肌及腋窝内容物Ⅰ~Ⅲ水平的整块切除，而全乳切除术保留胸肌及腋窝淋巴结。B-04试验首次证实，无论是否合并腋窝淋巴结转移，乳房切除术的解剖范围对患者25年随访总体生存率无显著影响；在临床淋巴结阳性或阴性患者中，无病生存率与局部无复发生存率均无统计学差异，提示限制性手术可实现有效的局部控制。这些发现使接受乳房切除术患者的并发症发生率显著降低。

随后的NSABP B-06试验及米兰试验进一步确立了保乳治疗（BCT）在早期乳腺癌患者中的肿瘤学安全性。研究显示，接受改良根治术、肿块切除术联合腋窝淋巴结清扫术（ALND），以及肿块切除术联合ALND序贯全乳放疗的Ⅰ~Ⅱ期乳腺癌患者，20年总体生存率与无病生存率均相当，接受全乳放疗组的20年同侧乳房肿瘤复发（IBTR）率显著低于未放疗组（14.3%：39.2%，$P<0.001$）[4, 5]。

同侧乳房肿瘤复发（ipsilateral breast tumor recurrence，IBTR）率与区域淋巴结状态及手术切缘情况密切相关。对于采用"切缘无肿瘤墨染"（no ink on tumor）标准的浸润性癌患者，临床腋窝淋巴结阴性患者与阳性患者的IBTR率分别为5%与9%[6, 7]，而扩大切缘范围并未显著降低复发风险[8]。对导管原位癌（ductal carcinoma in situ，DCIS）患者行保乳治疗时，切缘宽度2mm可使IBTR风险最小化，进一步扩大切除无显著获益[9]。若经二次切除仍无法获得阴性切缘，则须行乳房切除术以实现局部控制。

3.3 乳房切除术适应证

尽管保乳治疗（breast-conserving therapy，BCT）是众多早期乳腺癌患者的优选方案，但以下情况仍需行乳房切除术：同侧多灶性乳腺癌、T4期病变（定义为肿瘤直接侵犯胸壁和/或皮肤伴溃疡或皮肤结节）或炎性乳腺癌（inflammatory breast cancer，IBC）[10]（图3.1）。其他传统适应证包括肿瘤-乳房体积比不佳、携带BRCA1/BRCA2等高危基因突变、既往接受过乳腺/胸壁放疗，以及存在放疗禁忌证（如妊娠）等。虽然在上述情况下乳房切除术是主要治疗手段，但特定情况下仍可能成功实施BCT。

传统认为多象限多灶性乳腺癌（即多中心性病变）是BCT的禁忌证，因历史回顾性研究显示其局部区域复发率高达40%[11-13]。ACOSOG Z11102（联盟）的前瞻性试验表明，适当筛选的多灶性肿瘤患

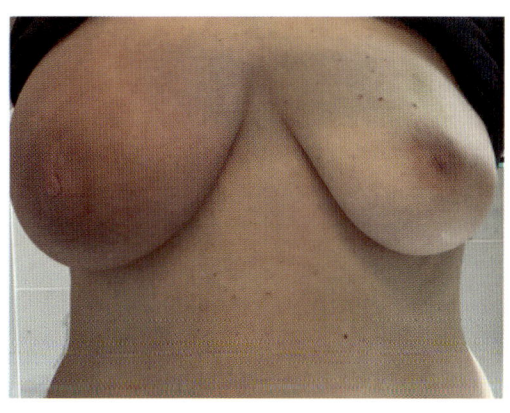

图3.1 炎性乳腺癌

者可通过同侧乳房至少一次的手术切除来实现保乳治疗，同时不影响美容效果[14, 15]，但需更长期的随访以评估局部复发风险。尽管 BCT 在多灶性乳腺癌患者中具有可行性，但再次切除仍无法获得阴性切缘者改行乳房切除术的比例因病理类型而异：浸润癌为 7.1%，至少一处为浸润性小叶癌者达 12.5%[14]。接受新辅助化疗后，多灶性病变患者 3 年局部复发率较单灶患者更高（9.6%：7.1%，$P=0.002$），但该差异与手术方式及是否达到病理完全缓解无关[16]。对于浸润灶间存在广泛导管原位癌（DCIS）的多中心性病变，乳房切除术仍为标准推荐。此外，对于为规避多次手术风险而倾向一次性治疗的多灶性乳腺癌患者，亦建议优先选择乳房切除术。

对于局部进展期乳腺癌，术前新辅助化疗（neoadjuvant chemotherapy，NAC）的应用显著拓宽了保乳治疗的适应证范围。原来因肿瘤-乳房体积比不佳而无法行保乳手术的患者，经 NAC 后约 75% 可成功转化为保乳手术候选者[17-20]。对于肿瘤-乳房体积比欠佳但强烈要求保乳且需接受系统化疗的患者，经严格筛选后成功实施 BCT 的概率也较高。以下情况仍不建议保乳：预计术后美学效果不可接受者，或系统治疗后肿瘤降期不充分者。

传统观点认为，对 BCT 术后同侧乳房复发（IBTR）应行挽救性乳房切除术，主要基于重复保乳的肿瘤学安全性考量及再程放疗风险。前瞻性研究显示，BCT 术后 20 年 IBTR 率为 9%~20%[4, 5, 21-23]。虽无随机试验直接比较挽救性切除术与二次保乳+再程放疗的疗效，但回顾性研究显示两者 10 年总生存率（65.7%：58.0%，P 无统计学意义）与病因特异性生存率（73.1%：61.1%，P 无统计学意义）相当[24, 25]。值得注意的是，选择二次保乳的患者多具有低级别、小肿瘤及良好生物学特征，提示需严格筛选低复发风险患者。对于年轻、高危乳腺癌 BCT 术后复发者，乳房切除术仍为标准选择[26]。若选择二次保乳+再程放疗，需充分评估既往放疗区域术后重建的并发症风险[27]。

BRCA1/BRCA2 突变携带者行预防性乳房切除术可使终生乳腺癌风险降低 90%~95%[28, 29]。该突变在普通人群发生率约 1/300，德系犹太人群高达 1/40。BRCA1 与 BRCA2 携带者至 80 岁累积乳腺癌风险分别为 72%（95%CI：65%~79%）和 69%（95%CI：61%~77%），并且多早发（BRCA1：30~40 岁；BRCA2：40~50 岁）[30]。BRCA1 携带者首次乳腺癌后对侧乳腺患癌风险显著高于 BRCA2（40%：26%，$P=0.001$），故建议双侧预防性切除。美国国家综合癌症网络（NCCN）指南推荐在多学科讨论框架下，对高危基因突变者权衡预防性切除与强化影像随访[31]。目前，中外显率基因突变尚缺乏足够证据支持预防性手术。

3.4 乳房切除术分类

乳房切除术的术式选择应基于综合肿瘤学特征、患者意愿及术者经验。在目前的临床实践中，主要术式包括未行即刻重建患者采用的传统全乳切除术（total mastectomy），以及拟行即刻重建患者适用的保留皮肤乳房切除术（skin-sparing mastectomy，SSM）与保留乳头乳晕复合体乳房切除术（nipple-sparing mastectomy，NSM）。不同术式局部复发率与组织保留程度呈正相关，但总体复发率处于可接受范围，经严格筛选的适应证患者可选择保留性术式。

该术式标志着20世纪初根治性手术向微创的首次转变[32, 33]，核心操作包括完整切除乳腺实质、覆盖皮肤及乳头-乳晕复合体，同时保留胸肌。由于术区皮肤广泛切除，全乳切除术后通常不实施即刻重建。主要适应证涵盖炎性乳腺癌（IBC）及其他需要扩大皮肤切除范围的T4肿瘤。回顾性研究显示，经新辅助化疗（NAC）降期的T4患者行即刻重建具有安全性[34, 35]，但术后并发症发生率显著高于未重建组（31.3%∶2.6%，$P=0.006$）[35]。鉴于需要二次手术处理的并发症风险以及可能延误辅助放疗，建议T4肿瘤患者（尤其IBC患者），即使NAC后成功降期仍首选全乳切除术。

SSM通过保留乳房皮肤袋（skin envelope）实现即刻假体或自体组织移植重建，术后美学效果得到显著改善（图3.2，图3.3）。该术式经乳晕周围小切口切除全部腺体组织，最大限度地保留皮肤及乳房下皱襞（inframammary fold）[36, 37]。传统SSM需切除乳头-乳晕复合体，但可在重建后期行乳头再造。腋窝处理可根据临床分期选择经同切口或独立切口进行操作。理想适应证为无即刻重建禁忌证者，如无皮肤或真皮淋巴管浸润的IBC/T4肿瘤。

目前尚无前瞻性试验直接比较保留皮肤乳房切除术（SSM）与传统全乳切除术的疗效，但多项回顾性研究证实SSM在0~Ⅲ期乳腺癌中的肿瘤学安全性。早期研究显示，经严格筛选的适应证患者行SSM联合即刻重建，局部复发率（local

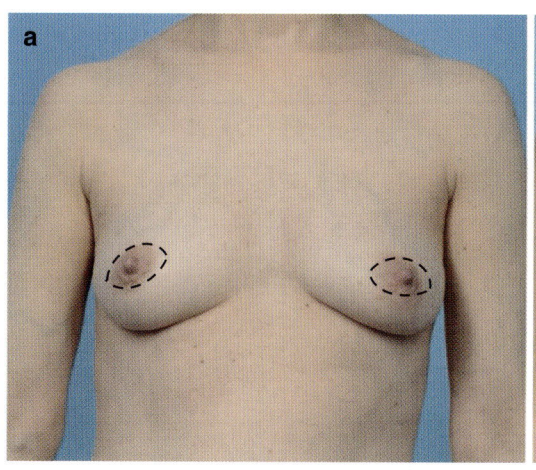 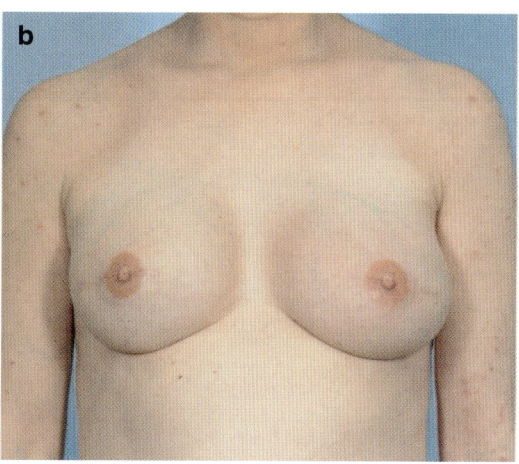

图3.2 双侧保留皮肤的乳房切除联合胸大肌前内置物重建及乳头纹身。（a）术前基线（状态）；（b）重建后11个月的美容效果

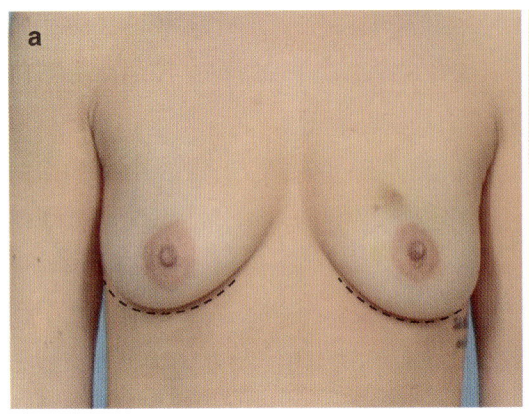 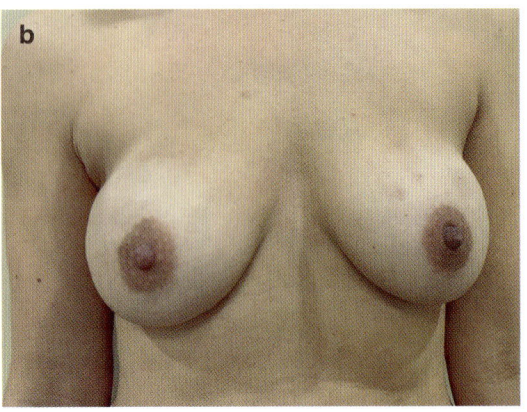

图3.3 经乳晕周围切口行双侧保留皮肤的乳房切除联合自体组织重建。(a)术前基线（状态）；(b)重建后6个月的美容效果

recurrence，LR）为4.0%~6.2%，与传统非保留皮肤术式相当[38-41]。一项纳入1 810例的前瞻性队列研究显示，SSM术后中位随访53个月，0~ⅡA期与ⅡB~Ⅲ期患者LR率分别为0.2%和1.6%[42]。优异的局部控制效果归因于辅助治疗实施率显著高于历史研究（对照研究[40, 41, 43-47]）。校正临床TNM分期后，SSM与传统术式的校正后无病生存率（adjusted DFS）与总生存率（OS）均无统计学差异。

对于经严格筛选的乳腺癌患者而言，与全乳切除术相比，保留皮肤乳房切除术（SSM）具有更高的安全性且能获得更优的美容效果。采用该术式时，应建立包括经验丰富的乳腺外科医师、整形外科医师以及放疗科和肿瘤内科医师在内的多学科团队，不仅有助于确保患者选择的严谨性，还可为乳房重建时机的选择与辅助治疗方案的制订提供科学依据。

保留乳头-乳晕复合体乳房切除术（nipple-sparing mastectomy，NSM）是保留皮肤乳房切除术的一种特殊术式，特点在于完整保留包括乳头-乳晕复合体在内的皮肤被覆结构（图3.4，图3.5）。与传统乳房切除术相比，NSM不仅能获得更佳的美容效果，还可明显改善患者的心理健康，提高生活质量[48, 49]。目前美国国立综合癌症网络（NCCN）指南提出，对于符合预防性乳房切除指征或乳腺癌治疗需求的患者，若术中评估乳晕后组织切缘无肿瘤残留且肿瘤距乳头基底≥1cm，可考虑实施NSM[50]。尽管各机构筛选标准存在差异，但NSM的理想适应证通常包括乳房体积较小且无下垂、体重指数（BMI）较低、无吸烟史等[51]。绝对禁忌证涵盖临床确诊的乳头受累（如Paget病）或术前影像学提示存在乳头/皮肤浸润征象，具体包括肿瘤距乳头基底<1cm，距乳头-乳晕复合体1cm范围内存在提示导管内癌向乳头延伸的钙化灶[52]。相对禁忌证则包括既往放疗史、吸烟史及乳房体积较大（C罩杯及以上），此类因素可能增加术后乳头坏死风险。

随着适用范围的拓展，治疗性NSM

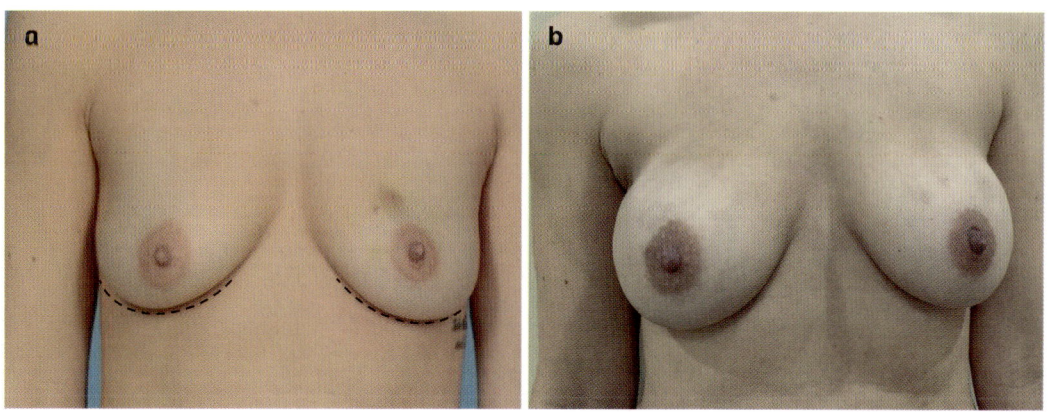

图 3.4 经乳房下皱襞切口行双侧保留乳头的乳房切除联合胸大肌前内置物重建。(a) 术前基线（状态）；(b) 重建后 10 个月的美容效果

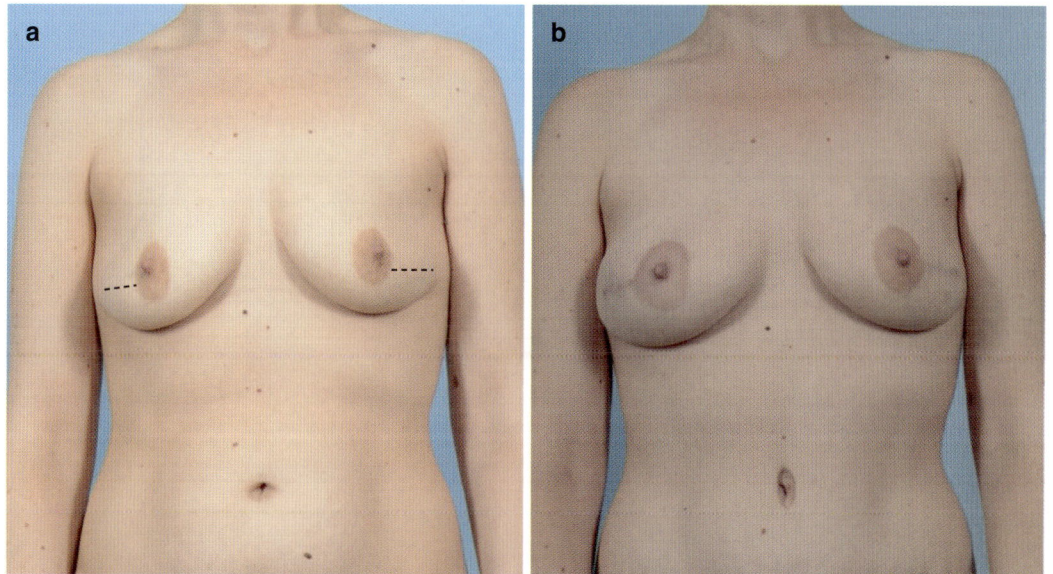

图 3.5 双侧保留乳头的乳房切除术联合自体组织重建。(a) 术前基线（状态）(b) 重建后 6 个月的美容效果

的临床应用日趋广泛[53-57]，多项大规模研究证实了其肿瘤学安全性。一项针对接受乳房切除术治疗的浸润性乳腺癌患者（$n=2\,207$，其中大部分为Ⅰ~Ⅱ期）的系统评价与荟萃分析显示，NSM 与改良根治术/保留皮肤乳房切除术的局部复发（LR）风险差异为 0.4%，无统计学显著性。在随访时间分层分析中，NSM 术后 <3 年、3~5 年及 >5 年的局部复发率分别为 5.4%、1.4% 与 11.4%；同期乳头-乳晕复合体局部复发率分别为 2.1%、1.5% 及 3.4%[58]。另一项针对 T1~3 期乳腺癌患者行 NSM 的前瞻性大样本研究（中位随访时间 85 个月）表明，术后 5 年乳头-乳晕复合体局部复发累积发生率为 3.5%，而胸壁或乳房皮肤（非乳头区域）局部复发率为 3.4%[59]。

无论是否发生乳头-乳晕复合体复发，患者的10年无远处转移生存率与总生存率均处于较高水平。

随着临床适应证的拓展，NSM 逐渐应用于接受新辅助化疗（neoadjuvant chemotherapy，NAC）的局部晚期乳腺癌患者。2015年的数据显示，接受 NSM 联合即刻乳房重建的Ⅲ期乳腺癌患者比例达10.7%，多为经 NAC 治疗后成功实现肿瘤降期的病例[60]。然而，对新辅助化疗背景下 NSM 的长期肿瘤学安全性仍需进一步评估。现有证据表明，NAC 后行 NSM 的术后并发症发生率较低，并且不会延误辅助治疗的启动[61]，但仍有待更多研究数据予以佐证。

在高危人群（如 BRCA1/2 基因突变携带者、具有乳腺癌或非典型增生家族史者）中，预防性 NSM 的临床应用亦呈上升趋势，与多项研究证实其局部复发率（LR）及术后并发症发生率较低的证据积累密切相关[62,63]。仍需针对此类人群开展长期随访研究，以明确 NSM 对生存预后的影响。

虽然 NSM 的适用范围逐步扩大，但对局部复发及全身转移风险极高的患者仍应审慎选择，包括 T4 期肿瘤患者，以及经临床检查或影像学评估无法可靠排除乳头隐匿性病灶者[53]。近期研究数据显示，治疗性 NSM 术后需二次手术处理的并发症的发生率达9.4%[53]，在制订个体化治疗方案时，需充分权衡此类风险对患者预后的潜在影响。

3.5 乳房切除术后放疗

乳房切除术后，多数病理检查证实腋窝淋巴结阴性的患者无须放疗，但对于局部复发（locoregional recurrence，LRR）风险极高者仍需考虑放疗。乳房切除术后放疗（post-mastectomy radiation therapy，PMRT）的目标是通过杀灭胸壁残留病灶以降低 LRR 及全身转移风险。美国国立综合癌症网络（NCCN）建议对肿瘤直径>5cm 或淋巴结阴性但切缘阳性的患者实施 PMRT[50]。此外，对腋窝淋巴结阳性数≥4者常规推荐 PMRT，因研究证实腋窝高淋巴结负荷是乳房切除术后 LRR 的最重要预测因素[64,65]。对于腋窝淋巴结转移数目有限（1~3）的患者，PMRT 的应用因机构而异，应结合高危因素综合评估，包括转移灶较大、年轻、肿瘤体积大、组织学分级高、存在淋巴脉管浸润（lymphovascular invasion，LVI）以及 HER2 阳性或三阴性受体状态等[66]。美国临床肿瘤学会（ASCO）、美国放射肿瘤学会（ASTRO）及美国外科肿瘤学会（SSO）建议对1~3枚淋巴结转移患者接受 PMRT 的临床获益进行多学科讨论评估[67]。关于新辅助化疗（NAC）后临床淋巴结分期降期为阴性的患者是否需要区域淋巴结照射，本章后续内容将予以详述。

3.6 早期乳腺癌腋窝处理策略

腋窝淋巴结是否存在转移是评估浸润性乳腺癌预后的重要指标。随着精准分期技术的普及，腋窝处理模式近几十年来经历了重大变革。对于临床淋巴结阴性（clinically node-negative）的早期浸润性乳腺癌患者，前哨淋巴结活检（sentinel lymph node biopsy，SLNB）已取代腋窝淋巴结清扫（axillary lymph node dissection，ALND），成为评估腋窝淋巴结状态的标准术式。对于接受乳房切除术的导管原位癌（ductal carcinoma in situ，DCIS）患者，若存在术后升级为浸润性癌的风险因素，可同期行 SLNB[68]。

选择性腋窝分期评估基于以下解剖学原理：整个乳腺的淋巴引流集中于有限数量的腋窝淋巴结，即前哨淋巴结（SLN），其病理状态可预测非前哨淋巴结的肿瘤转移情况。前哨淋巴结活检（SLNB）技术通过注射染色剂（异硫蓝、亚甲蓝或专利蓝）、放射性胶体（锝-99m）或联合使用两者（即"双重示踪法"）进行淋巴定位。对于拟行乳房切除术的患者，推荐采用皮内或乳晕后蓝染剂注射法[69]。当使用锝-99m时，需在术中使用 γ 探测器定位放射"热点"，将放射性绝对计数最高的淋巴结以及所有放射性计数超过该最高值10%的淋巴结均判定为前哨淋巴结。临床研究显示，对于存在多个前哨淋巴结的患者，SLNB 可识别 98.3% 的阳性淋巴结[70]。在初始手术治疗场景中，该技术成功率可达 96%，假阴性率（FNR，即前哨淋巴结阴性但非前哨淋巴结在 ALND 中阳性）为 7%[71]。

NSABP B-04 试验[4]首次证实，对于临床淋巴结阴性患者，常规行腋窝淋巴结清扫术（ALND）并不能提高生存获益。该研究将 1 079 例临床腋窝淋巴结阴性患者随机分至三组：根治性乳房切除术组、全乳切除未行 ALND 但术后接受腋窝放疗组，以及全乳切除仅当出现临床阳性淋巴结时行 ALND 组。另将 586 例临床淋巴结阳性患者随机分配至根治性乳房切除术组或全乳切除联合放疗组。20 年随访显示，无论淋巴结阴性或阳性患者，各组总生存率均相当；对于淋巴结阳性患者，与放疗相比，ALND 也未能显著改善无病生存率，与未行腋窝手术组无显著差异。这些重要发现证实残留淋巴结转移灶并不影响生存结局，提示 ALND 及其相关并发症[72]——包括淋巴水肿、肩关节功能障碍、运动/感觉神经病变及腋窝综合征等——在保证肿瘤学安全性的前提下可予以避免。

1994 年，Giuliano 团队基于黑色素瘤研究证据[73, 74]，首次报道了乳腺癌淋巴定位及选择性淋巴结切除术的可行性。欧洲肿瘤研究所（米兰）[75]与 NSABP B-32 研究[76]通过随机对照临床试验（表 3.1）进一步验证了该理念，比较了前哨淋巴结活检（SLNB）联合或不联合 ALND 的生存率与腋窝复发率。两项研究均显示，长期随访后各组总生存率（OS）、无病生存率（DFS）相当，腋窝复发率均处于较低水平。这些里程碑式研究确立了 SLNB 替代常规 ALND 对临床淋巴结阴性乳腺癌患者进行安全预后评估的临床价值。更多证据表明 SLNB 阴性后远期腋窝复发较为罕见：一项回顾性研究纳入 1997—2000 年治疗的 1 529 例患者（中位获取前哨淋巴

表 3.1 临床淋巴结阴性且前哨淋巴结阴性的早期乳腺癌患者行前哨淋巴结活检的随机试验（基于 Kaplan-Meier 法的生存分析）

研究	治疗组	例数	总生存率（95% CI）[a]	P 值	无病生存率（95% CI）[a]	P 值	以腋窝复发为首发事件的	P 值
NSABP B-32	SLNB 联合 ALND	1 975	91.8%（90.4%~93.3%）未校正 HR vs. 单独 SLNB：1.20（0.96~1.50）	0.12	82.4% 未校正 HR vs. 单独 SLNB：1.05（0.90~1.22）（80.5%~84.4%）	0.54	8	0.22
	单独 SLNB[b]	2 011	90.3%（88.8%~91.8%）		81.5%（79.6%~83.4%）		14	
Milan	SLNB 联合 ALND	257	89.7%（85.5%~93.8%）	0.15	88.8%（84.6%~92.9%）	0.52	0	0.17
	SLNB 单独[b]	259	93.5%（90.3%~96.8%）		89.9%（85.9%~93.9%）		2	

[a] NSABP B-32 试验报告 8 年随访结果，米兰（IEO）试验提供 10 年随访数据 *
[b] 若术中检出前哨淋巴结阳性，则行补充性腋窝淋巴结清扫术（ALND）

结 3 枚），中位随访 10.8 年，结果显示首次腋窝复发率为 0.9%（13/1 529），15 年累积复发率为 0.9%（95% CI：0.5~1.6）；在 13 例腋窝复发患者中，62%（7/13）发生于术后 5 年内[77]。

随后的前瞻性研究为临床淋巴结阴性且前哨淋巴结（sentinel lymph node，SLN）转移负荷较低患者的腋窝处理策略提供了依据，具体处理方案需依据手术方式而定。基于国际乳腺癌研究组（IBCSG）23-01 试验证据[78]，接受乳房切除术且 SLN 存在 1~2 个微转移灶（≤ 2mm）的患者，可免行腋窝淋巴结清扫（axillary lymph node dissection，ALND）（表 3.2）。当发现 SLN 宏转移或微转移时，AMAROS 试验结果表明接受区域淋巴结放疗的患者可免行 ALND[79]。两项试验入组人群主要为接受保乳治疗（breast-conserving therapy，BCT）的患者，包含部分乳房切除术病例。经过 10 年随访，两组在无病生存期（disease-free survival，DFS）和腋窝复发率方面均未见显著差异。对于符合保乳手术联合全乳放疗（BCT）指征的患者，上述研究及具有里程碑意义的美国外科医师学会肿瘤组（ACOSOG）Z0011 试验[80]证实，无论转移灶大小，存在 1~2 枚阳性 SLN 的患者均可安全避免 ALND 及其相关并发症。

IBCSG 23-01 与 AMAROS 试验结果

表 3.2 临床淋巴结阳性而前哨淋巴结阳性的早期乳腺癌患者行前哨淋巴结活检的随机试验

研究名称	治疗组	前哨淋巴结阳性病例数	接受乳房切除术病例数	中位随访时间	10年总生存率（%）	10年无病生存率（%）	腋窝复发率（%）
IBCSG 23-01	前哨淋巴结活检	469	44	9.7年	76.8	74.9	1.7
	腋窝淋巴结清扫	465	42	–	–	74.9	0.4
AMAROS	腋窝淋巴结清扫	744	127	10年	93.3	86.9	1.8
	腋窝放疗	681	121	–	92.5	82.7	0.9
Z-0011	前哨淋巴结活检	446	0	9.3年	86.3	80.2	1.1
	腋窝淋巴结清扫	445	0	–	83.6	78.2	0.5

a IBCSG 23-01 试验仅纳入仅存在 SLN 微转移的患者；AMAROS 和 Z0011 试验则纳入了存在 SLN 宏转移和微转移的患者。

表明，对于适合接受辅助全身治疗的早期临床淋巴结阴性乳腺癌患者，若接受乳房切除术时前哨淋巴结（sentinel lymph node，SLN）受累程度较轻，则可安全避免腋窝淋巴结清扫（axillary lymph node dissection，ALND）及其相关并发症[81~83]。需要注意的是，并非所有接受乳房切除术且 SLN 阳性的患者均需接受腋窝放疗。建议对接受乳房切除术后放疗且存在 1~2 枚阳性 SLN 的患者进行腋窝多学科评估，综合考虑免行 ALND 的可行性。

3.7 腋窝降期

术前系统治疗的目标是使不可手术的乳腺癌降期，并且新辅助化疗（NAC）的适应证已逐步扩展[84]。目前，美国国家综合癌症网络（NCCN）建议对炎性乳腺癌（IBC）、T4 肿瘤或 N2-N3 期患者应用 NAC，无论 NAC 疗效如何，均需行腋窝淋巴结清扫术（ALND）。然而，对于早期乳腺癌伴临床 N1 期患者，NAC 可能导致腋窝临床降期。此时可考虑行前哨淋巴结活检（SLNB），若未发现残留癌证据，则可避免 ALND 相关并发症。HER2 阳性（HER2+）及激素受体阴性/HER2 阴性（HR-/HER2-，三阴性）亚型患者的腋窝降期可能性最高。

近 10 年来，新辅助治疗（NAC）背景下前哨淋巴结活检（SLNB）的应用价值受到广泛关注。多项大型前瞻性试验评估了初始临床淋巴结阳性（cN+）且接受 NAC

治疗患者的 SLNB 假阴性率（FNR），通过常规腋窝淋巴结清扫术（ALND）验证残留腋窝病灶的比例[85-88]。结果显示，SLNB 的检出率较高（79.5%~92.7%），假阴性率为 11.9%~14.2%；若采用双示踪技术（放射性标记胶体联合亚甲蓝染色）并获取 ≥ 3 枚前哨淋巴结，假阴性率可降至 10% 以下。

ACOSOG Z1071 试验评估了临床分期 T0~4 且经活检证实为 N1~2 期肿瘤患者接受前哨淋巴结活检（SLNB）的假阴性率（FNR）。84% 的入组患者在新辅助化疗（NAC）后转为临床淋巴结阴性（cN0），但该状态并非入组必要条件（表 3.3）。在检出 ≥ 2 枚前哨淋巴结的 649 例患者中，FNR 达 12.6%，超过预设阈值（10%），因此不推荐将 SLNB 作为 NAC 后腋窝淋巴结清扫术（ALND）的替代方案。同样，前哨淋巴结新辅助化疗（SENTINA）试验作为一项前瞻性四组多中心研究，专门评估初始临床淋巴结阳性（cN+）经 NAC 转为 cN0（占原始队列 83%）患者的 SLNB 假阴性率。两项研究均发现，采用双示踪剂标测法及检出 ≥ 3 枚前哨淋巴结可有效降低 FNR；Z1071 试验还支持切除术前标记的转移淋巴结。美国国家综合癌症网络（NCCN）现行指南推荐，对于 NAC 后转为 cN0 且通过双示踪剂标测检出至少 3 枚前哨淋巴结的患者可采用 SLNB 方案[50]。

目前研究证据表明，在接受新辅助化疗（NAC）后获得淋巴结病理完全缓解（pCR）的患者中，41% 可避免腋窝淋巴结清扫术（ALND）[89]。淋巴结 pCR 率因肿瘤亚型而异：激素受体阴性/HER2 阳性（HR-/HER2+）及 HER2 阳性（HER2+）亚型患者最高（70%~80%），而激素受体阳性/HER2 阴性（HR+/HER2-）患者最低（0~50%）[90-96]。关于通过前哨淋巴结活检（SLNB）或 ALND 确认 NAC 后达到淋巴结 pCR 的患者，区域淋巴结照射（RNI）能否改善浸润性乳腺癌无复发生

表 3.3 ACOSOG Z1071 试验与 SENTINA 试验报告的新辅助化疗后前哨淋巴结活检假阴性率（FNR）比较

研究特征	Z1071	P	SENTINA	P
总体假阴性率	12.6%[a]		14%	
前哨淋巴结活检术技术改进相关的假阴性率				
检出 1 枚前哨淋巴结	31%	–	24%	Ref
检出 2 枚前哨淋巴结	21%	Ref	19%	0.008*
≥ 3 枚前哨淋巴结检出	9.1%	0.007	4.9%	
单示踪剂定位	20%	Ref	16%	Ref
双示踪剂定位	10.8%	0.052	8.6%	0.145
检出 ≥ 3 枚前哨淋巴结的比例[b]	57%		27%	

存率（IBC-RFS）的问题，将由NSABP B-51（美国国家外科辅助乳腺与肠道项目）随机临床试验予以解答[97]。该研究目前正在进行中：对于临床T1~3期、经活检证实为N1期且获得淋巴结pCR的乳腺癌患者，若接受乳房切除术，将被随机分配至全胸壁和RNI组或无放疗组；接受保乳手术的患者则随机分配至全乳放疗（含瘤床加量）联合RNI组或单纯全乳放疗组。

与初诊手术不同，新辅助化疗后若前哨淋巴结存在≥1处宏观或微观转移灶时，需要行腋窝淋巴结清扫术[50]。在此临床情形下，区域淋巴结综合照射的获益不明确，但前瞻性ALLIANCE A011202试验结果将进一步阐明[98]。该研究对接受新辅助化疗后仍有临床T1~3/N1且前哨淋巴结阳性的患者，随机给予乳腺/胸壁联合区域淋巴结综合照射（是否联合腋窝清扫），主要目的在于评估存在残留未清扫腋窝病灶患者的无浸润性乳腺癌复发生存率。若证实放疗可达到非劣效性，新辅助化疗后残留淋巴结病变患者对腋窝清扫的需求可能进一步降低。

最新证据表明，初诊时腋窝淋巴结转移有限或新辅助化疗疗效良好的患者无须常规行腋窝淋巴结清扫术，标志着乳腺癌多学科治疗模式取得重大进展。随着前瞻性循证依据的累积，针对不同亚群患者的腋窝手术去强化策略必将持续推进。

3.8 小结

保乳手术的肿瘤安全性已在早期乳腺癌患者中得到证实，近期证据显示该术式亦可应用于新辅助化疗后肿瘤降期的局部晚期患者。对乳腺病灶负荷较重（如T4期肿瘤、皮肤受累及炎性乳腺癌）的患者，全乳切除后不重建仍是标准术式，此类患者的局部控制依赖皮肤全层及腺体组织的完整切除。尽管多数新诊断乳腺癌患者适宜行保乳治疗，但许多患者仍选择全乳切除以降低局部复发风险。此时若无禁忌证，应与患者就即刻重建进行充分沟通。与传统全乳切除术相比，保留皮肤与保留乳头-乳晕复合体的全乳切除术，虽局部复发风险略高，但能显著改善美容效果。

前哨淋巴结活检的常规应用使21世纪腋窝分期体系获得了革命性进展。该技术适用于初诊时临床腋窝阴性患者，近来亦拓展至新辅助化疗后临床分期由N1降为N0的患者。虽然多数患者在当代诊疗模式下可安全豁免腋窝清扫，但对新辅助化疗后分期未降期或存在任何程度前哨淋巴结转移的患者，仍需常规实施该术式。

参考文献

1. Halsted WS. I. The results of radical operations for the cure of carcinoma of the breast. Ann Surg. 1907,46(1):1–19.
2. Welch HG, Prorok PC, O'Malley AJ, Kramer BS. Breast-cancer tumor size, overdiagnosis, and mammography screening effectiveness. N Engl J Med. 2016,375(15):1438–47.
3. Cancer Facts & Figures 2020 Atlanta: American Cancer Society; 2020 [Available from: https://www.cancer.org/research/cancer-facts-statistics/all-cancer-facts-figures/cancer-facts-figures-2020.html.

4. Fisher B, Jeong JH, Anderson S, Bryant J, Fisher ER, Wolmark N. Twenty-five-year follow-up of a randomized trial comparing radical mastectomy, total mastectomy, and total mastectomy followed by irradiation. N Engl J Med. 2002,347(8):567–75.
5. Veronesi U, Cascinelli N, Mariani L, et al. Twenty-year follow-up of a randomized study comparing breast-conserving surgery with radical mastectomy for early breast cancer. N Engl J Med. 2002,347(16):1227–32.
6. Wapnir IL, Anderson SJ, Mamounas EP, et al. Prognosis after ipsilateral breast tumor recurrence and locoregional recurrences in five National Surgical Adjuvant Breast and Bowel Project node-positive adjuvant breast cancer trials. J Clin Oncol. 2006,24(13):2028–37.
7. Anderson SJ, Wapnir I, Dignam JJ, et al. Prognosis after ipsilateral breast tumor recurrence and locoregional recurrences in patients treated by breast-conserving therapy in five National Surgical Adjuvant Breast and Bowel Project protocols of node-negative breast cancer. J Clin Oncol. 2009,27(15):2466–73.
8. Moran MS, Schnitt SJ, Giuliano AE, et al. Society of Surgical Oncology-American Society for Radiation Oncology consensus guideline on margins for breast-conserving surgery with whole-breast irradiation in stages I and II invasive breast cancer. Ann Surg Oncol. 2014,21(3):704–16.
9. Morrow M, Van Zee KJ, Solin LJ, et al. Society of Surgical Oncology-American Society for Radiation Oncology-American Society of Clinical Oncology Consensus Guideline on Margins for Breast-Conserving Surgery With Whole-Breast Irradiation in Ductal Carcinoma In Situ. J Clin Oncol. 2016,34(33):4040–6.
10. AJCC. Cancer Staging Manual. Chicago, IL: American Joint Committee on Cancer; 2018.
11. Wilson LD, Beinfield M, McKhann CF, Haffty BG. Conservative surgery and radiation in the treatment of synchronous ipsilateral breast cancers. Cancer. 1993,72(1):137–42.
12. Kurtz JM, Jacquemier J, Amalric R, et al. Breast-conserving therapy for macroscopically multiple cancers. Ann Surg. 1990,212(1):38–44.
13. Leopold KA, Recht A, Schnitt SJ, et al. Results of conservative surgery and radiation therapy for multiple synchronous cancers of one breast. Int J Radiat Oncol Biol Phys. 1989,16(1):11–6.
14. Rosenkranz KM, Ballman K, McCall L, et al. The feasibility of breast-conserving surgery for multiple ipsilateral breast cancer: an initial report from ACOSOG Z11102 (alliance) trial. Ann Surg Oncol. 2018,25(10):2858–66.
15. Rosenkranz KM, Ballman K, McCall L, et al. Cosmetic outcomes following breast-conservation surgery and radiation for multiple ipsilateral breast cancer: data from the alliance Z11102 study. Ann Surg Oncol. 2020,27(12):4650–61.
16. Ataseven B, Lederer B, Blohmer JU, et al. Impact of multifocal or multicentric disease on surgery and locoregional, distant and overall survival of 6,134 breast cancer patients treated with neoadjuvant chemotherapy. Ann Surg Oncol. 2015,22(4):1118–27.
17. Petruolo O, Sevilimedu V, Montagna G, Le T, Morrow M, Barrio AV. How often does modern neoadjuvant chemotherapy downstage patients to breast-conserving surgery? Ann Surg Oncol. 2020,28(1):287–94.
18. Golshan M, Cirrincione CT, Sikov WM, et al. Impact of neoadjuvant chemotherapy in stage II-III triple negative breast cancer on eligibility for breast-conserving surgery and breast conservation rates: surgical results from CALGB 40603 (Alliance). Ann Surg. 2015,262(3):434–9. discussion 8–9
19. Golshan M, Cirrincione CT, Sikov WM, et al. Impact of neoadjuvant therapy on eligibility for and frequency of breast conservation in stage II-III HER2-positive breast cancer: surgical results of CALGB 40601 (Alliance). Breast Cancer Res Treat. 2016,160(2):297–304.
20. Golshan M, Loibl S, Wong SM, et al. Breast conservation after neoadjuvant chemotherapy

21. van Dongen JA, Voogd AC, Fentiman IS, et al. Long-term results of a randomized trial comparing breast-conserving therapy with mastectomy: European Organization for Research and Treatment of Cancer 10801 trial. J Natl Cancer Inst. 2000,92(14):1143–50.
22. Poggi MM, Danforth DN, Sciuto LC, et al. Eighteen-year results in the treatment of early breast carcinoma with mastectomy versus breast conservation therapy: the National Cancer Institute Randomized Trial. Cancer. 2003,98(4):697–702.
23. Arriagada R, Lê MG, Rochard F, Contesso G. Conservative treatment versus mastectomy in early breast cancer: patterns of failure with 15 years of follow-up data. Institut Gustave-Roussy Breast Cancer Group. J Clin Oncol. 1996,14(5):1558–64.
24. Yoshida A, Takahashi O, Okumura Y, et al. Prognosis after mastectomy versus repeat lumpectomy in patients with ipsilateral breast cancer recurrence: a propensity score analysis. Eur J Surg Oncol. 2016,42(4):474–80.
25. Alpert TE, Kuerer HM, Arthur DW, Lannin DR, Haffty BG. Ipsilateral breast tumor recurrence after breast conservation therapy: outcomes of salvage mastectomy vs. salvage breast-conserving surgery and prognostic factors for salvage breast preservation. Int J Radiat Oncol Biol Phys. 2005,63(3):845–51.
26. Montagne L, Hannoun A, Hannoun-Levi JM. Second conservative treatment for second ipsilateral breast tumor event: a systematic review of the different re-irradiation techniques. Breast. 2020,49:274–80.
27. Cordeiro PG, Snell L, Heerdt A, McCarthy C. Immediate tissue expander/implast breast reconstruction after salvage mastectomy for cancer recurrence following lumpectomy/irradiation. Plast Reconstr Surg. 2012,129(2):341–50.
28. Carbine NE, Lostumbo L, Wallace J, Ko H. Risk-reducing mastectomy for the prevention of primary breast cancer. Cochrane Database Syst Rev. 2018,4(4):Cd002748.
29. Domchek SM, Friebel TM, Singer CF, et al. Association of risk-reducing surgery in BRCA1 or BRCA2 mutation carriers with cancer risk and mortality. JAMA. 2010,304(9):967–75.
30. Kuchenbaecker KB, Hopper JL, Barnes DR, et al. Risks of breast, ovarian, and contralateral breast cancer for BRCA1 and BRCA2 mutation carriers. JAMA. 2017,317(23):2402–16.
31. NCCN Guidelines Version 1.2020 Breast Cancer Risk Reduction. National Comprehensive Cancer Network; 2020.
32. Maddox WA, Carpenter JT Jr, Laws HL, et al. A randomized prospective trial of radical (Halsted) mastectomy versus modified radical mastectomy in 311 breast cancer patients. Ann Surg. 1983,198(2):207–12.
33. Staunton MD, Melville DM, Monterrosa A, Thomas JM. A 25-year prospective study of modified radical mastectomy (Patey) in 193 patients. J R Soc Med. 1993,86(7):381–4.
34. Wang M, Chen H, Wu K, Ding A, Zhang P, Zhang M. Post-mastectomy immediate breast reconstruction is oncologically safe in well-selected T4 locally advanced breast cancer: a large population-based study and matched case-control analysis. Breast Cancer Res Treat. 2019,176(2):337–47.
35. Simpson AB, McCray D, Wengler C, et al. Immediate reconstruction in inflammatory breast cancer: challenging current care. Ann Surg Oncol. 2016,23(Suppl 5):642–8.
36. Freeman BS. Subcutaneous mastectomy for benign breast lesions with immediate or delayed prosthetic replacement. Plast Reconstr Surg Transplant Bull. 1962,30:676–82.
37. Toth BA, Lappert P. Modified skin incisions for mastectomy: the need for plastic surgical input in preoperative planning. Plast Reconstr Surg. 1991,87(6):1048–53.
38. Downes KJ, Glatt BS, Kanchwala SK, et al.

Skin-sparing mastectomy and immediate reconstruction is an acceptable treatment option for patients with high-risk breast carcinoma. Cancer. 2005,103(5):906–13.
39. Foster RD, Esserman LJ, Anthony JP, Hwang ES, Do H. Skin-sparing mastectomy and immediate breast reconstruction: a prospective cohort study for the treatment of advanced stages of breast carcinoma. Ann Surg Oncol. 2002,9(5):462–6.
40. Medina-Franco H, Vasconez LO, Fix RJ, et al. Factors associated with local recurrence after skin-sparing mastectomy and immediate breast reconstruction for invasive breast cancer. Ann Surg. 2002,235(6):814–9.
41. Newman LA, Kuerer HM, Hunt KK, et al. Presentation, treatment, and outcome of local recurrence afterskin-sparing mastectomy and immediate breast reconstruction. Ann Surg Oncol. 1998,5(7):620–6.
42. Yi M, Kronowitz SJ, Meric-Bernstam F, et al. Local, regional, and systemic recurrence rates in patients undergoing skin-sparing mastectomy compared with conventional mastectomy. Cancer. 2011,117(5):916–24.
43. Carlson GW, Page A, Johnson E, Nicholson K, Styblo TM, Wood WC. Local recurrence of ductal carcinoma in situ after skin-sparing mastectomy. J Am Coll Surg. 2007,204(5):1074–8. discussion 8–80
44. Garwood ER, Moore D, Ewing C, et al. Total skin-sparing mastectomy: complications and local recurrence rates in 2 cohorts of patients. Ann Surg. 2009,249(1):26–32.
45. Kroll SS, Khoo A, Singletary SE, et al. Local recurrence risk after skin-sparing and conventional mastectomy: a 6-year follow-up. Plast Reconstr Surg. 1999,104(2):421–5.
46. Spiegel AJ, Butler CE. Recurrence following treatment of ductal carcinoma in situ with skin-sparing mastectomy and immediate breast reconstruction. Plast Reconstr Surg. 2003,111(2):706–11.

47. Vaughan A, Dietz JR, Aft R, et al. Scientific Presentation Award. Patterns of local breast cancer recurrence after skin-sparing mastectomy and immediate breast reconstruction. Am J Surg. 2007,194(4):438–43.
48. Romanoff A, Zabor EC, Stempel M, Sacchini V, Pusic A, Morrow M. A comparison of patient-reported outcomes after nipple-sparing mastectomy and conventional mastectomy with reconstruction. Ann Surg Oncol. 2018,25(10):2909–16.
49. Wei CH, Scott AM, Price AN, et al. Psychosocial and sexual well-being following nipple-sparing mastectomy and reconstruction. Breast J. 2016,22(1):10–7.
50. NCCN Guidelines Version 5.2020 Breast Cancer. National Comprehensive Cancer Network; 2020.
51. Tousimis E, Haslinger M. Overview of indications for nipple sparing mastectomy. Gland Surg. 2018,7(3):288–300.
52. Moo TA, Sanford R, Dang C, Morrow M. Overview of breast cancer therapy. PET Clin. 2018,13(3):339–54.
53. Valero MG, Muhsen S, Moo TA, et al. Increase in utilization of nipple-sparing mastectomy for breast cancer: indications, complications, and oncologic outcomes. Ann Surg Oncol. 2020,27(2):344–51.
54. Agarwal S, Agarwal S, Neumayer L, Agarwal JP. Therapeutic nipple-sparing mastectomy: trends based on a national cancer database. Am J Surg. 2014,208(1):93–8.
55. Krajewski AC, Boughey JC, Degnim AC, et al. Expanded indications and improved outcomes for nipple-sparing mastectomy over time. Ann Surg Oncol. 2015,22(10):3317–23.
56. de Alcantara FP, Capko D, Barry JM, Morrow M, Pusic A, Sacchini VS. Nipple-sparing mastectomy for breast cancer and risk-reducing surgery: the Memorial Sloan-Kettering Cancer Center experience. Ann Surg Oncol. 2011,18(11):3117–22.
57. Moo TA, Pinchinat T, Mays S, et al. Oncologic outcomes after nipple-sparing mastectomy. Ann

58. De La Cruz L, Moody AM, Tappy EE, Blankenship SA, Hecht EM. Overall survival, disease-free survival, local recurrence, and nipple-areolar recurrence in the setting of nipple-sparing mastectomy: a meta-analysis and systematic review. Ann Surg Oncol. 2015,22(10):3241–9.
59. Wu ZY, Kim HJ, Lee JW, et al. Breast cancer recurrence in the nipple-areola complex after nipple-sparing mastectomy with immediate breast reconstruction for invasive breast cancer. JAMA Surg. 2019,154(11):1030–7.
60. Wong SM, Chun YS, Sagara Y, Golshan M, Erdmann-Sager J. National patterns of breast reconstruction and nipple-sparing mastectomy for breast cancer, 2005–2015. Ann Surg Oncol. 2019,26(10):3194–203.
61. Bartholomew AJ, Dervishaj OA, Sosin M, et al. Neoadjuvant chemotherapy and nipple-sparing mastectomy: timing and postoperative complications. Ann Surg Oncol. 2019,26(9):2768–72.
62. Valero MG, Moo TA, Muhsen S, et al. Use of bilateral prophylactic nipple-sparing mastectomy in patients with high risk of breast cancer. Br J Surg. 2020; https://doi.org/10.1002/bjs.11616.
63. Heemskerk-Gerritsen BA, Menke-Pluijmers MB, Jager A, et al. Substantial breast cancer risk reduction and potential survival benefit after bilateral mastectomy when compared with surveillance in healthy BRCA1 and BRCA2 mutation carriers: a prospective analysis. Ann Oncol. 2013,24(8):2029–35.
64. Recht A, Gray R, Davidson NE, et al. Locoregional failure 10 years after mastectomy and adjuvant chemotherapy with or without tamoxifen without irradiation: experience of the Eastern Cooperative Oncology Group. J Clin Oncol. 1999,17(6):1689–700.
65. Overgaard M, Jensen MB, Overgaard J, et al. Postoperative radiotherapy in high-risk postmenopausal breast-cancer patients given adjuvant tamoxifen: Danish Breast Cancer Cooperative Group DBCG 82c randomised trial. Lancet. 1999,353(9165):1641–8.
66. Morrow M, Van Zee KJ, Patil S, et al. Axillary dissection and nodal irradiation can be avoided for most node-positive Z0011-eligible breast cancers: a prospective validation study of 793 patients. Ann Surg. 2017,266(3):457–62.
67. Recht A, Comen EA, Fine RE, et al. Postmastectomy Radiotherapy: An American Society of Clinical Oncology, American Society for Radiation Oncology, and Society of Surgical Oncology Focused Guideline Update. Ann Surg Oncol. 2017,24(1):38–51.
68. Lyman GH, Temin S, Edge SB, et al. Sentinel lymph node biopsy for patients with early-stage breast cancer: American Society of Clinical Oncology clinical practice guideline update. J Clin Oncol. 2014,32(13):1365–83.
69. Valero MG, Golshan M. Management of the axilla in early breast cancer. Cancer Treat Res. 2018,173:39–52.
70. Chung A, Yu J, Stempel M, Patil S, Cody H, Montgomery L. Is the "10% rule" equally valid for all subsets of sentinel-node-positive breast cancer patients? Ann Surg Oncol. 2008,15(10):2728–33.
71. Kim T, Giuliano AE, Lyman GH. Lymphatic mapping and sentinel lymph node biopsy in early-stage breast carcinoma: a metaanalysis. Cancer. 2006,106(1):4–16.
72. Norton S. Chapter 104. Lymphedema. In: Kuerer HM, editor. Kuerer's Breast Surgical Oncology. New York: McGraw-Hill; 2010. p. 1067–80.
73. Giuliano AE, Kirgan DM, Guenther JM, Morton DL. Lymphatic mapping and sentinel lymphadenectomy for breast cancer. Ann Surg. 1994,220(3):391–8. discussion 8–401
74. Krag DN, Weaver DL, Alex JC, Fairbank JT. Surgical resection and radiolocalization of the sentinel lymph node in breast cancer using a gamma probe. Surg Oncol. 1993,2(6):335–9. discussion 40
75. Veronesi U, Paganelli G, Viale G, et al. A ran-

domized comparison of sentinel-node biopsy with routine axillary dissection in breast cancer. N Engl J Med. 2003,349(6):546–53.

76. Krag DN, Anderson SJ, Julian TB, et al. Sentinel-lymph-node resection compared with conventional axillary-lymph-node dissection in clinically node-negative patients with breast cancer: overall survival findings from the NSABP B-32 randomised phase 3 trial. Lancet Oncol. 2010,11(10):927–33.

77. Matsen C, Villegas K, Eaton A, et al. Late axillary recurrence after negative sentinel lymph node biopsy is uncommon. Ann Surg Oncol. 2016,23(8):2456–61.

78. Galimberti V, Cole BF, Zurrida S, et al. Axillary dissection versus no axillary dissection in patients with sentinel-node micrometastases (IBCSG 23–01): a phase 3 randomised controlled trial. Lancet Oncol. 2013,14(4):297–305.

79. Donker M, van Tienhoven G, Straver ME, et al. Radiotherapy or surgery of the axilla after a positive sentinel node in breast cancer (EORTC 10981–22023 AMAROS): a randomised, multicentre, open-label, phase 3 non-inferiority trial. Lancet Oncol. 2014,15(12):1303–10.

80. Giuliano AE, Hunt KK, Ballman KV, et al. Axillary dissection vs no axillary dissection in women with invasive breast cancer and sentinel node metastasis: a randomized clinical trial. JAMA. 2011,305(6):569–75.

81. Galimberti V, Cole BF, Viale G, et al. Axillary dissection versus no axillary dissection in patients with breast cancer and sentinel-node micrometastases (IBCSG 23–01): 10-year follow-up of a randomised, controlled phase 3 trial. Lancet Oncol. 2018,19(10):1385–93.

82. Solá M, Alberro JA, Fraile M, et al. Complete axillary lymph node dissection versus clinical follow-up in breast cancer patients with sentinel node micrometastasis: final results from the multicenter clinical trial AATRM 048/13/2000. Ann Surg Oncol. 2013,20(1):120–7.

83. Rutgers E, Donker M, Poncet C, et al. Abstract GS4–01: Radiotherapy or surgery of the axilla after a positive sentinel node in breast cancer patients: 10 year follow up results of the EORTC AMAROS trial (EORTC 10981/22023). Cancer Res. 2019,79(4 Supplement):GS4–01-GS4-.

84. King TA, Morrow M. Surgical issues in patients with breast cancer receiving neoadjuvant chemotherapy. Nat Rev Clin Oncol. 2015,12(6):335–43.

85. Boughey JC, Suman VJ, Mittendorf EA, et al. Sentinel lymph node surgery after neoadjuvant chemotherapy in patients with node-positive breast cancer: the ACOSOG Z1071 (Alliance) clinical trial. JAMA. 2013,310(14):1455–61.

86. Kuehn T, Bauerfeind I, Fehm T, et al. Sentinel-lymph-node biopsy in patients with breast cancer before and after neoadjuvant chemotherapy (SENTINA): a prospective, multicentre cohort study. Lancet Oncol. 2013,14(7):609–18.

87. Boileau JF, Poirier B, Basik M, et al. Sentinel node biopsy after neoadjuvant chemotherapy in biopsy-proven node-positive breast cancer: the SN FNAC study. J Clin Oncol. 2015,33(3):258–64.

88. Classe JM, Loaec C, Gimbergues P, et al. Sentinel lymph node biopsy without axillary lymphadenectomy after neoadjuvant chemotherapy is accurate and safe for selected patients: the GANEA 2 study. Breast Cancer Res Treat. 2019,173(2):343–52.

89. Montagna G, Mamtani A, Knezevic A, Brogi E, Barrio AV, Morrow M. Selecting node-positive patients for axillary downstaging with neoadjuvant chemotherapy. Ann Surg Oncol. 2020,27(11):4515–22.

90. Pilewskie M, Morrow M. Axillary nodal management following neoadjuvant chemotherapy: a review. JAMA Oncol. 2017,3(4):549–55.

91. Boughey JC, McCall LM, Ballman KV, et al. Tumor biology correlates with rates of breast-conserving surgery and pathologic complete response after neoadjuvant chemotherapy for breast cancer: findings from the ACOSOG

Z1071 (Alliance) Prospective Multicenter Clinical Trial. Ann Surg. 2014,260(4):608–14. discussion 14–6

92. Zhang GC, Zhang YF, Xu FP, et al. Axillary lymph node status, adjusted for pathologic complete response in breast and axilla after neoadjuvant chemotherapy, predicts differential disease-free survival in breast cancer. Curr Oncol. 2013,20(3):e180–92.

93. Kim JY, Park HS, Kim S, Ryu J, Park S, Kim SI. Prognostic nomogram for prediction of axillary pathologic complete response after neoadjuvant chemotherapy in cytologically proven node-positive breast cancer. Medicine (Baltimore). 2015,94(43):e1720.

94. Mamtani A, Barrio AV, King TA, et al. How often does neoadjuvant chemotherapy avoid axillary dissection in patients with histologically confirmed nodal metastases? results of a prospective study. Ann Surg Oncol. 2016,23(11):3467–74.

95. T ALT, AlSayed A, Alawadi S, et al. A multicenter prospective phase II trial of neoadjuvant epirubicin, cyclophosphamide, and 5-fluorouracil (FEC100) followed by cisplatin-docetaxel with or without trastuzumab in locally advanced breast cancer. Cancer Chemother Pharmacol. 2016,77(1):147–53.

96. Diego EJ, McAuliffe PF, Soran A, et al. Axillary staging after neoadjuvant chemotherapy for breast cancer: a pilot study combining sentinel lymph node biopsy with radioactive seed localization of pre-treatment positive axillary lymph nodes. Ann Surg Oncol. 2016,23(5):1549–53.

97. Standard or Comprehensive Radiation Therapy in Treating Patients With Early-Stage Breast Cancer Previously Treated With Chemotherapy and Surgery. National Library of Medicine; 2013.

98. Alliance A011202: A Randomized Phase III Trial Comparing Axillary Lymph Node Dissection to Axillary Radiation in Breast Cancer Patients (cT1–3 N1) Who Have Positive Sentinel Lymph Node Disease After Receiving Neoadjuvant Chemotherapy. National Library of Medicine; 2019.

4 保留性乳房切除术的肿瘤学安全性及技术进展

编者：Paolo Veronesi, Francesca Magnoni, Antonio Toesca
译者：尹永硕

4.1 引言

皮肤保留乳房切除术（Skin-sparing mastectomy，SSM）及乳头保留乳房切除术（nipple-sparing mastectomy，NSM）标志着改良根治性乳房切除术（modified-radical mastectomy，MRM）的重大革新。随着保留皮肤和/或乳头-乳晕复合体（nipple-areolar complex，NAC）等新手术技术的应用，对乳腺癌采取保乳治疗的趋势不断增强，显著提升了乳腺癌患者对手术方式的接受度[1]。

Umberto Veronesi 提出"保留性乳房切除术"，用于定义 SSM 与 NSM，核心在于强调手术美学维度而非单纯技术层面，并将乳房外形维护确立为核心治疗目标："……保留性乳房切除术初看似存在逻辑悖论，但若将'保留'定义为形体完整性的维持，则此术语恰如其分……"[1] 该术式的确立显著改善了乳腺癌患者的生活质量。在乳房外科向形体美学方向演进的过程中，同步开展的相关研究亦证实了此类保留性手术的肿瘤学安全性，从而形成了技术革新与科学验证相互促进的发展格局。

4.2 保留性乳房切除术的历史沿革

近 20 年来，对保留性乳房切除术的广泛认可深刻改变了乳腺癌患者的手术治疗格局，其中乳头保留乳房切除术（NSM）逐渐取代皮肤保留乳房切除术（SSM）成为优选方案。多项研究表明，NSM 联合即刻重建能显著提高患者满意度及美学效果[2-5]。

P. Veronesi (✉)
IEO, European Institute of Oncology, IRCCS,
Division of Breast Cancer Surgery, Milan, Italy

Department of Oncology and Hemato-Oncology,
Faculty of Medicine, University of Milan, Milan, Italy
e-mail: paolo.veronesi@ieo.it

F. Magnoni · A. Toesca
IEO, European Institute of Oncology, IRCCS,
Division of Breast Cancer Surgery, Milan, Italy

© The Author(s), under exclusive license to Springer Nature Switzerland AG 2023
R. Vidya, H. Becker (eds.), *Prepectoral Breast Reconstruction*,
https://doi.org/10.1007/978-3-031-15590-1_4

乳房切除术通常适用于多中心性或局部晚期乳腺癌患者，应用比例因诊疗中心及地域差异存在显著差别[1]。该术式应用比例的提升，部分归因于乳房重建技术的进步与普及，以及乳腺影像学诊断精度的提高。乳腺 MRI 高灵敏度检测的广泛应用，使得 16% 患者检出额外病灶，且未影响局部复发率或生存风险[6]，在筛查及分期中对多灶性/多中心性肿瘤的检出率具有重要价值[7]。然而，COMICE 随机对照试验表明，MRI 在保守治疗与乳房切除术的决策选择中作用有限[8]。值得关注的是，术前接受乳腺 MRI 检查的患者选择乳房切除术的比例显著高于未行乳腺 MRI 检查者（43%：28%）[1, 9, 10]。

对于肿瘤体积较大、多中心性浸润癌、广泛导管内成分或多中心性纯导管原位癌患者，SSM 或 NSM 已成为必要术式[1]。尤其是乳腺体积较小或中等的多中心性癌患者，为确保切缘阴性常需实施乳房切除术。保留性乳房切除术可彻底清除全部乳腺组织（NSM 中，即使保留乳头-乳晕复合体亦能去除所有导管结构），同时实现理想美学效果。在此背景下，即刻乳房重建技术致力于塑造形态自然的乳房外形，最大限度缓解患者的心理创伤[1]。

保留乳头-乳晕复合体（NAC）对维持乳房自然形态至关重要，与非 NSM 术式相比，能显著提升患者术后生活质量[11-13]。然而，保留乳头的肿瘤学安全性仍存争议[1]。研究证实，SSM 中皮肤被膜的保留未增加肿瘤学风险，其复发率与传统全乳切除术相当[14-22]，现已被列为标准术式，并且不增加局部复发风险[23]。

在 NSM 操作中，必须彻底清除乳头区乳管结构[24]，仅保留乳头后方表皮及真皮层。尽管如此，因乳头后方可能残留微小导管组织的生物学特性，其远期局部复发风险仍受学界关注[25]。术前 NAC 临床受累及乳晕后切缘阳性是 NSM 的主要禁忌证。目前临床常规采用术中冰冻切片评估 NAC 状态，其特异性与阳性预测值达 100%，阴性预测值为 83%[1]。

近年来的重大进展包括胚系 BRCA 基因突变的发现。此类乳腺癌高危人群的识别，显著提升了预防性单侧/双侧乳房切除术的实施率，亦推动了 NSM 的临床需求[26]。预防性乳房切除术通过完全切除乳腺体实现风险最小化，而同期重建则兼顾美学效果。基于现有证据与指南更新[27]，采用 NSM 联合即刻重建既能保留皮肤及 NAC 结构，又可实现良好肿瘤控制与美学效果[26, 27]。

4.3 手术技术

保留皮肤乳房切除术（SSM）与保留乳头乳房切除术（NSM）均需分阶段实施腺体剥离与重建手术，NSM 需额外保留乳头-乳晕复合体（NAC）。1991 年，Toth 和 Lappert 首次提出 SSM 术式[28]，核心理念在于最大化保留皮肤以优化美学效果并实现即刻重建。该术式通过环绕 NAC 的梭形切口移除全部乳腺体及 NAC，同时完整保留皮肤被膜与自然乳房下皱襞结构[23, 29]。

Freeman 提出的 NSM 术式[30]在完全

切除乳腺腺体组织的基础上，完整保留皮肤被膜与 NAC。无论 SSM 或 NSM，保留皮肤被膜均为内置物或自体组织移植等即刻乳房重建技术创造了有利条件[23]。该技术的操作要点包括严格遵循解剖边界完整切除乳腺实质，同时保护皮肤被膜与乳房下皱襞以优化即刻重建效果。

术者应确保完全切除腺体组织并精细制备皮瓣：于腺体与皮下脂肪层间的浅筋膜层识别 Cooper 韧带，在此相对无血管层面谨慎进行剥离；精准把握皮下脂肪去除量，同时维持充足的皮瓣血供，尽量降低坏死风险[31]。

乳晕后间隙剥离更具技术挑战性：既要彻底清除所有乳腺导管，又需保护乳头血供系统[32]。在将腺体与胸大肌分开的过程中，若无肿瘤累及应保留筋膜结构[1]。对于乳房体积较大者，往往需结合皮肤缩减技术以塑造自然下垂形态[33,34]。

乳房皮肤切口应依据肿瘤位置及乳房形态进行选择[31]，最常采用外上象限线形切口，但基于不同临床特征亦可个性化调整。文献中已提出多种保留乳头乳晕术式（NSM）的切口设计方案。针对不同乳房体积、乳晕大小及下垂分型，可采用一系列非标准切口术式。Corso 团队对 100 例乳腺癌患者的 117 次手术进行回顾性分析[35]，详细分类包括：①半乳晕切口，适用于罩杯 A—B 型且无下垂，乳晕中—大的乳房；②环形乳晕切口，适用于罩杯 A—B 型伴 Ⅰ—Ⅱ 度下垂且乳晕小的乳房，尤其适合乳房组织量过多但下垂轻微者；③垂直切口，适用于罩杯 C—D 型伴 Ⅱ—Ⅳ 度下垂的乳房；④倒 T 形切口，适用于罩杯 D 型伴 Ⅲ—Ⅳ 度下垂的乳房。研究未发现临床病理参数、并发症发生率及手术满意度，与乳房下垂程度、体积等特征存在显著相关性，证实这些术式是对传统保留乳头-乳晕术式的改良，兼具多样性与安全性[35]。

乳房重建可由接受过肿瘤整形培训的乳腺外科医师独立完成，或由乳腺外科与整形外科团队协作实施[36-38]。

随着手术个性化需求的增加，机器人辅助乳房切除术作为开放手术的替代方案被引入，可在远离皮肤切口区域实现精准解剖[39]。机器人辅助保留乳头-乳晕的乳房切除术（RNSM）旨在改善传统开放式手术视野局限的缺点，通过腋中线切口实现更清晰的组织层面显露与深部操作。该技术在遵循标准乳房切除原则（全乳腺整体切除、解剖层次完整）的基础上，追求更优的操作精准性与美学效果[40,41]，同时可降低乳头-乳晕复合体损伤的风险。

机器人辅助乳房切除术首见于 2015 年[40]，其优势与局限性已在前瞻及随机试验中进行了评估[41,42]。多项研究证实其安全性与可行性，短期随访显示并发症发生率低且无局部复发[43-45]。第 15 届圣加仑国际乳腺癌会议将其纳入部分患者可选术式[46]，目前已有共识文件[47-51]及国际联合研究方案[52]正在推进，以验证其长期疗效。

为评估机器人辅助术式远期预后，一项对比该术式与传统开放手术的前瞻性随机对照试验已完成,结果即将发表[42]。

机器人辅助保留乳头-乳晕的乳房切除术（RNSM）已由多位先驱医师完成技术探索。韩国机器人内镜微创乳腺外科研究组（KoREaBSG）报道了8家机构11名经规范培训外科医师的早期经验[53]。研究表明学习曲线快速稳定，第二代术者在先驱医师的带教下获益更显著。作为新术式，RNSM需建立完善的培训体系，规范流程包括掌握传统的保留乳头-乳晕的乳房切除术（CNSM）、机器人模拟操作训练、尸体解剖实操及专家术式带教。

2019年，一项围术期数据分析显示[54]，2014年6月至2019年1月共进行94例RNSM手术（治疗或预防性），所有病例均获技术成功，并发症发生率极低，仅4例（4%）需再次手术或假体取出，另有13%患者出现仅需观察的轻微并发症。该数据与传统开放式NSM联合重建的大型单中心经验相当[55, 56]。

与开放式手术相比，RNSM的视觉系统优势与切口设计优化可提升操作精准度。手术机器人的机械臂在开放手术中拉钩无法到达的角度仍可灵活操作，采用高分辨率成像系统可清晰辨识组织层次。腋中线切口不仅被完美隐藏，更可优化血管保护——乳头血供主要依赖源自胸廓内动脉、肋间前动脉及胸外侧动脉的皮下穿支，而非腋动脉或肋间后动脉分支[57]。

Toesca等的首项RNSM与CNSM对比研究为Ⅲ期、开放标签、单中心随机对照试验（RCT），主要终点为手术并发症与生活质量，次要终点为肿瘤学结局[58]。结果显示，RNSM组在乳房形态满意度、心理适应、躯体功能及性健康评分均显著高于CNSM组（P值分别为<0.0001、<0.0001、0.0005和<0.0001），术后12个月各项评分仍维持稳定（P=0.12、0.93、1.00），而CNSM组显著下降（P=0.02、0.005、0.02）。RNSM组的总体躯体形象量表评分显著占优（20.7±13.8：9.9±5.1，P<0.0001）。中位随访28.6个月，未见局部复发[58]。

最新中位随访42.0个月的分析显示，两组无病生存率（P=0.910）与总生存率（P=0.760）无统计学差异，RNSM组未发生乳头复发而CNSM组出现1例（数据于2022年9月18~21日在意大利全国ACOI大会上公布）。该RCT入组始于2017年，肿瘤学结果随访期仍较短，但RNSM组中位随访42个月无局部复发数据令人鼓舞。国际荟萃研究（SORI研究）显示了相似的肿瘤学结局[59]。

尽管如此，仍需以无病生存率为主要终点的随机对照试验结合高级别证据来证明机器人辅助手术在远期肿瘤学结局上不劣于传统手术。韩国研究组正计划开展相关随机对照试验以评估无病生存率。虽然早期研究提示安全性可控，但仍需更大样本研究佐证。

在胸肌前重建中，虽基于肿瘤学考虑必须维持正确的浅层结构，但需要普外科医师与整形外科医师密切协作以最大限度避免切除过于激进，保障皮瓣血供。为降低皮瓣或乳头-乳晕复合体的坏死风险，应系统评估组织灌注状态。既往放疗史、吸烟史更可能会导致皮肤血供受损，肥胖及免疫功能抑制亦增加并发症风险。此外，接受直接胸肌前假体重建者需具备足够脂肪储备，以满足脂肪移植需求[60]。

4.4 并发症

保乳术式的术后并发症包括皮瓣坏死、血肿、血清肿、切口裂开、假体脱失等[31, 61]。多项研究表明，切口类型、辅助化疗/放疗、初始瘤灶大小、淋巴结受累及吸烟等，与保留乳头－乳晕的乳房切除术后并发症相关[4, 31, 62]。乳头－乳晕复合体坏死较为常见[31]，其存活率是保乳手术关键评估指标[1]。欧洲肿瘤研究院的研究显示，合并症、吸烟、切口类型、皮瓣厚度及重建方式等，均影响乳头乳晕－复合体坏死的发生率[63]。

Headon 等[64]对 12 358 例保留乳头乳晕的乳房切除术的荟萃分析显示，总体并发症发生率（22.3%）与传统保乳术式相当，但乳头坏死风险增加（5.9%）。乳房体积过大、下垂、吸烟、术前放疗及乳晕切口，被证实为乳头坏死的独立危险因素[63]。

欧洲肿瘤研究院对 1 989 例患者的大型单中心研究显示[56]，导管原位癌组乳头－乳晕复合体坏死率为 2.2%，浸润癌组为 3.5%，稍低于既往报道。

4.5 肿瘤安全性研究现状

美国外科学院国家癌症数据库与美国癌症协会联合研究指出，保留乳头－乳晕的乳房切除术（NSM）在进展期患者尤其接受新辅助化疗人群中的应用呈上升趋势，但尚缺乏充分证据证实其肿瘤学安全性[65]。乳头－乳晕复合体作为潜在复发风险区域，其保留与否直接关系到保乳术式的肿瘤安全性[1]。两项大型多中心随机试验表明，乳房切除术联合放疗与广泛局部切除的远期生存率相当，提示保留乳头－乳晕复合体对总生存率无显著影响[66, 67]。

欧洲肿瘤研究院对 2002~2007 年的 934 例保乳术后患者的研究显示[68, 69]，中位随访 50 个月时 5 年总生存率达 96.4%（浸润癌患者 95.5%，导管原位癌患者 100%），浸润癌患者 5 年累计乳房相关事件发生率为 14.7%。该生存数据与传统术式（保留皮肤全乳切除术、象限切除联合辅助放疗）相当，证实保乳技术在安全性及美容效果上的优势[66, 70]。

后续研究表明，保留皮肤的手术具备肿瘤安全性，保留皮肤的全乳切除术（SSM）的局部复发率（5%~6%）与改良根治术相近[71, 72]。9 项研究对 3 739 例患者进行荟萃分析，结果显示，SSM 组局部复发率与非 SSM 组无统计学差异，且远处转移发生率更低[19]。

目前的争论聚焦于保留乳头－乳晕复合体是否增加局部复发风险[1]。多项前瞻性试验正在评估 NSM 的肿瘤安全性。美国国家综合癌症网络（NCCN）推荐对经多学科团队严格筛选的早期、生物学特征良好、无乳头溢液及 Paget 病患者采用该术式[73]。

文献显示，接受 NSM 的乳腺癌患者的乳头-乳晕复合体受累率为 8%~33%[23, 72, 74, 75]。2012 年，Veronesi 在综述中提示该数据为 0~18%，局部复发多位于皮肤，发生率为 0~20.8%[1]。Gerber 研究对比了改良根治术、SSM 与 NSM 组患者（中位随访 59 个月），局部复发率分别为 8%、6%、5%，总生存率组间无差异[72]。

迄今为止，多项研究（随访 10~101 个月）显示保乳术式局部复发率较低[69, 72, 76]：SSM 组中位随访 25~78.1 个月，局部复发率为 5.5%~6.2%[22, 77]；NSM 组随访 10~60 个月，局部复发率为 0~4.6%[76-82]。

欧洲肿瘤研究院对浸润性癌及原位癌患者进行了大样本研究[56]，中位随访近 8 年。结果显示，NSM 对经严格筛选的患者具有肿瘤学安全性。浸润癌患者局部复发率为 5.3%，原位癌组为 4%，其中乳头-乳晕复合体复发占 1.8%；浸润癌患者 5 年总生存率为 96.1%，原位癌组达 99.2%。

Wu 等[83]分析了 944 例（962 次 NSM）浸润性乳腺癌患者，39 例发生乳头-乳晕复合体复发。多灶性/多中心病灶、激素受体阴性、高组织学分级及广泛导管内成分是通过多因素分析得出的独立风险因素，但复发组与无复发组的无远处转移生存率及总生存率无差异，并且经恰当治疗后预后良好[84]。

在涉及 3 015 例乳房切除术的 14 项研究中，系统评价表明[85]，NSM 与 SSM 组的局部复发率（3.9% : 3.3%，$P=0.45$）及死亡率均无统计学差异（$P=0.34$）。

Memorial Sloan Kettering 癌症中心于 2009 年发表的一项早期研究的样本量不足[86]，但后续 467 例治疗性 NSM 的回顾性分析显示[23]，与 2011 年前相比，乳腺癌 NSM 实施率显著提升（58% : 77%，$P<0.001$）。中位随访 39.4 个月时，449 例中仅 4 例局部复发，并且均未累及乳头-乳晕复合体。

最新纳入 588 例 NSM（83% 双侧）的回顾性研究[61]中，针对乳腺癌患者的 399 例手术结果显示，半数复发患者为三阴性或淋巴结阳性，但无一例累及乳头-乳晕复合体。

近期多项研究提示有必要拓展 NSM 适应证，如新辅助化疗后[87]或肿瘤毗邻乳头[88]等。Wu 等[87]分析了 310 例新辅助化疗后患者（319 次 NSM）发现，中位随访 63 个月 ± 22 个月时 38 例局部复发（6 例乳头乳晕复合体复发），多因素分析提示术后 Ki67>10%（HR=4.245，95%CI：1.865~9.663，$P=0.001$）是独立危险因素。

Kim 等[88]对肿瘤—乳头距离 ≤ 2cm（47.4%），甚至 ≤ 1cm（27.5%）的 251 例 NSM 研究发现，中位随访 68 个月时局部复发率为 4.4%，浸润癌患者 5 年总生存率为 98.0%，原位癌患者达 100%，乳头-乳晕复合体复发仅 0.4%。

4.6 美容效果与心理获益

保留乳头-乳晕的乳房切除术（NSM）对患者心理健康、性生活与社交健康具有重要影响。研究表明，与延迟重建的保留皮肤全乳切除术（SSM）相比，NSM 手术保留了乳头-乳晕复合体（NAC），可显著提高患者对手术的接受度，提升自我形象满意度与自尊水平[89]，尽管多数病例会出现乳头感觉显著或完全丧失[31]。

Yueh 等[90] 报道 10 例 NSM 患者术后美学效果优异（满意度评分 7.6/10），但乳头敏感度评分较低（2.8/10）。Petit 等[68] 的研究显示，美学满意度评分中位数为 8/10，乳头敏感度为 2/10，仅 15% 患者术后 1 年敏感度轻微恢复。Djohan 的研究[91] 显示，141 例患者中的 67 例 NAC 保留合理敏感度，乳房体积大、体重指数高及假体容量大的患者的满意度降低。

2016 年，Sisco 等经系统回顾[92] 指出，NSM 术后 NAC 感觉正常者比例为 10%~43%。

4.7 小结

Umberto Veronesi 教授提出的"从最大可耐受治疗向最小有效治疗演进"[93]，体现了乳腺外科领域逐步保守化的趋势。保乳手术是这一理念的典型实践，其肿瘤学安全性已在多项研究中得到验证。文献表明，在严格多学科评估下，NSM 联合即刻个性化重建用于乳腺癌治疗，或作为 BRCA 突变携带者的预防性手术时，具备肿瘤学安全性，但需更多长期随访数据佐证对特定乳腺癌患者的安全性。

4.8 要点

- 新一代保乳术式（保留皮肤和/或乳头乳晕复合体）显著提高了乳腺癌患者对治疗的接受度。
- 保留皮肤-乳房切除术（SSM）与保留乳头乳房切除术（NSM）作为改良根治术的革新术式，体现了患者对形体完整性的诉求。
- Veronesi 提出的"保乳手术"理念，强调在 SSM/NSM 中形体美学与手术技术同等重要，能显著改善患者术后身心健康。
- 近 20 年来，因 NSM 联合即刻重建在肿瘤治疗与风险预防中的优异美容效果与满意度，其已逐渐取代 SSM 成为优选术式。
- SSM/NSM 应遵循腺体切除联合重建的手术流程（NSM 额外需保留 NAC），耗时较传统术式倍增。
- 依据肿瘤位置与乳房形态差异，NSM 可采取多种新切口设计。
- 机器人辅助乳房切除术作为开放手术的补充，满足个性化需求，近年来逐步应用于临床。
- 保乳手术（尤其保留 NAC）的肿瘤学安全性，仍需多学科团队根据严格临床标准审慎评估。
- 如大量研究所示，保留乳头乳房切除术（NSM）联合即刻个性化重建术的适应证选择，应依据特定临床标准由多学科专家小组进行讨论。

未来需更多研究拓展 NSM 适应证并

提供充分的长期安全性证据。

致谢 感谢 Linda Ann Cairns 对本章节文稿编辑工作的支持，以及 Maria Grazia Villardita 的编辑协助。

利益冲突 作者声明无利益冲突。

参考文献

1. Veronesi U, Stafyla V, Petit JY, Veronesi P. Conservative mastectomy: extending the idea of breast conservation. Lancet Oncol. 2012,13(7):e311–7. https://doi.org/10.1016/S1470–2045(12)70133-X.
2. Moyer HR, Ghazi B, Daniel JR, Daniel JR, Gasgarth R, Carlson GW. Nipple-sparing mastectomy: technical aspects and aesthetic outcomes. Ann Plast Surg. 2012,68:446e450.
3. Frey JD, Alperovich M, Levine JP, Choi M, Karp NS. Does smoking history confer a higher risk for reconstructive complications in nipplesparing mastectomy? Breast J. 2017,23:415e420.
4. Radovanovic Z, Radovanovic D, Golubovic A, Ivkovic-Kapicl T, Bokorov B, Mandic A. Early complications after nipple-sparing mastectomy and immediate reconstruction with silicone prosthesis: results of 214 procedures. Scand J Surg. 2010,99:115e118.
5. Wengler CA, Valente SA, Al-Hilli Z, Woody NM, Muntean JH, Abraham J, et al. Determinants of short and long term outcomes in patients undergoing immediate breast reconstruction following neoadjuvant chemotherapy. J Surg Oncol. 2017,116:797e802.
6. Houssami N, Ciatto S, Macaskill P, Lord SJ, Warren RM, Dixon JM, et al. Accuracy and surgical impact of magnetic resonance imaging in breast cancer staging: systematic review and meta-analysis in detection of multifocal and multicentric cancer. J Clin Oncol. 2008,26:3248–58.
7. Corso G, Magnoni F, Provenzano E, Girardi A, Iorfida M, De Scalzi AM, et al. Multicentric breast cancer with heterogeneous histopathology: a multidisciplinary review. Future Oncol. 2020,16(8):395–412. https://doi.org/10.2217/fon-2019–0540.
8. Turnbull L, Brown S, Harvey I, Olivier C, Drew P, Napp V, et al. Comparative effectiveness of MRI in breast cancer (COMICE) trial: a randomised controlled trial. Lancet. 2010,375:563–71.
9. Barchie MF, Clive KS, Tyler JA, Sutcliffe JB, Kirkpatrick AD, Bell LM, et al. Standardized pretreatment breast MRI-accuracy and influence on mastectomy decisions. J Surg Oncol. 2011,104: 741–5.
10. Miller BT, Abbott AM, Tuttle TM. The influence of preoperative MRI on breast cancer treatment. Ann Surg Oncol. 2012,19:536–40.
11. Weber WP, Haug M, Kurzeder C, Bjelic-Radisic V, Koller R, Reitsamer R, et al. Oncoplastic breast consortium consensus conference on nipple-sparing mastectomy. Breast Cancer Res Treat. 2018,172(3):523–37. https://doi.org/10.1007/s10549–018–4937–1.
12. Bailey CR, Ogbuagu O, Baltodano PA, Simjee UF, Manahan MA, Cooney DS, et al. Quality-of life outcomes improve with nipple-sparing mastectomy and breast reconstruction. Plast Reconstr Surg. 2017,140(2):219–26.
13. Metcalfe KA, Cil TD, Semple JL, Xuan Li LD, Baghcr S, Zhong T, et al. Long-term psychosocial functioning in women with bilateral prophylactic mastectomy: does preservation of the nipple-areolar complex make a difference? Ann Surg Oncol. 2015,22(10):3324–30.
14. Eldor L, Spiegel A. Breast reconstruction after bilateral prophylactic mastectomy in women at high risk for breast cancer. Breast J. 2009,15(Suppl 1):S81–9.
15. Lostumbo L, Carbine NE, Wallace J. Prophylactic mastectomy for the prevention of breast cancer. Cochrane Database Syst Rev. 2010,(11):CD002748. https://doi.org/10.1002/14651858.CD002748.pub3.
16. Morrow M, Mehrara B. Prophylactic mastectomy and the timing of breast reconstruction. Br J

Surg. 2009,96(1):1–2.
17. Peled AW, Irwin CS, Hwang ES, Ewing CA, Alvarado M, Esserman LJ. Total skin-sparing mastectomy in BRCA mutation carriers. Ann Surg Oncol. 2014,21(1):37–41.
18. Peled AW, Foster RD, Stover AC, et al. Outcomes after total skin-sparing mastectomy and immediate reconstruction in 657 breasts. Ann Surg Oncol. 2012,19(11):3402–9.
19. Lanitis S, Tekkis PP, Sgourakis G, Dimopoulos N, Al Mufti R, Hadjiminas DJ. Comparison of skin-sparing mastectomy versus non-skin-sparing mastectomy for breast cancer: a meta-analysis of observational studies. Ann Surg. 2010,251(4):632–9.
20. Kroll SS, Schusterman MA, Tadjalli HE, Singletary SE, Ames FC. Risk of recurrence after treatment of early breast cancer with skin-sparing mastectomy. Ann Surg Oncol. 1997,4(3):193–7.
21. Kroll SS, Khoo A, Singletary SE, Ames FC, Wang BG, Reece GP, et al. Local recurrence risk after skin-sparing and conventional mastectomy: a 6-year follow-up. Plast Reconstr Surg. 1999,104(2):421–5.
22. Newman LA, Kuerer HM, Hunt KK, Kroll SS, Ames FC, Ross MI, et al. Presentation, treatment, and outcome of local recurrence after skin-sparing mastectomy and immediate breast reconstruction. Ann Surg Oncol. 1998,5(7):620–6.
23. Valero MG, Muhsen S, Moo TA, Zabor EC, Stempel M, Pusic A, et al. Increase in utilization of nipple-sparing mastectomy for breast cancer: indications, complications, and oncologic outcomes. Ann Surg Oncol. 2020,27(2):344–51. https://doi.org/10.1245/s10434–019–07948-x.
24. Tokin C, Weiss A, Wang-Rodriguez J, Blair SL. Oncologic safety of skin-sparing and nipple-sparing mastectomy: a discussion and review of the literature. Int J Surg Oncol. 2012,2012:921821. https://doi.org/10.1155/2012/921821.
25. De La Cruz L, Moody AM, Tappy EE, Blankenship SA, Hecht EM. Overall survival, disease-free survival, local recurrence, and nipple-areolar recurrence in the setting of nipple-sparing mastectomy: a meta-analysis and systematic review. Ann Surg Oncol. 2015,22(10):3241–9. https://doi.org/10.1245/s10434–015–4739–1.
26. Jakub JW, Peled AW, Gray RJ, Greenup RA, Kiluk JV, Sacchini V, et al. Oncologic safety of prophylactic nipple-sparing mastectomy in a population with BRCA mutations. JAMA Surg. 2018,153:123.
27. Corso G, Magnoni F. Hereditary breast cancer: translation into clinical practice of recent American Society of Clinical Oncology, American Society of Radiation Oncology, and Society of Surgical Oncology recommendations [published online ahead of print, 2020 Sep 3]. Eur J Cancer Prev. 2020,10.1097/CEJ.0000000000000624. https://doi.org/10.1097/CEJ.0000000000000624.
28. Toth BA, Lappert P. Modified skin incisions for mastectomy: the need for plastic surgical input in preoperative planning. Plast Reconstr Surg. 1991,87(6):1048–53.
29. Carlson GW. Skin sparing mastectomy: anatomic and technical considerations. Am Surg. 1996,62(2):151–5.
30. Freeman BS. Subcutaneous mastectomy for benign breast lesions with immediate or delayed prosthetic replacement. Plast Reconstr Surg Transplant Bull. 1962,30:676–82.
31. Galimberti V, Vicini E, Corso G, Morigi C, Fontana S, Sacchini V, et al. Nipple-sparing and skin-sparing mastectomy: review of aims, oncological safety and contraindications. Breast. 2017,34 Suppl 1(Suppl 1):S82–4. https://doi.org/10.1016/j.breast.2017.06.034.
32. Franceschini G, Masetti R. What the surgeons should know about the bilateral prophylactic mastectomy in BRCA mutation carriers. Eur J Breast Health. 2019,15:135–6.
33. Larson DL, Basir Z, Bruce T. Is oncologic safety compatible with a predictably viable mastectomy skin flap? Plast Reconstr Surg. 2011,127:27–33.

34. Nava MB, Ottolenghi J, Pennati A, Spano A, Bruno N, Catanuto G, et al. Skin/nipple sparing mastectomies and implant-based breast reconstruction in patients with large and ptotic breast: oncological and reconstructive results. Breast. 2012,21(3):267–71. https://doi.org/10.1016/j.breast.2011.01.004.
35. Corso G, De Lorenzi F, Vicini E, Pagani G, Veronesi P, Sargenti M, et al. Nipple-sparing mastectomy with different approaches: surgical incisions, complications, and cosmetic results. Preliminary results of 100 consecutive patients at a single center. J Plast Reconstr Aesthet Surg. 2018,71(12):1751–60. https://doi.org/10.1016/j.bjps.2018.07.022.
36. Petit J, Rietjens M, Garusi C. Breast reconstructive techniques in cancer patients: which ones, when to apply, which immediate and long term risks? Crit Rev Oncol Hematol. 2001,38:231–9.
37. Masetti R, Di Leone A, Franceschini G, Magno S, Terribile D, Fabbri MC, et al. Oncoplastic techniques in the conservative surgical treatment of breast cancer: an overview. Breast J. 2006,12(5 suppl 2):S174–80.
38. Kollias J, Davies G, Bochner MA, Gill PG. Clinical impact of oncoplastic surgery in a specialist breast practice. ANZ J Surg. 2008,78:269–72.
39. Toesca A, Peradze N, Galimberti V, et al. Robotic nipple-sparing mastectomy and immediate breast reconstruction with implant: first report of surgical technique. Ann Surg. 2017,266(2):e28–30. Epub 2015
40. Toesca A, Manconi A, Peradze N, et al. 1931 preliminary report of robotic nipple-sparing mastectomy and immediate breast reconstruction with implant. Eur J Cancer. 2015,51(3):S309.
41. Toesca A, Peradze N, Manconi A, Manconi A, Intra M, Gentilini O, et al. Robotic nipple-sparing mastectomy for the treatment of breast cancer: feasibility and safety study. Breast. 2017,31:51–6.
42. NIH U.S. National Library of Medicine. ClinicalTrials.gov https://clinicaltrials.gov/ct2/show/NCT03440398.
43. Lai HW, Wang CC, Lai YC, Chen CJ, Lin SL, Chen ST, et al. The learning curve of robotic nipple sparing mastectomy for breast cancer: an analysis of consecutive 39 procedures with cumulative sum plot. Eur J Surg Oncol. 2019,45(2):125–33. https://doi.org/10.1016/j.ejso.2018.09.021.
44. Lai HW, Chen ST, Lin SL, Chen CJ, Lin YL, Pai SH, et al. Robotic nipple-sparing mastectomy and immediate breast reconstruction with gel implant: technique, preliminary results and patient-reported cosmetic outcome. Ann Surg Oncol. 2019,26(1):42–52. https://doi.org/10.1245/s10434-018-6704-2. Epub 2018 Aug 14
45. Sarfati B, Honart JF, Leymarie N, Rimareix F, Al Khashnam H, Kolb F. Robotic da Vinci xi-assisted nipple-sparing mastectomy: first clinical report. Breast J. 2018,24(3):373–6. https://doi.org/10.1111/tbj.12937. Epub 2017 Dec 18
46. Morigi C. Highlights from the 15th St Gallen international breast cancer conference 15–18 March, 2017, Vienna: tailored treatments for patients with early breast cancer. Ecancermedicalscience. 2017,11:732.
47. Margenthaler JA. Robotic mastectomy-program malfunction? JAMA Surg. 2020,155(6):461–2.
48. Kopkash K, Sisco M, Poli E, Seth A, Pesce C. The modern approach to the nipple-sparing mastectomy. J Surg Oncol. 2020,122:29–35.
49. Selber JC. Robotic nipple-sparing mastectomy: the next step in the evolution of minimally invasive breast surgery. Ann Surg Oncol. 2019,26(1):10–1.
50. Struk S, Qassemyar Q, Leymarie N, Honart J-F, Alkhashnam H, De Fremicourt K, et al. The ongoing emergence of robotics in plastic and reconstructive surgery. Ann Chir Plast Esthet. 2018,63(2):105–12.
51. Toesca A, Peradze N, Manconi A, Nevola Teixeira LF. Reply to the letter to the editor "Robotic-assisted Nipple Sparing Mastectomy: a feasibility study on cadaveric models" by

Sarfati B. et al. J Plast Reconstr Aesthet Surg. 2017,70(4):558–60.
52. NIH U.S. National Library of Medicine. ClinicalTrials.gov (https://clinicaltrials.gov/ct2/show/NCT04108117).
53. Ryu JM, Kim JY, Choi HJ, Ko B, Kim J, Cho J, et al. Robot-assisted nipple-sparing mastectomy with immediate breast reconstruction: an initial experience of the Korea Robot-endoscopy Minimal Access Breast Surgery Study Group (KoREa-BSG). Ann Surg. 2022,275(5):985–91. https://doi.org/10.1097/SLA.0000000000004492.
54. Toesca A, Invento A, Massari G, Girardi A, Peradze N, et al. Update on the feasibility and Progress on robotic breast surgery. Ann Surg Oncol. 2019,26:3046. https://doi.org/10.1245/s10434–019–07590–7.
55. Botteri E, Gentilini O, Rotmensz N, Veronesi P, Ratini S, Fraga-Guedes C, et al. Mastectomy without radiotherapy: outcome analysis after 10 years of follow-up in a single institution. Breast Cancer Res Treat. 2012,134(3):1221–8.
56. Galimberti V, Morigi C, Bagnardi V, Corso G, Vicini E, Kahler Ribeiro Fontana S, et al. Oncological outcomes of nipple-sparing mastectomy: a single-center experience of 1989 patients. Ann Surg Oncol. 2018,25(13):3849–57. https://doi.org/10.1245/s10434–018–6759–0.
57. Dm O'D, Prescher A, Pallua N. Vascular reliability of nipple-areola complex-bearing pedicles: an anatomical microdissection study. Plast Reconstr Surg. 2007,119(4):1167–77.
58. Toesca A, Sangalli C, Maisonneuve P, Massari G, Girardi A, Baker JL, et al. A randomized trial of robotic mastectomy versus open surgery in women with breast cancer or BrCA mutation. Ann Surg. 2022,276(1):11–9. https://doi.org/10.1097/SLA.0000000000004969. Epub 2021 Jun 9
59. Prospective Study of MAstectomy With Reconstruction Including Robot Endoscopic Surgery (MARRES). https://clinicaltrials.gov/ct2/show/NCT04585074. Accessed 12 Jan 2023.
60. Sigalove S, Maxwell GP, Sigalove NM, Storm-Dickerson TL, Pope N, Rice J, Gabriel A. Prepectoral implant-based breast reconstruction: rationale, indications, and preliminary results. Plast Reconstr Surg. 2017,139(2):287–94. https://doi.org/10.1097/PRS.0000000000002950.
61. Mergenthaler JA, Gan C, Yan Y, Cyr AE, Tenenbaum M, Hook D, et al. Oncologic safety and outcomes in patients undergoing nipple-sparing mastectomy. J Am Coll Surg. 2020,230(4):535–41. https://doi.org/10.1016/j.jamcollsurg.2019.12.028.
62. Colwell AS, Tessler O, Lin AM, Liao E, Winograd J, Cetrulo CL, et al. Breast reconstruction following nipple-sparing mastectomy: predictors of complications, reconstruction outcomes, and 5-year trends. Plast Reconstr Surg. 2014,133:496e506.
63. Lohsiriwat V, Rotmensz N, Botteri E, Intra M, Veronesi P, Martella S, et al. Do clinicopathological features of the cancer patient relate with nipple areolar complex necrosis in nipple-sparing mastectomy? Ann Surg Oncol. 2013,20(3):990e6. https://doi.org/10.1245/s10434–012–2677–8.
64. Headon HL, Kasem A, Mokbel K. The oncological safety of nipple-sparing mastectomy: a systematic review of the literature with a pooled analysis of 12,358 procedures. Arch Plast Surg. 2016,43(4):328e38. https://doi.org/10.5999/aps.2016.43.4.328.
65. Wong SM, Chun YS, Sagara Y, Golshan M, Erdmann-Sager J. National patterns of breast reconstruction and nipple-sparing mastectomy for breast cancer, 2005–2015. Ann Surg Oncol. 2019,26:3194–203.
66. Fisher B, Anderson S, Bryant J, Margolese RG, Deutsch M, Fisher ER, et al. Twenty-year follow-up of a randomized trial comparing total mastectomy, lumpectomy, and lumpectomy plus irradiation for the treatment of invasive breast cancer. N Engl J Med. 2002,347:1233–41.
67. Salgarello M, Visconti G, Barone-Adesi L.

Nipple-sparing mastectomy with immediate implant reconstruction: cosmetic outcomes and technical refinements. Plast Reconstr Surg. 2010,126:1460–71.
68. Petit JY, Veronesi U, Orecchia R, Rey P, Martella S, Didier F, et al. Nipple sparing mastectomy with nipple sparing areola intraoperative radiotherapy: one thousand and one cases of five years experience at the European Institute of Oncology of Milan (EIO). Breast Cancer Res Treat. 2009,117:333–8.
69. Petit JY, Veronesi U, Orecchia R, Curigliano G, Rey PC, Botteri E, et al. Risk factors associated with recurrence after nipple-sparing mastectomy for invasive and intraepithelial neoplasia. Ann Oncol. 2012,23(8):2053–8.
70. Veronesi U, Cascinelli N, Mariani L, Greco M, Saccozzi R, Luini A, et al. Twenty-year follow-up of a randomized study comparing breast-conserving surgery with radical mastectomy for early breast cancer. N Engl J Med. 2002,347:1227–32.
71. Yi M, Kronowitz SJ, Meric-Bernstam F, Feig BW, Symmans WF, Lucci A, et al. Local, regional and systemic recurrence rates in patients undergoing skin sparing mastectomy compared with conventional mastectomy. Cancer. 2011,117:916–24.
72. Gerber B, Krause A, Dieterich M, Kundt G, Reimer T. The oncological safety of skin sparing mastectomy with conservation of the nipple-areola complex and autologous reconstruction: an extended follow-up study. Ann Surg. 2009,249:461–8.
73. National Comprehensive Cancer Network (NCCN). NCCN guidelines version 6.2020. Invasive breast cancer. https://www.nccn.org/professionals/physician_gls/pdf/breast.pdf. Accessed 12 December 2020.
74. Crowe JP, Patrick RJ, Yetman RJ, Djohan R. Nipple-sparing mastectomy update: one hundred forty-nine procedures and clinical outcomes. Arch Surg. 2008,143(11):1106–10. (discussion 10)
75. Lagios MD, Gates EA, Westdahl PR, Richards V, Alpert BS. A guide to the frequency of nipple involvement in breast cancer. a study of 149 consecutive mastectomies using a serial sub-gross and correlated radiographic technique. Am J Surg. 1979,138(1):135–42.
76. de Alcantara FP, Capko D, Barry JM, Morrow M, Pusic A, Sacchini VS. Nipple-sparing mastectomy for breast cancer andrisk-reducing surgery: the memorial Sloan-Kettering cancer center experience. Ann Surg Oncol. 2011,18(11):3117–22.
77. Carlson GW, Styblo TM, Lyles RH, Jones G, Murray DR, Staley CA, et al. The use of skin sparing mastectomy in the treatment of breast cancer: the Emory experience. Surg Oncol. 2003,12(4):265–9.
78. Orzalesi L, Casella D, Santi C, Cecconi L, Murgo R, Rinaldi S, et al. Nipple sparing mastectomy: surgical and oncological outcomes from a national multicentric registry with 913 patients (1006 cases) over a six year period. Breast. 2016,25:75–81.
79. Coopey SB, Tang R, Lei L, Freer PE, Kansal K, Colwell AS, et al. Increasing eligibility for nipplesparing mastectomy. Ann Surg Oncol. 2013,20(10):3218–22.
80. Krajewski AC, Boughey JC, Degnim AC, Jakub JW, Jacobson SR, Hoskin TL, et al. Expanded indications and improved outcomes for nipple-sparing mastectomy over time. Ann Surg Oncol. 2015,22(10):3317–23.
81. Boneti C, Yuen J, Santiago C, et al. Oncologic safety of nipple skin-sparing or total skin-sparing mastectomies with immediate reconstruction. J Am Coll Surg. 2011,212(4):686–93. (discussion 93–5)
82. Lohsiriwat V, Martella S, Rietjens M, Botteri E, Rotmensz N, Mastropasqua MG, et al. Paget's disease as a local recurrence after nipple-sparing mastectomy: clinical presentation, treatment, outcome, and risk factor analysis. Ann Surg Oncol. 2012,19(6):1850–5.

83. Wu ZY, Kim HJ, Lee JW, Chung IY, Kim JS, Lee SB, et al. Breast cancer recurrence in the nipple-areola complex after nipple-sparing mastectomy with immediate breast for invasive breast cancer. JAMA Surg. 2019,154:1030e1037.
84. Wu ZY, Ko B. Recurrence at nipple-areola complex and safety of nipple-sparing mastectomy-reply. JAMA Surg. 2020,155(4):365. https://doi.org/10.1001/jamasurg.2019.5478.
85. Agha RA, Al Omran Y, Wellstead G, Sagoo H, Barai I, Rajmohan S, et al. Systematic review of therapeutic nipple-sparing versus skin-sparing mastectomy. BJS Open. 2019,3:135e145.
86. Garcia-Etienne CA, Cody Iii HS, Disa JJ, Cordeiro P, Sacchini V. Nipple-sparing mastectomy: initial experience at the memorial Sloan-Kettering cancer center and a comprehensive review of literature. Breast J. 2009,15(4):440–9.
87. Wu ZY, Kim HJ, Lee JW, Chung IY, Kim JS, Lee SB, et al. Oncologic outcomes of nipple-sparing mastectomy and immediate reconstruction after neoadjuvant chemotherapy for breast cancer. Ann Surg. 2020, https://doi.org/10.1097/SLA.0000000000003798. Online ahead of print
88. Kim S, Lee S, Bae Y, Lee S. Nipple-sparing mastectomy for breast cancer close to the nipple: a single institution's 11-year experience. Breast Cancer. 2020,27(5):999–1006. https://doi.org/10.1007/s12282–020–01104–0.
89. Didier F, Radice D, Gandini S, Bedolis R, Rotmensz N, Maldifassi A, et al. Does nipple preservation in mastectomy improve satisfaction with cosmetic results, psychological adjustment, body image and sexuality? Breast Cancer Res Treat. 2009,118(3):623e33. https://doi.org/10.1007/s10549–008–0238–4.
90. Yueh JH, Houlihan MJ, Slavin SA, Lee BT, Pories SE, Morris DJ. Nipple-sparing mastectomy: evaluation of patient satisfaction, aesthetic results, and sensation. Ann Plast Surg. 2009,62: 586–90.
91. Djohan R, Gage E, Gatherwright J, Pavri S, Firouz J, Bernard S, et al. Patient satisfaction following nipple-sparing mastectomy and immediate breast reconstruction: an 8-year outcome study. Plast Reconstr Surg. 2010,125:818–299.
92. Sisco M, Yao KA. Nipple-sparing mastectomy: a contemporary perspective. J Surg Oncol. 2016,113(8):883e90. https://doi.org/10.1002/jso.24209.
93. Veronesi U, Stafyla V, Luini A, Veronesi P. Breast cancer: from "maximum tolerable" to "minimum effective" treatment. Front Oncol. 2012,2:125. https://doi.org/10.3389/fonc.2012.00125.

5　胸肌前乳房重建：选择标准与患者考量

编者：Hani Sbitany, Sharat Chopra, Raghavan Vidya, Hilton Becker
译者：王新昭

5.1　引言

全球每年新诊断乳腺癌近百万例，仅英国就年新增约 55 900 例[1]。随着合成材料（Vicryl®、钛或 TIGR® 网）与生物材料（ADM）应用于假体重建，传统胸肌后假体重建正逐步被创伤更小的胸肌前重建技术取代。胸肌前间隙指乳房皮肤与胸壁肌肉间的潜在腔隙[2]，用于放置 ADM 与假体。在该技术中，假体置于胸大肌与前锯肌浅面，保留胸壁肌肉的自然解剖位置[3]，可规避放疗引发的胸壁纤维化与挛缩（导致上肢活动受限及假体移位），并减少术后疼痛，防止动态畸形，提升满意度与美观度[4-6]。

通过严格筛选患者并规范技术操作，胸肌前重建可实现较低的并发症发生率与较高的满意度。需充分评估术前/术中风险因素（因假体邻近皮瓣致血供相对不足），以保障手术安全。

5.2　术前选择考量

5.2.1　患者标准

胸肌前假体重建适用于符合假体置入重建条件的患者（图 5.1）。

相对禁忌证包括：肥胖（BMI ≥ 35）、糖尿病控制不佳、免疫功能低下及吸烟者——此类因素易导致皮瓣血供障碍，增加皮瓣坏死及假体外露风险。其他禁忌证包括皮肤质量差（如胶原缺陷、乳腺癌或霍奇金淋巴瘤胸部放疗史）[7]。放疗后

适合	可考虑提供	禁忌
• BMI 20~35，无糖尿病史，无吸烟史 • 美国麻醉医师协会（ASA）分级1级 • 无既往放疗史 • 肿瘤可切除	• BMI 35~40，糖尿病控制良好，既往有吸烟史 • ASA 分级2级 • 既往放疗：评估显示最小辐射损伤 • 新辅助化疗后肿瘤可切除	• 病理性肥胖（BMI>40） • 糖尿病控制不佳 • ASA 3/4级 • 目前吸烟 • 慢性免疫抑制 • 既往放疗：评估显示明显辐射损伤 • 肿瘤侵犯皮肤、胸壁

图 5.1　术前选择注意事项

延迟性皮肤纤维化会使包膜挛缩、假体失败的发生率增高并影响美观[8]。对此类患者，建议选择自体组织重建。

对于需行乳房切除术后放疗（PMRT）的患者，胸肌前重建仍具可行性：虽并发症风险略高，但与全肌下重建+放疗的情况差不多[9]。此外，放疗后延期重建的成功率较高（因皮瓣血管适应性增强）[10]。既往行胸肌后假体重建并出现明显的肌肉疼痛、紧缩或动态畸形者，通过延期胸肌前重建可有效缓解症状并矫正畸形[10]。

5.2.2　肿瘤特异性考量

除上述标准外，应于术前对肿瘤位置与组织学进行评估。肿瘤侵犯胸壁或毗邻胸大肌为胸肌前重建禁忌证，此类患者局部复发风险较高[7,11]，可考虑胸肌后重建，以便通过触诊早期发现复发征象。

炎性乳腺癌或Ⅳ期乳腺癌、进展性腋窝病变及病灶不可切除者，同样不适于胸肌前重建，此类患者常需创伤较大的辅助治疗，不利于重建预后。

图 5.2 总结了胸肌前重建患者选择标准。

5.3　术中注意事项

5.3.1　术中皮瓣血供评估

皮瓣灌注不良可导致坏死、愈合障碍并继发感染，最终造成假体外露。术中准确评估皮瓣血供是手术成功关键，可通过经验判断或仪器检测来实现。

患者筛选需重点评估皮肤弹性、既往放疗史、糖尿病与吸烟史等影响因素[7]。乳腺数字化X线检查[12]或MRI可辅助评估皮肤厚度[13]。

观察皮瓣厚度时应注意[14,15]：创缘出血活跃、未暴露真皮层及良好毛细血管再充盈均提示血供良好。术中可检测皮瓣

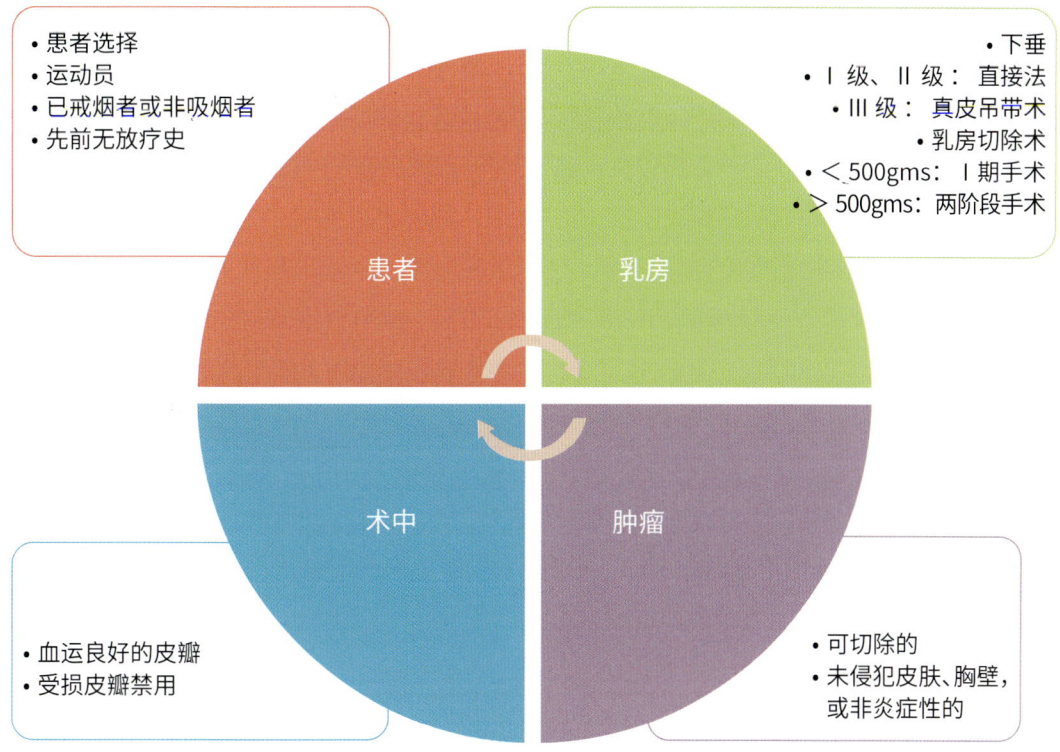

图5.2 胸大肌前乳房重建：选择标准与患者相关考量

pH 值辅助判断[16~18]。

疑有血供不佳时，可使用影像评估技术：术前行吲哚菁绿血管造影测量流量，激光辅助荧光血管造影系统（LA-ICG）具有更高敏感性与特异性[19~21]。

切口规划应避免损伤皮瓣血供，优先选择外缘切口或乳房下皱襞切口[22]，乳头周围切口因可能破坏血供应尽量避免。

5.3.2 美容考量

假体波纹是胸肌前重建常见的并发症，文献报道发生率为0~35%[10, 23, 24]，使用盐水假体较使用硅胶假体更易出现。采用以下技术可减少该现象：初次置入扩张器时减量填充100mL可形成更紧密的囊腔，降低假体移位风险；对BMI<21的纤瘦患者，可缩小基底部囊腔容积以优化切口闭合，从而减少术后波纹的形成[25]。

假体类型选择至关重要，使用硅胶假体术后出现波纹的发生率明显低于使用盐水假体[26]。适当的皮瓣厚度与患者体重，亦影响术后波纹显现[25, 26]。

自体脂肪移植是矫正波纹的有效手段，尤其适用于乳房上极[27]。因该区域完全依赖保留皮瓣与ADM提供组织量，上极充填尤为关键。

5.4 术后注意事项

5.4.1 感染

胸肌前重建缺乏肌肉覆盖，皮肤破损

易导致ADM及假体外露。疑似感染患者需门诊密切随访并口服抗生素。若假体濒临外露，则需住院行静脉抗生素治疗、急诊清创（必要时假体取出）。既往假体置入术后感染需急诊手术处理（生物膜形成风险高），其常对抗菌治疗反应差[28, 29]。

一项对51例患者（84侧乳房）的研究显示，平均随访11.1个月±5.8个月时蜂窝织炎发生率为5%，需冲洗清创率为2.4%。另一项对54例两阶段胸肌前重建患者的回顾性研究发现，放疗侧感染率（18.8%）显著高于未放疗侧（7.7%）[30]。

De vita等对34例聚氨酯假体NSM患者的研究（随访4月）未见感染事件[31]。而Singla研究显示感染率为15%（轻微11.5%，严重3.8%），可能与15.3%的血清肿发生率相关（易继发浅表感染）[32]。

5.5 小结

随着乳房重建需求的增长，兼顾美学与肿瘤安全性的新型重建技术得到持续发展。皮下全乳切除术的普及，进一步提升了胸肌前假体重建的应用价值。胸肌前假体重建（联合合成补片或ADM）可为假体提供充分的浅层软组织覆盖，疗效与胸肌后假体重建相当，但需融合术前、术中及术后多维策略。尤其需通过多学科讨论审慎评估肿瘤学因素（如原发灶特征、治疗史等），严格患者筛选以规避并发症风险。

术中技术要点包括：
- 精准的皮瓣血供评估（结合经验性触诊与吲哚菁绿激光血管造影等技术以优化灌注评估）。
- 规范腺体切除操作。

该术式优点明显，包括可消除动态畸形，减轻术后疼痛，基于ADM构建自然乳房形态，患者满意度高。通过上述规范化管理，术者可有效降低并发症风险，为患者提供理想的重建效果。

参考文献

1. Cancer Research U.K. Breast Cancer Statistics, Available at: http://www.cancerresearchuk.org/health-professional/cancer-statistics/statistics-by-cancer-type/breast-cancer. Accessed: October 25, 2021.
2. Vidya R, Iqbal FM. Breast anatomy: Time to classify the subpectoral and prepectoral spaces. Clin Anat. 2017,30(4):434–5. https://doi.org/10.1002/ca.22878. Epub 2017 April 8. P.M.I.D.: 28318062
3. Becker H, Lind JG 2nd, Hopkins EG, et al. Immediate implant-based prepectoral breast reconstruction using a vertical incision. Plast Reconstr Surg Glob Open. 2015,3(6):e412.
4. Sigalove S, Maxwell GP, Sigalove NM, et al. Prepectoral implant-based breast reconstruction: rationale, indications, and preliminary results. Plast Reconstr Surg. 2017,139(2):287–94.
5. Becker H, Fregosi N. The impact of animation deformity on quality of life in post-mastectomy reconstruction patients. Aesthet Surg J. 2017,37(5):531–6.
6. Gabriel A, Sigalove S, Sigalove NM, et al. Prepectoral revision breast reconstruction for treatment of implant-associated animation deformity: a review of 102 reconstructions. Aesthet Surg J. 2018,38(5):519–26.
7. Vidya R, Berna G, Sbitany H, Nahabedian M, Becker H, Reitsamer R, Rancati A, Macmillan D, Cawthorn S. Prepectoral implant-based

breast reconstruction: a joint consensus guide from U.K., European and U.S.A. breast and plastic reconstructive surgeons. Ecancermedicalscience. 2019,13:927. https://doi.org/10.3332/ecancer.2019.927. PMID: 31281424; PMCID: PMC6592711

8. Barry M, Kell MR. Radiotherapy and breast reconstruction: a meta-analysis. Breast Cancer Res Treat. 2011,127(1):15–22. https://doi.org/10.1007/s10549–011–1401-x. Epub 2011 February 20. P.M.I.D.: 21336948

9. Sbitany H, Gomez-Sanchez C, Piper M, et al. Prepectoral breast reconstruction in the setting of postmastectomy radiation therapy: an assessment of clinical outcomes and benefits. Plast Reconstr Surg. 2019,143(1):10–20.

10. Sbitany H, Piper M, Lentz R. Prepectoral breast reconstruction: a safe alternative to submuscular prosthetic reconstruction following nipple-sparing mastectomy. Plast Reconstr Surg. 2017,140(3):432–43. https://doi.org/10.1097/PRS.0000000000003627.

11. Buchanan CL, Dorn PL, Fey J, et al. Locoregional recurrence after mastectomy: incidence and outcomes. J Am Coll Surg. 2006,203(4):469–74.

12. Rancati AO, Angrigiani CH, Hammond DC, et al. Direct to implant reconstruction in nipple-sparing mastectomy: patient selection by preoperative digital mammogram. Plast Reconstr Surg Glob Open. 2017,5(6):e1369. https://doi.org/10.1097/GOX.0000000000001369.

13. Frey JD, Salibian AA, Choi M, Karp NS. Mastectomy flap thickness and complications in nipple-sparing mastectomy: objective evaluation using magnetic resonance imaging. Plast Reconstr Surg Glob Open. 2017,5(8):e1439. https://doi.org/10.1097/GOX.0000000000001439.

14. Pafitanis G, Raveendran M, Myers S, Ghanem AM. Flowmetry evolution in microvascular surgery: a systematic review. J Plast Reconstr Aesthet Surg. 2017,70(9):1242–51. https://doi.org/10.1016/j.bjps.2017.05.010.

15. Jeon FHK, Varghese J, Griffin M, Butler PE, Ghosh D, Mosahebi A. Systematic review of methodologies used to assess mastectomy flap viability. BJS Open. 2018,2(4):175–84. https://doi.org/10.1002/bjs5.61.

16. Raskin DJ, Erk Y, Spira M, Melissinos EG. Tissue pH monitoring in microsurgery: a preliminary evaluation of continuous tissue pH monitoring as an indicator of perfusion disturbances in microvascular free flaps. Ann Plast Surg. 1983,11(4):331–9. https://doi.org/10.1097/00000637–198310000–00013.

17. Dunn RM, Kaplan IB, Mancoll J, Terzis JK, Trengove-Jones G. Experimental and clinical use of pH monitoring of free tissue transfers. Ann Plast Surg. 1993,31(6):539–45. https://doi.org/10.1097/00000637–199312000–00011.

18. Warner KG, Durham-Smith G, Butler MD, Attinger CE, Upton J, Khuri SF. Comparative response of muscle and subcutaneous tissue pH during arterial and venous occlusion in musculocutaneous flaps. Ann Plast Surg. 1989,22(2):108–16. https://doi.org/10.1097/00000637–198902000-00005. PMID: 2735706

19. Mirhaidari SJ, Beddell GM, Orlando MV, Parker MG, Pedersen JC, Wagner DS. A prospective study of immediate breast reconstruction with laser-assisted indocyanine green angiography. Plast Reconstr Surg Glob Open. 2018,6(9):e1774. https://doi.org/10.1097/GOX.0000000000001774.

20. Phillips BT, Lanier ST, Conkling N, et al. Intraoperative perfusion techniques can accurately predict mastectomy skin flap necrosis in breast reconstruction: results of a prospective trial. Plast Reconstr Surg. 2012,129:778e–88e. https://doi.org/10.1097/PRS.0b013e31824a2ae8.

21. Mattison GL, Lewis PG, Gupta SC, et al. S.P.Y. imaging use in postmastectomy breast reconstruction patients: preventative or overly conservative? Plast Reconstr Surg. 2016,138:15e–21e. https://doi.org/10.1097/PRS.0000000000002266.

22. Frey JD, Salibian AA, Levine JP, Karp NS,

Choi M. Incision choices in nipple-sparing mastectomy: a comparative analysis of outcomes and evolution of a clinical algorithm. Plast Reconstr Surg. 2018,142:826e–35e. https://doi.org/10.1097/PRS.0000000000004969.

23. Downs RK, Hedges K. An alternative technique for immediate direct-to-implant breast reconstruction-a case series. Plast Reconstr Surg Glob Open. 2016,4(7):e821.

24. Casella D, Bernini M, Bencini L, et al. Ti-Loop® Bra mesh used for immediate breast reconstruction: comparison of retropectoral and subcutaneous implant placement in a prospective single-institution series. Eur J Plast Surg. 2014,37:599–604.

25. Salibian AH, Harness JK, Mowlds DS. Staged suprapectoral expander/implant reconstruction without acellular dermal matrix following nipple-sparing mastectomy. Plast Reconstr Surg. 2017,139(1):30–9. https://doi.org/10.1097/PRS.0000000000002845.

26. Isaac KV, Murphy BD, Beber B, et al. The reliability of anthropometric measurements used preoperatively in aesthetic breast surgery. Aesthet Surg J. 2016,36(4):431–7.

27. Sbitany H. Important considerations for performing prepectoral breast reconstruction. Plast Reconstr Surg. 2017,140(6S Prepectoral Breast Reconstruction):7S–13S. https://doi.org/10.1097/PRS.0000000000004045. PMID: 29166342

28. Vidya R, Masià J, Cawthorn S, et al. Evaluation of the effectiveness of the prepectoral breast reconstruction with Braxon dermal matrix: first multicenter European report on 100 cases. Breast J. 2017,23(6):670–6. https://doi.org/10.1111/tbj.12810.

29. Chopra S, Al-Ishaq Z, Vidya R. The journey of prepectoral breast reconstruction through time. World J Plast Surg. 2021,10(2):3–13. https://doi.org/10.29252/wjps.10.2.3. PMID: 34307092; PMCID: PMC8290458

30. Elswick SM, Harless CA, Bishop SN, et al. Prepectoral implant-based breast reconstruction with postmastectomy radiation therapy. Plast Reconstr Surg. 2018,142(1):1–12. https://doi.org/10.1097/PRS.0000000000004453.

31. De Vita R, Buccheri EM, Villanucci A, Pozzi M. Breast reconstruction actualized in nipple-sparing mastectomy and direct-to-implant, prepectoral polyurethane positioning: early experience and preliminary results. Clin Breast Cancer. 2019,19(2):e358–63. https://doi.org/10.1016/j.clbc.2018.12.015.

32. Singla A, Singla A, Lai E, Caminer D. Subcutaneously placed breast implants after a skin-sparing mastectomy: do we always need A.D.M.? Plast Reconstr Surg Glob Open. 2017,5(7):e1371. https://doi.org/10.1097/GOX.0000000000001371. PMID: 28831335; PMCID: PMC5548558

6 保留皮肤和乳头乳房切除胸肌前重建中的腋窝分期

编者：Marios-Konstantinos Tasoulis, Gerald Gui
译者：龙厚隆　田西朋

6.1 引言

在多模态管理时代，保乳手术已被证实是早期乳腺癌的安全治疗选项[1,2]。时序趋势分析显示，保乳手术比例显著增高的同时全乳切除率下降[3]，这与肿瘤整形技术的革新[4]及新辅助系统治疗的应用[5]密切相关。保乳手术在可行时可提供自然的乳房形态且耐受放疗，但全乳切除术仍是重要手段——常见肿瘤学适应证包括多象限多灶性病灶、保乳术中发现切缘阳性及既往保乳联合放疗后局部复发。遗传检测的普及和对遗传易感性认知的深入，也促使预防性乳房切除术数量增加。

随着更保守术式（具等效肿瘤学预后）的发展与标准化[6~10]，保留皮肤和乳头的全乳切除术逐渐成为主要术式，适用于多数需全腺体切除患者。其优势不仅在于肿瘤安全性，还在于可最大限度地利用保留的皮肤结构进行即刻乳房重建：原生皮肤提供自然覆盖（避免供区组织拼合外观），保留乳头则保留了乳房特征。保留乳头-乳晕复合体（NAC）不仅保留了乳房特征，亦有助于提高患者对重建乳房的接受度。

多数接受保留皮肤乳房切除术患者后续需行乳头再造，但该技术存在局限性：乳头凸度丧失，难以复现乳晕平滑肌皱褶感及 Montgomery 腺的缺失等[11]，放疗可加重上述缺陷。有基于此，三维文饰技术（尽管可能因放疗或褪色需二次修复）提升了美学效果[12,13]——保留 NAC 的患者的满意度显著高于再造组患者[14]。

尽管自体组织重建有所进展，假体重建仍是全乳切除术后最常见重建方式[15]。近十年来，技术改良推动假体放置层次由传统胸肌后转向胸肌前平面[16]。保留皮肤/乳头的全乳切除联合胸肌前重建常与腋窝分期操作同期完成。

M.-K. Tasoulis · G. Gui (✉)
Breast Surgery Unit, The Royal Marsden NHS Foundation Trust, London, UK
e-mail: Marios.Tasoulis@rmh.nhs.uk;
Gerald.Gui@rmh.nhs.uk

© The Author(s), under exclusive license to Springer Nature Switzerland AG 2023
R. Vidya, H. Becker (eds.), *Prepectoral Breast Reconstruction*,
https://doi.org/10.1007/978-3-031-15590-1_6

6.2 保留皮肤及乳头的全乳切除胸肌前重建：手术规划

保留皮肤和乳头的全乳切除胸肌前重建（PPBR）的手术规划始于术前评估，需综合考量表 6.1 所列参数。应结合患者主观意愿详细评估原乳房形态特征、对称性诉求、身高、体重及躯干软组织条件。需测量胸骨切迹至乳头距离、乳头至乳房下皱襞（IMF）距离，中线至乳头距离，乳房横径、纵径及凸度等，配合术前医学摄影留存影像资料。

确定乳房横径时，可用游标卡尺或卷尺测量乳房外侧缘至内侧边界水平投影距离（图 6.1a）；确定乳房纵径时，则应测量自乳房下皱襞至乳房轮廓最上点的垂直投影距离（图 6.1b）。乳房凸度定义为胸壁（或后侧乳腺边界）至乳房最大凸度点（通常为乳头位置）的矢状投影距离，其后方参考线为胸骨切迹垂线（图 6.1c）。乳房纵横径决定了重建用假体的大小，而凸度结合患者偏好是假体选择的另一关键维度。基底径固定不变的情况下，凸度决定了容积水平，直接影响重建乳房的正视投影形态与自然乳沟外观。

表 6.1 保留皮肤和乳头的乳房切除胸肌前重建术前规划要点

分类	参数项目
一般情况	患者 BMI 与体型；日常活动强度（职业、休闲、运动）；合并症（吸烟、糖尿病、高血压、凝血障碍）
肿瘤特征	治疗性或风险降低性手术；单/双侧；肿瘤范围（含恶性微钙化分布）；肿瘤与皮肤的距离及肿瘤与乳头的距离；既往或计划放疗；局部进展期或炎性乳腺癌
局部条件	乳房体积、形态、下垂度；皮肤质量（含弹性）；躯干–髋部形态特征；既有瘢痕；健侧乳房条件及对称化要求
患者意愿	对手术获益、风险及并发症的认知；预期目标；二次手术及维护需求；知情确认

除决定乳房重建体积的宽度、高度及凸度外，假体的形状（圆形或解剖型）对乳房形态亦有影响。假体选择与重建乳房形态的关联复杂，并非单纯由高、宽、凸度测量数据决定。解剖型与圆形假体在上极形态及乳头至乳房下皱襞距离等特征上存在差异。与盐水填充假体（双腔或单纯盐水）相比，硅凝胶假体的黏弹性及形态稳定性亦是影响重建效果的重要参数。这

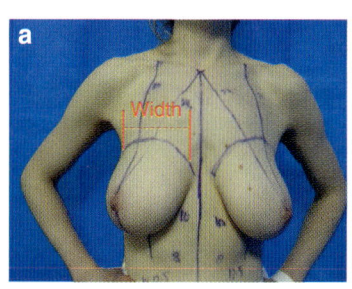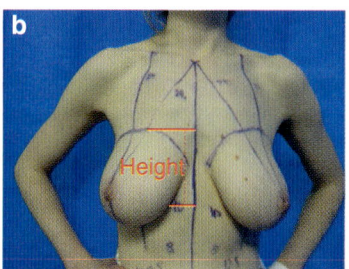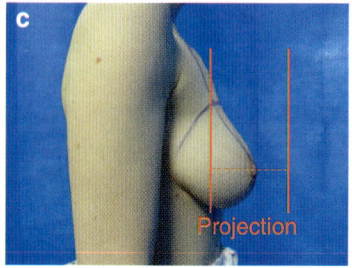

图 6.1 术前标记及测量的演示，（a）乳房宽度，（b）乳房高度，（c）乳房突出度

属手术规划核心内容,需纳入假体选择并与患者共同决策。例如,偏好上极饱满凸度者或更适合圆形假体,而解剖型假体可塑造容量更充盈的下极自然轮廓。胸罩上方区域的曲线坡度(即"社交外观")由假体凸度决定。弹性体特性会影响与前胸壁皮瓣的固着效果:毛面设计旨在促进组织粘连以降低旋转风险,而光面假体组织黏附较弱。圆形假体兼具光面与毛面类型,表面纹理亦是形态选择的影响因素之一。现有研究提示,假体表面粗糙度与发生乳房假体相关间变性大细胞淋巴瘤(BIA-ALCL)的风险存在潜在关联[17, 18]。虽然总体风险较低[17],但该因素可能促使部分女性拒绝毛面假体而选择圆形假体。

若重建乳房的预期宽度与高度相近,解剖型假体与圆形假体的差异效应可能更隐匿,因术后早期形态主要由凸度及上极坡度决定。中期乳房形态取决于覆盖假体的软组织顺应性及囊腔稳定性,使假体维持术中预设位置,此即单阶段(含即刻)假体重建手术需在初次术中构建稳定无张力囊腔的缘由——若乳房切除后无法实现囊腔稳定,则需采用两阶段法。

6.3 术前标记

术前评估及体表标记应在患者取立位/坐位下完成,使用卷尺及手术标记笔标记胸骨切迹、中线、乳房正中线及乳房下皱襞等关键解剖标志。乳房正中线始于锁骨固定点(锁骨内侧端5cm处或锁骨中点),向尾端延长经乳头至乳房下皱襞及其外侧。此外,描绘乳房轮廓(含乳房上缘起始点及下皱襞)有助于界定切除范围并控制"囊腔",对即刻重建尤其是保留皮肤乳房切除术(PPBR)至关重要(图 6.2)。即使拟行单侧切除,亦应标记双侧乳房以优化对称性。

6.4 术中准备

患者取仰卧位,双肩外展。无论单侧或双侧手术,消毒铺巾均需暴露双侧乳房。术区皮肤准备范围自颈根部延伸至上腹部(脐部除外)。摆放体位及铺巾应确保术中可按需将患者体位调整为坐位。手术台需具备体位调节功能,便于术中对比乳房形状、位置及维度(尤其在需匹配健侧时)。

纤维光源或头灯有助于深部照明(尤其经下皱襞切口时)。术中应谨慎操作,

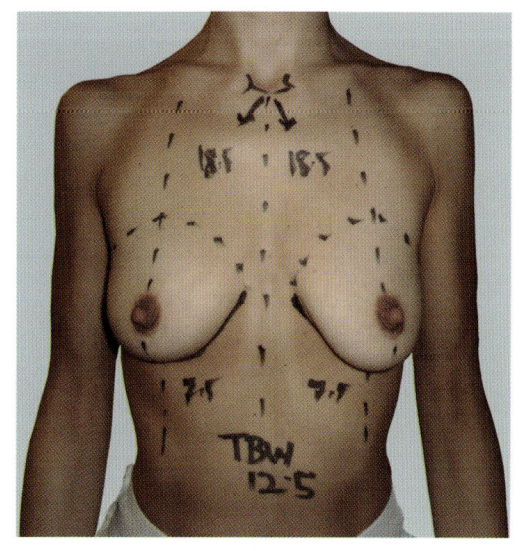

图 6.2 患者取站立位时的术前标记。标记内容包括胸骨切迹、中线、乳房子午线、乳房下皱襞及乳房轮廓。测量内容包括胸骨切迹 — 乳头距离、乳头 — 中线距离和乳房横径

避免牵拉或电刀所致皮瓣热损伤，使用电刀解剖时推荐绝缘器械。

6.4.1 保留皮肤乳房切除术：切口设置

规划切除乳头的乳房切除术时，切口设计通常需包含乳头-乳晕复合体（NAC）（图6.3）。若联合假体重建，围绕NAC的椭圆形切口通常位于乳房赤道区的水平瘢痕（图6.4）。另一种策略是设计椭圆切口仅切除乳头而保留乳晕。水平切口可向外侧延伸为乳房切除术入路（图6.5）。此类切口亦可垂直走行[19]（图6.3d），整合入乳房切除术垂直切口或乳房悬吊切口。无论何种方式，切口乳晕段可纳入后期乳头重建规划。包含乳头的垂直切口（无论是否保留NAC）可能使重建乳房赤道区瘢痕更隐匿，但需谨慎设计，以避免瘢痕超出胸罩线（图6.6）。

既往瘢痕可能需纳入乳房切除切口范围，尤其是既往保乳术后前切缘受累或局部复发需切除瘢痕组织时（图6.3e）。若肿瘤邻近皮肤表层，切口设计应覆盖受累区域。肿瘤侵及Cooper韧带导致的皮肤收缩非皮肤切除指征，而皮肤直接受累则为局部晚期表现。

假体重建往往难以实现乳房自然下垂。必要时，乳房切除重建方案需考虑通过对侧乳房手术来调整对称性（图6.6）。

6.4.2 保留乳头乳房切除术：切口设置

保留乳头乳房切除术可通过多种切口完成（图6.7）。最常用者为经乳房下皱襞（IMF）切口（图6.7a），适用于中小体积乳房，因瘢痕藏于IMF内而美学效果佳（图6.8）。对于较大的乳房，外侧皱襞切口可充分暴露术野，并便于必要时同期行腋窝手术（图6.7b）。乳房下皱襞与外侧皱襞切口的优势在于切口完美避开乳房体表面[20]。尤其IMF切口位于天然皮纹线处，愈合良好，文献显示其裂开风险较低（尤其在放疗后）[21]，且缺血及总体并发症发生率更低[22-24]。

放射状切口亦常用于保留乳头手术（图6.7c~e），潜在优势在于：若术后发现乳头切缘受累，可延展切口切除NAC而无须过多牺牲皮肤。外侧放射状切口（图6.7c）可能与乳头缺血风险较低相关[25,26]。垂直放射状切口（图6.7d、e）并发症发生率亦较低[22]并且具有美学优势——后续手术可整合切口使其形似乳房悬吊术瘢痕。乳晕周围切口（伴或不伴放射状延伸）（图6.7f~i，图6.9）亦有报道，但可能增加乳头坏死[24,25]及其他并发症的风险[22,23]。

保留皮肤乳房切除术的肿瘤学和重建原则同样适用于保留乳头术式。近期乳晕周围切口（如原保乳手术遗留瘢痕）需特别关注：不仅影响乳头血供，二次瘢痕形成可能导致缺血高风险的组织桥形成。新近环乳晕瘢痕可能成为NAC保留禁忌，但远期瘢痕（如既往保乳术或乳房悬吊术后）则不然。

6.4.3 皮瓣剥离与腺体切除

切开后轻柔提起皮肤及皮下脂肪组

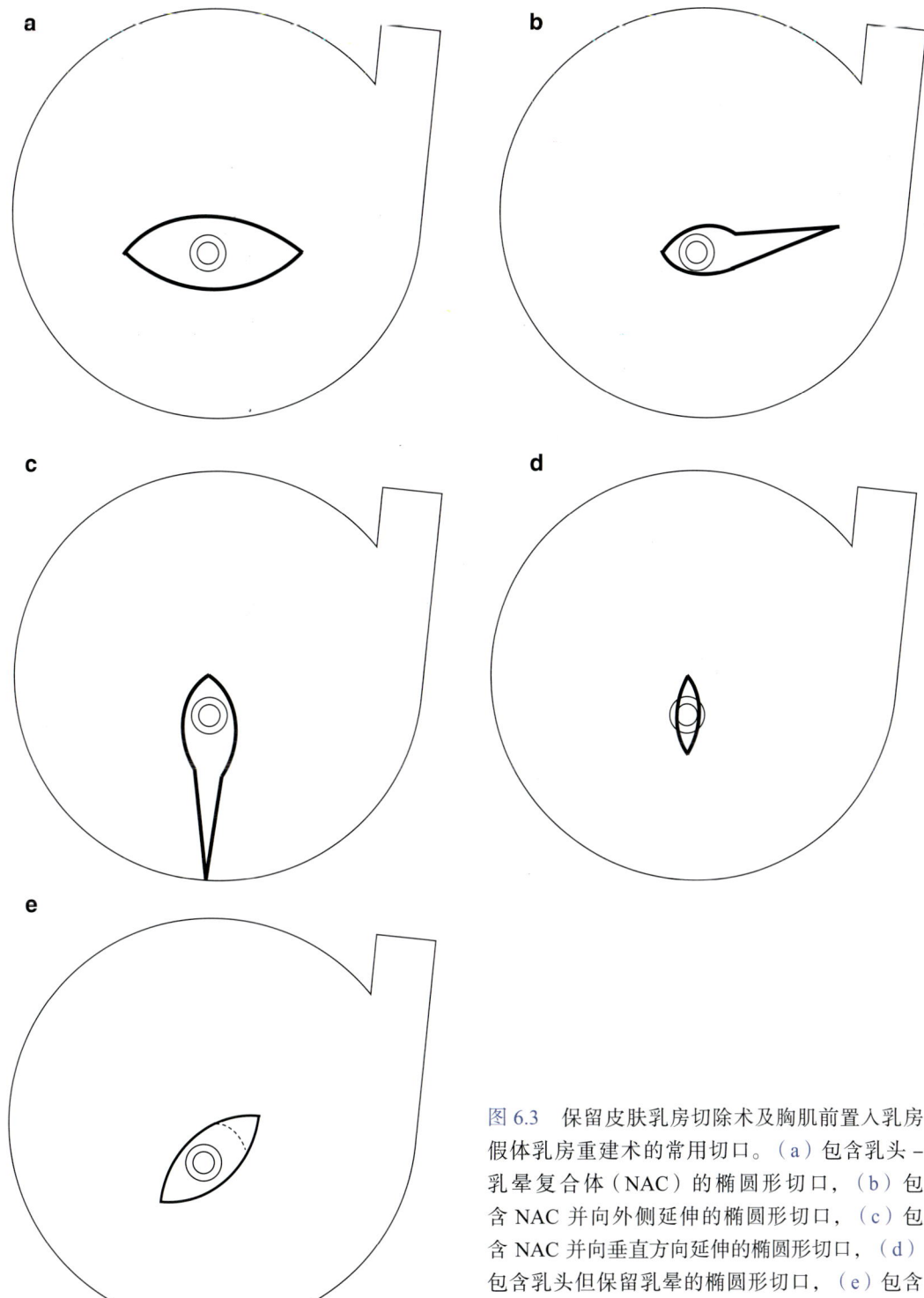

图 6.3 保留皮肤乳房切除术及胸肌前置入乳房假体乳房重建术的常用切口。(a) 包含乳头－乳晕复合体（NAC）的椭圆形切口，(b) 包含 NAC 并向外侧延伸的椭圆形切口，(c) 包含 NAC 并向垂直方向延伸的椭圆形切口，(d) 包含乳头但保留乳晕的椭圆形切口，(e) 包含 NAC 及既往保乳手术瘢痕的椭圆形切口

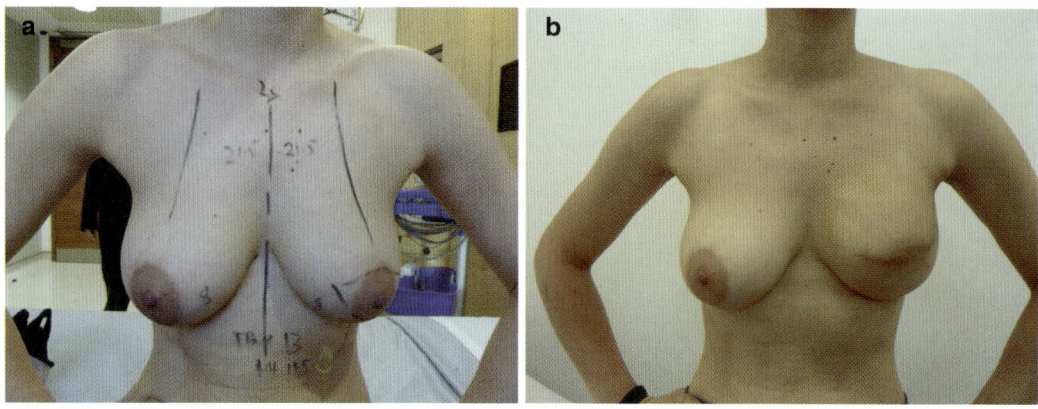

图 6.4 保留乳头乳房切除术及胸肌前假体乳房重建术的术前标记。（a）采用水平椭圆形切口包含乳头乳晕复合体的术前标记；（b）术后美容效果

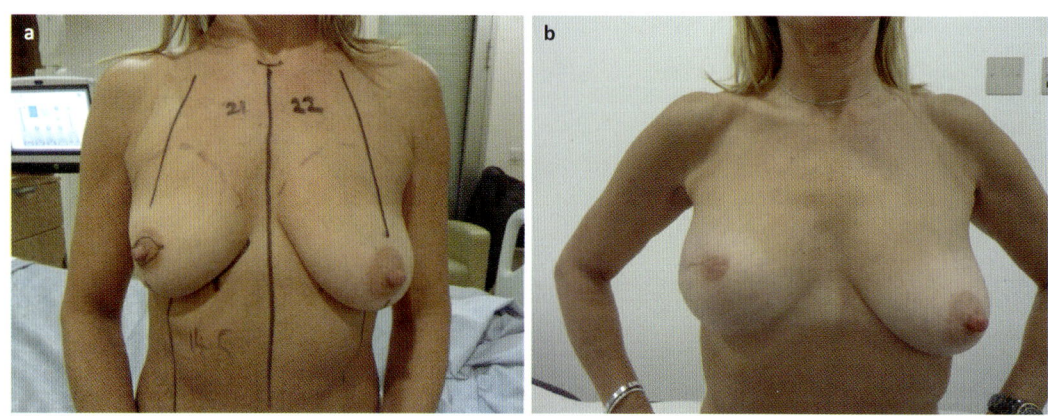

图 6.5 保留乳头 – 乳晕的水平椭圆形切口术前标记。（a）术前标记；（b）术后美容效果

织，沿"肿瘤整形平面"进行分离（即 Cooper 韧带界定的腺体实质与皮下脂肪组织间层面，图 6.10），目的在于最大限度地切除乳房腺体。皮瓣厚度存在个体差异，建议术中间断评估分离平面。精细操作以控制囊腔形成范围，保留乳房下皱襞（IMF）并避免过度分离至外侧非腺体皮下组织，对保留皮肤乳房切除术（PPBR）的成功尤为关键。须保留真皮下血管丛完整性以维持皮瓣血供。完成肿瘤整形平面分离后，将腺体自胸壁剥离。整个手术过程中应避免过度牵拉皮瓣以减少潜在损伤。

在保留乳头术式中，乳晕后组织可通过环切或乳头外翻法切除。肿瘤手术中，乳晕后组织常需送术中快速病理检查来评估癌灶，以指导进一步切除。冰冻切片法最常用于术中评估，其假阴性率为 1%～9.2%[27-30]。是否同期切除乳头须结合患者知情同意审慎决策。若术中或术后需处理乳头切缘阳性问题，则凸显保留乳头术式患者筛选及切口选择的重要性。例如，需二次切除 NAC 的 IMF 切口患者可能形

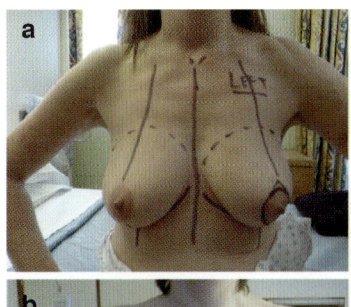
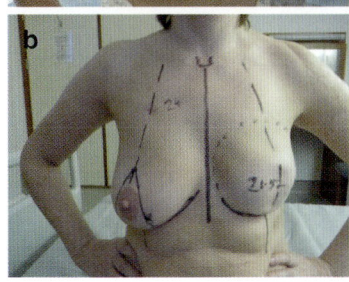
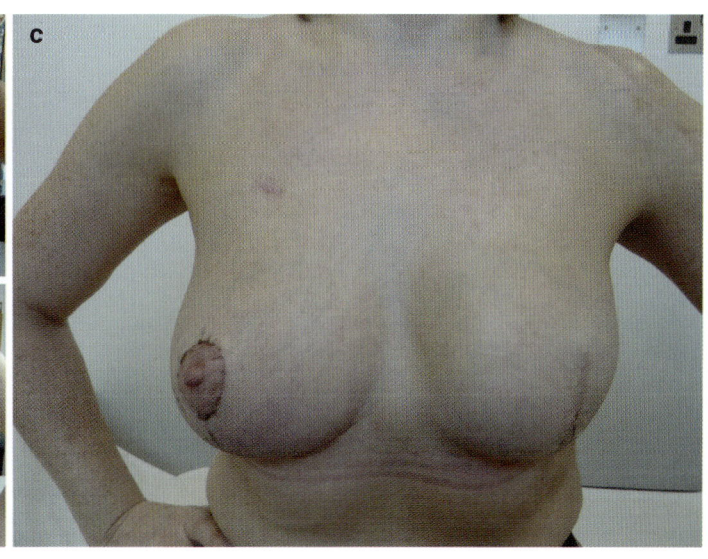

图6.6 （a）采用垂直椭圆形切口的保留乳头－乳晕复合体的乳房切除术前标记；（b）作为Ⅱ期手术，对侧对称化手术的Wise模式术前标记；（c）双侧手术后的美容效果

成缺血风险较高的组织桥（尤其假体较小者），此类情况应作为术前告知内容纳入共同决策流程。

采用保留乳头术式时，乳晕后腺体盘状残留不可避免。切除腺体时将中断经腋动脉分支（胸上动脉、胸肩峰动脉、胸外侧动脉、肩胛下动脉）、胸廓内动脉及肋间血管穿支至乳头的血供，此时乳头存活依赖真皮下血管丛（经乳晕下丛达乳头），故分离NAC时须维持真皮下血管丛完整性。精细操作应包括主动保留肋间动脉前穿支——因腋尾部或腋窝手术常损及腋血管分支（图6.11）。

静脉回流对乳头存活同等重要。影响静脉回流的术中因素包括缝合张力、假体体积/扩张囊充注量及敷料外部压迫。远离乳头的切口（如外侧或IMF入路）较环乳晕切口对静脉回流的影响更小，因术后肿胀更易造成静脉（而非小动脉）闭塞。

乳房切除中可采用多种分离技术，包括剪刀/手术刀锐性分离或常规电刀操作。采用保留乳头术式时，推荐在NAC周围行锐性分离以避免血管丛热损伤。水分离术作为一种新技术逐渐应用于皮瓣制备[31-34]，特别适用于经IMF等远端切口的保留乳头手术，因其可在低牵张力状态下完成腺体切除。应区分术野注射与水分离术：后者通过在肿瘤整形平面的灌注产生的静水压来分离皮下脂肪，扩展浅层间隙并牵张Cooper韧带（联结腺体与皮肤结构）。该技术可减少术中出血但存在学习曲线，尤适用于NAC与乳晕后结构分离及肌间平面剥离。

腺体切除后须严格止血，但应避免过度破坏皮瓣血管网。建议放置引流管（建立皮下隧道，以防逆行感染），出口位置避开敷料区并确保患者舒适。多采用密闭负压引流系统，引流时间尚无统一规定[35, 36]。尽

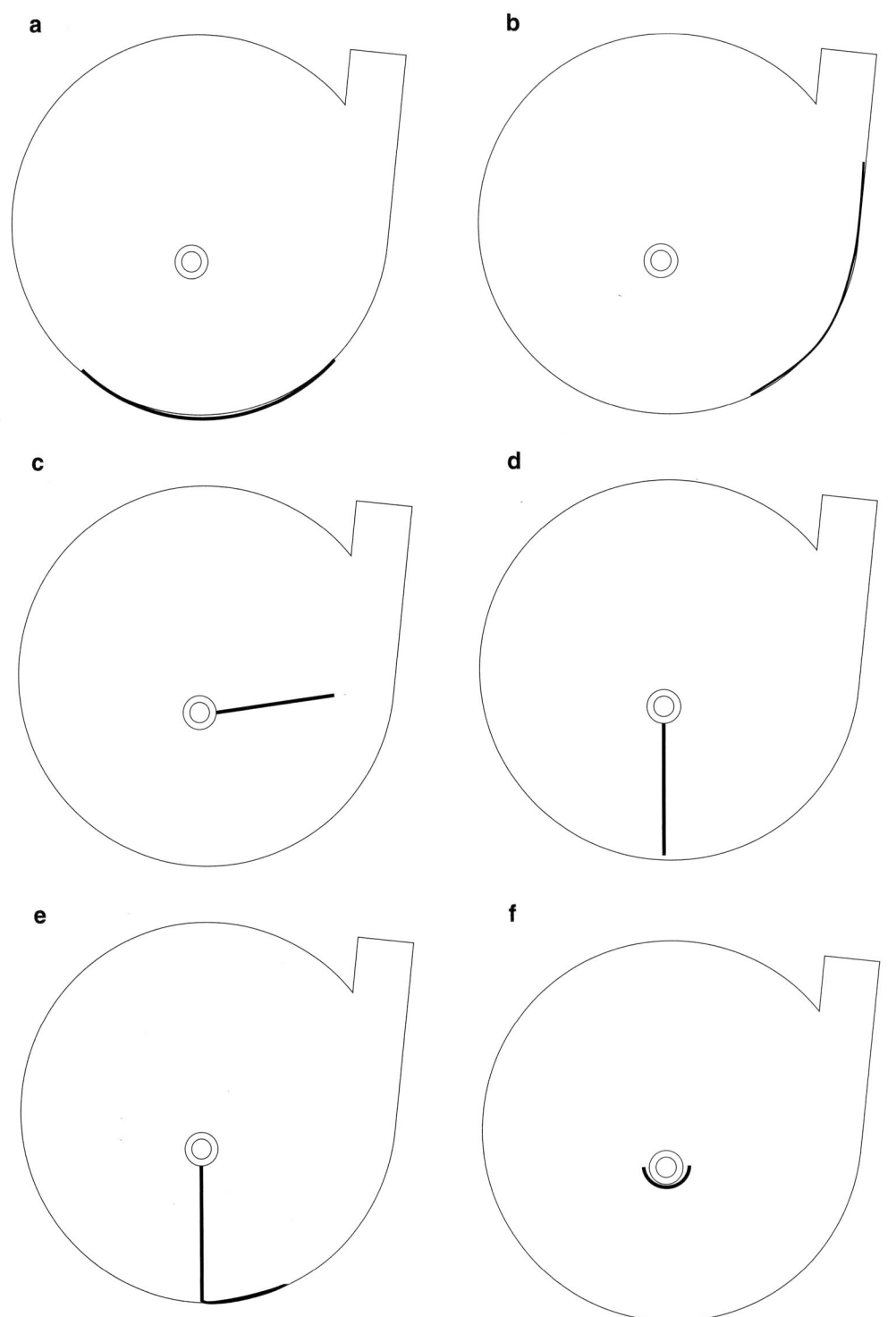

图 6.7 保留乳头乳房切除术及胸肌前假体乳房重建术的常用切口。(a) 乳房下皱襞切口;(b) 乳房外侧皱襞切口;(c) 外侧放射状切口;(d) 垂直放射状切口;(e) 带外侧延伸的垂直放射状切口;(f) 乳晕周围切口

6 保留皮肤和乳头乳房切除胸肌前重建中的腋窝分期

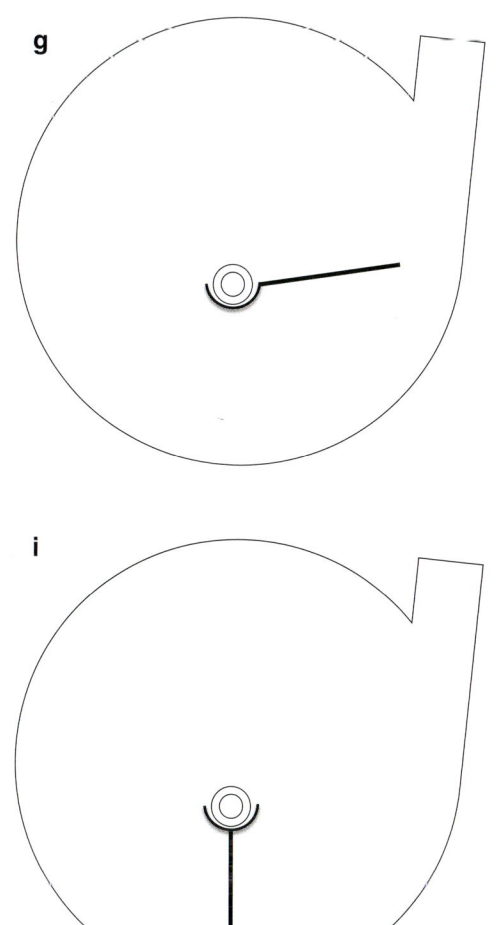

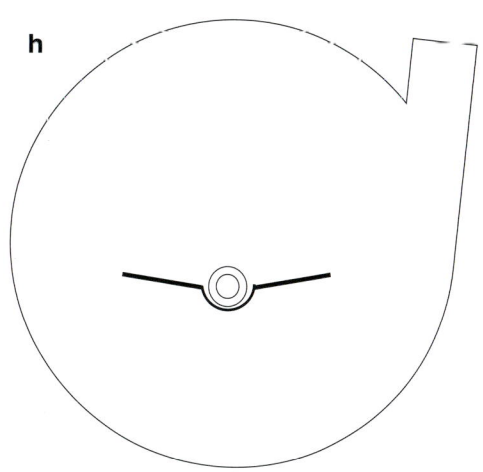

图 6.7（续）（g）带外侧延伸的乳晕周围切口；（h）带内外侧延伸的乳晕周围切口；（i）带垂直延伸的乳晕周围切口

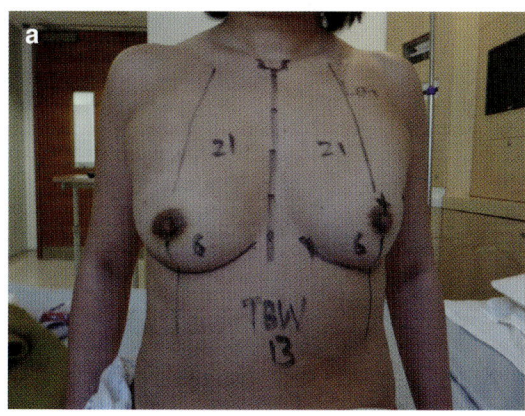
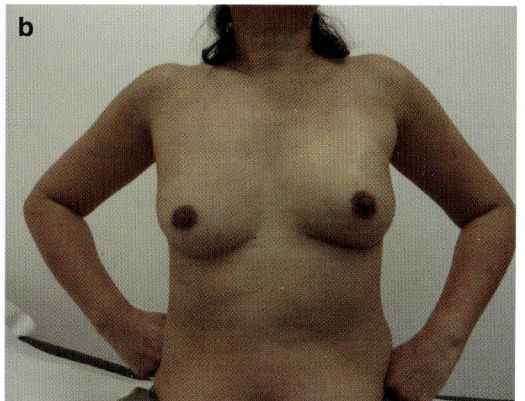

图 6.8 采用乳房下皱襞切口的保留乳头乳房切除术术前标记。（a）术前标记；（b）术后美容效果

管无引流乳房切除术已有报道[37]，但缺乏保留皮肤/乳头术式及PPBR的相关数据支持。

完成切除及重建后，切口可覆盖纱布敷料、防水贴膜（加垫/无垫）或特殊敷料（如羧甲基纤维素银[38]、负压敷料[39,40]）。现有证据未显示何种敷料系统更具优势，应根据既往敷料过敏史、感染风险及患者舒适度等个体化选择。

6.4.4 保留皮肤及乳头乳房切除术与胸肌前乳房重建的感染预防

乳房切除和胸肌前乳房重建（PPBR）术后手术部位感染（SSI），可引发假体感染、取出，以及住院时间延长、二次手术、多次返院等并发症。假体并发症的远期影响显著——即使成功保留假体，后续软组织质量低下及需手术干预的包膜挛缩风险

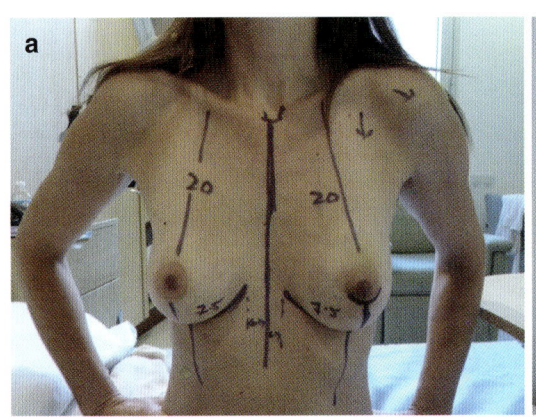
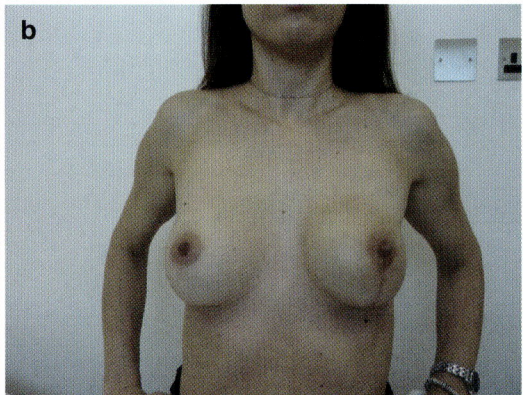

图6.9 带垂直放射状延伸的乳晕周围切口术前标记。（a）术前标记；（b）术后美容效果

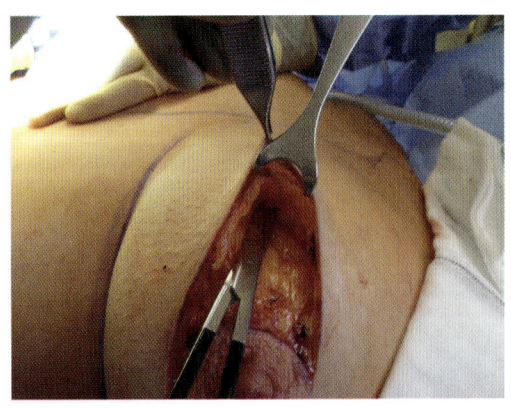

图6.10 "肿瘤整形"分离平面

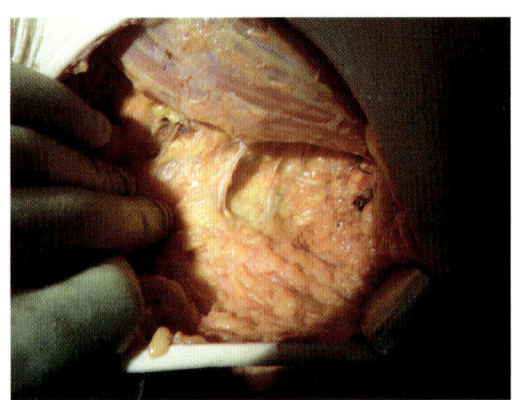

图6.11 仔细分离以保留胸外侧动脉穿支及肋间神经分支

亦增加，因此SSI防控至关重要。目前虽无降低SSI风险的标准方案，但建议措施包括：常规筛查并治疗甲氧西林敏感及耐药金黄色葡萄球菌（MSSA及MRSA），预防性应用抗生素，酒精制剂术区准备，层流空气系统，预防术中低体温，假体置入期减少人员流动，最小化假体接触，双层手套操作。上述建议已被整合为操作性核查清单[41]，旨在为手术团队提供关于SSI防控措施实施的便捷工具。

6.4.5 保留皮肤和乳头乳房切除与即刻假体乳房重建的腋窝分期

对于接受保留皮肤和乳头的乳房切除联合即刻假体乳房重建（PPBR）治疗浸润性或原位乳腺癌的患者，常规实施腋窝手术。前哨淋巴结活检（SLNB）是临床评估及影像学检查显示淋巴结阴性的患者进行腋窝分期的标准方案。虽然SLNB在降低风险的手术中也有应用[42]，但在乳腺癌高风险遗传基因携带者接受MRI筛查的时代，应谨慎权衡采用该术式时该亚组患者的获益与不良反应。SLNB仍存在虽小但明确的淋巴水肿、软组织并发症及持续性神经痛风险。对于腋窝淋巴结阳性者，腋窝淋巴结清扫术（ALND）是常规标准治疗方案。

6.4.6 前哨淋巴结活检

6.4.6.1 前哨淋巴结识别技术

目前已有多种前哨淋巴结识别方法，包括将蓝染料（异磺胺蓝、亚甲蓝或专利蓝）、放射性胶体（锝-99m）或二者（即"双示踪法"）注射至肿瘤旁乳腺实质或乳晕周围区域[43,44]，可根据可用性及术者偏好来选择，但双示踪法为优选方案，尤其适用于新辅助化疗后影像学显示完全缓解且接受SLNB的临床淋巴结阳性患者[45,46]。行腋窝清扫术时，通过标记和定位引导靶向切除活检证实存在转移的索引淋巴结可能降低假阴性率[47,48]。已报道多种标记夹闭淋巴结的术前定位方式[49]，包括导丝定位[50]、碘粒子标记[47]或其他非放射性定位器[51~53]。其他SLNB技术包括使用特殊红外光照射野的吲哚菁绿（ICG）染色[54~56]，以及采用手持磁力探针识别前哨淋巴结的超顺磁性氧化铁（SPIO）[56~59]。

6.4.6.2 切口

保留皮肤和乳头的乳房切除术中的前哨淋巴结活检通常经独立小切口实施，切口常位于腋窝毛发线下方，呈横形或稍倾斜状，需注意避免跨越腋前线。对于特定患者，腋窝手术可经乳房切除切口完成（图6.12）。尽管有时可将腋窝入路与乳房切除手术切口合并，但多数外科医师倾向采用独立切口，便于外侧乳房囊腔控制，并减少皮瓣牵拉以优化腋窝显露。若存在既往腋窝瘢痕，可沿用原切口并根据需要延长，以获得充分显露。

6.4.6.3 手术技术

行仔细钝性分离以识别前哨淋巴结。根据淋巴结识别方法，可在注射放射性同位素后借助手持γ探针引导向放射性淋

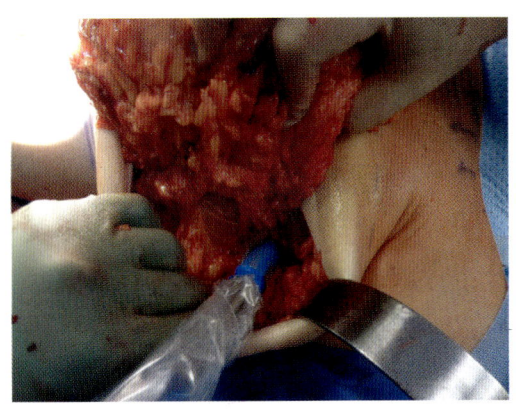

图 6.12 经乳房切除切口的前哨淋巴结活检操作

巴结的分离。若采用双示踪法（同位素＋蓝染料），可直视蓝染淋巴管并追踪至蓝染淋巴结。获取首个放射性（"热"）、蓝染或双染的前哨淋巴结后，需再次用 γ 探针探查其他放射性淋巴结；若存在更多蓝染淋巴管，应进一步追踪查找其他蓝染淋巴结。作为常规，放射性计数≥最高计数淋巴结 10% 的淋巴结均被视为前哨淋巴结并予切除。针对 ICG 或 SPIO 技术，须使用红外光或手持磁力探针引导分离，前哨淋巴结识别原则相同。前哨淋巴结多位于腋窝下部，胸外侧静脉旁。对于临床及影像学淋巴结阴性的患者，前哨淋巴结活检极少需要获取超过 4 枚淋巴结样本。

6.4.7 腋窝淋巴结清扫术

6.4.7.1 切口

若需行腋窝淋巴结清扫术（ALND），通常需另做切口，与前哨淋巴结活检（SLNB）类似，但可能需延长切口以便操作。同样需注意勿跨越腋前线。此外，"S"形切口可替代横切口或斜切口，既能提供良好术野暴露，又有利于后续闭合。对于有腋窝手术史的患者，可利用现有瘢痕切口，但可能需调整切口位置或修整瘢痕。从技术角度来说，ALND 可经乳房切除切口实施（如外侧乳腺皱襞或放射状外侧切口），但类似 SLNB，多数外科医师因相同原因仍倾向采用独立切口。

6.4.7.2 手术技术

因肿瘤学指征行 ALND 时，常规需要清扫Ⅰ、Ⅱ水平淋巴结（除特殊禁忌外）。手术通常始于辨认关键解剖结构，包括腋静脉、胸长神经及胸背神经血管束。随后在保护上述重要神经血管结构的前提下，清除腋窝脂肪组织。若技术上可行且肿瘤学条件允许，可保留肋间臂神经。经乳房切除切口行腋窝入路时，除肋间神经外，还可识别并保留下肋间神经外侧分支（图 6.11），以维持术后乳房隆起的触觉。完成 ALND 后应仔细触诊腋窝，切除残余淋巴结，重点探查胸背神经血管束与胸长神经处残留的淋巴组织。

6.5 要点

- 术前评估及患者站立位双侧皮肤标记，是保留皮肤和乳头乳房切除术的首要步骤。
- 术中患者体位摆放应便于调整为坐位，以评估重建效果及对称性。
- 行保留乳头乳房切除术时，选择下皱襞切口、外侧皱襞切口或放射状切口可降低乳头坏死风险。
- 乳腺癌患者行保留乳头乳房切除术时，需谨慎选择切口。

- 精细手术操作至关重要：在肿瘤整形平面上最大化切除乳腺体，同时保证皮瓣活性及皮肤血供，避免过度牵拉皮瓣。
- 在保留乳头的乳房切除术中，需精细解剖乳头-乳晕复合体（NAC）以保护乳晕下血管丛，对预防乳头缺血坏死至关重要。
- 锐性分离或水分离技术适用于NAC解剖，尤其在经远处切口实施乳房切除术时。
- 腋窝手术多经独立切口实施，但特定病例中也可经乳房切除相同切口完成。

参考文献

1. Fisher B, Anderson S, Bryant J, Margolese RG, Deutsch M, Fisher ER, et al. Twenty-year follow-up of a randomized trial comparing total mastectomy, lumpectomy, and lumpectomy plus irradiation for the treatment of invasive breast cancer. N Engl J Med. 2002,347(16):1233–41.
2. Veronesi U, Cascinelli N, Mariani L, Greco M, Saccozzi R, Luini A, et al. Twenty-year follow-up of a randomized study comparing breast-conserving surgery with radical mastectomy for early breast cancer. N Engl J Med. 2002,347(16):1227–32.
3. Kummerow KL, Du L, Penson DF, Shyr Y, Hooks MA. Nationwide trends in mastectomy for early-stage breast cancer. JAMA Surg. 2015,150(1):9–16.
4. Crown A, Wechter DG, Grumley JW. Oncoplastic breast-conserving surgery reduces mastectomy and postoperative re-excision rates. Ann Surg Oncol. 2015,22(10):3363–8.
5. Karakatsanis A, Tasoulis MK, Wärnberg F, Nilsson G, MacNeill F. Meta-analysis of neoadjuvant therapy and its impact in facilitating breast conservation in operable breast cancer. Br J Surg. 2018,105(5):469–81.
6. Simmons RM, Fish SK, Gayle L, La Trenta GS, Swistel A, Christos P, et al. Local and distant recurrence rates in skin-sparing mastectomies compared with non-skin-sparing mastectomies. Ann Surg Oncol. 1999,6(7):676–81.
7. Greenway RM, Schlossberg L, Dooley WC. Fifteen-year series of skin-sparing mastectomy for stage 0 to 2 breast cancer. Am J Surg. 2005,190(6):918–22.
8. Boneti C, Yuen J, Santiago C, Diaz Z, Robertson Y, Korourian S, et al. Oncologic safety of nipple skin-sparing or Total skin-sparing mastectomies with immediate reconstruction. J Am Coll Surg. 2011,212(4):686–93.
9. Smith BL, Tang R, Rai U, Plichta JK, Colwell AS, Gadd MA, et al. Oncologic safety of nipple-sparing mastectomy in women with breast cancer. J Am Coll Surg. 2017,225(3):361–5.
10. Wu Z-Y, Kim H-J, Lee J-W, Chung I-Y, Kim J-S, Lee S-B, et al. Breast cancer recurrence in the nipple-areola complex after nipple-sparing mastectomy with immediate breast reconstruction for invasive breast cancer. JAMA Surg. 2019,154(11):1030–7.
11. Paolini G, Firmani G, Briganti F, Sorotos M, Santanelli di Pompeo F. Guiding nipple-areola complex reconstruction: literature review and proposal of a new decision-making algorithm. Aesthet Plast Surg. 2021; https://doi.org/10.1007/s00266–020–02047–9.
12. Hammond JB, Teven CM, Bernard RW, Lucas HD, Casey WJ, Siebeneck ET, et al. 3D nipple-areolar tattoo: It's technique, outcomes, and utilization. Aesthet Plast Surg. 2021; https://doi.org/10.1007/s00266–020–01967-w.
13. Tomita S, Mori K, Yamazaki H. A survey on the safety of and patient satisfaction after nipple-areola tattooing. Aesthet Plast Surg. 2021; https://doi.org/10.1007/s00266–020–02018–0.
14. Satteson ES, Brown BJ, Nahabedian MY. Nipple-areolar complex reconstruction and patient satisfaction: a systematic review and meta-analysis. Gland Surg. 2017,6(1):4–13.

15. American Society of Plastic Surgery (ASPS): 2018 Plastic surgery statistics report; 2018
16. Tasoulis MK, Iqbal FM, Cawthorn S, MacNeill F, Vidya R. Subcutaneous implant breast reconstruction: time to reconsider? Eur J Surg Oncol. 2017,43(9):1636–46.
17. DeCoster RC, Lynch EB, Bonaroti AR, Webster JM, Butterfield TA, Evers BM, et al. Breast implant-associated anaplastic large cell lymphoma: an evidence-based systematic review. Ann Surg. 2021,273(3):449–58.
18. DeCoster RC, Clemens MW, Di Napoli A, Lynch EB, Bonaroti AR, Rinker BD, et al. Cellular and molecular mechanisms of breast implant-associated anaplastic large cell lymphoma. Plast Reconstr Surg. 2021,147(1):30e–41e.
19. Becker H, Lind JG 2nd, Hopkins EG. Immediate implant-based Prepectoral breast reconstruction using a vertical incision. Plast Reconstr Surg Glob Open. 2015,3(6):e412-e.
20. Kim JH, Chun YS, Park HK, Kim SE, Kim YW, Cheon YW. Inframammary fold incision can reduce skin flap necrosis in immediate breast reconstruction with implant and conjoined fascial flap. Ann Plast Surg. 2020,85(5):488–94.
21. Karunanayake M, Boghossian E, Govshievich A, Bernier C, Danino MA. A retrospective comparison study of the infra-mammary approach to the standard mastectomy scar in the 2nd stage of tissue expander to implant breast reconstruction. Ann Chir Plast Esthet. 2017,62(2):131–8.
22. Frey JD, Salibian AA, Levine JP, Karp NS, Choi M. Incision choices in nipple-sparing mastectomy: a comparative analysis of outcomes and evolution of a clinical algorithm. Plast Reconstr Surg. 2018,142(6):826e–35e.
23. Daar DA, Abdou SA, Rosario L, Rifkin WJ, Santos PJ, Wirth GA, et al. Is there a preferred incision location for nipple-sparing mastectomy? A systematic review and meta-analysis. Plast Reconstr Surg. 2019,143(5):906e–19e.
24. Park S, Yoon C, Bae SJ, Cha C, Kim D, Lee J, et al. Comparison of complications according to incision types in nipple-sparing mastectomy and immediate reconstruction. Breast (Edinburgh, Scotland). 2020,53:85–91.
25. Wijayanayagam A, Kumar AS, Foster RD, Esserman LJ. Optimizing the total skin-sparing mastectomy. Arch Surg. 2008,143(1):38–45.
26. Regolo L, Ballardini B, Gallarotti E, Scoccia E, Zanini V. Nipple sparing mastectomy: an innovative skin incision for an alternative approach. Breast (Edinburgh, Scotland). 2008,17(1):8–11.
27. Camp MS, Coopey SB, Tang R, Colwell A, Specht M, Greenup RA, et al. Management of positive sub-areolar/nipple duct margins in nipple-sparing mastectomies. Breast J. 2014,20(4):402–7.
28. D'Alonzo M, Pecchio S, Campisi P, De Rosa G, Bounous VE, Villasco A, et al. Nipple-sparing mastectomy: reliability of sub-areolar sampling and frozen section in predicting occult nipple involvement in breast cancer patients. Eur J Surg Oncol. 2018,44(11):1736–42.
29. Duarte GM, Tomazini MV, Oliveira A, Moreira L, Tocchet F, Worschech A, et al. Accuracy of frozen section, imprint cytology, and permanent histology of sub-nipple tissue for predicting occult nipple involvement in patients with breast carcinoma. Breast Cancer Res Treat. 2015,153(3):557–63.
30. Kneubil MC, Lohsiriwat V, Curigliano G, Brollo J, Botteri E, Rotmensz N, et al. Risk of Locoregional recurrence in patients with false-negative frozen section or close margins of Retroareolar specimen in nipple-sparing mastectomy. Ann Surg Oncol. 2012,19(13):4117–23.
31. Vargas CR, Koolen PG, Ho OA, Ricci JA, Tobias AM, Lin SJ, et al. Tumescent mastectomy technique in autologous breast reconstruction. J Surg Res. 2015,198(2):525–9.
32. Samper A, Blanch A. Improved subcutaneous mastectomy with hydrodissection of the subcutaneous space. Plast Reconstr Surg. 2003,112(2):694–5.
33. Folli S, Curcio A, Buggi F, Mingozzi M, Lelli D,

Barbieri C, et al. Improved sub-areolar breast tissue removal in nipple-sparing mastectomy using hydrodissection. Breast (Edinburgh, Scotland). 2012,21(2):190–3.

34. Tasoulis MK, Agusti A, Karakatsanis A, Montgomery C, Marshall C, Gui G. The use of Hydrodissection in nipple- and skin-sparing mastectomy: a retrospective cohort study. Plast Reconstr Surg Glob Open. 2019,7(11):e2495.

35. Phillips BT, Wang ED, Mirrer J, Lanier ST, Khan SU, Dagum AB, et al. Current practice among plastic surgeons of antibiotic prophylaxis and closed-suction drains in breast reconstruction: experience, evidence, and implications for postoperative care. Ann Plast Surg. 2011,66(5):460–5.

36. Scomacao I, Cummins A, Roan E, Duraes EFR, Djohan R. The use of surgical site drains in breast reconstruction: a systematic review. J Plast Reconstr Aesthet Surg. 2020,73(4):651–62.

37. Baker E, Piper J. Drainless mastectomy: is it safe and effective? Surgeon. 2017,15(5):267–71.

38. Struik GM, Vrijland WW, Birnie E, Klem T. A randomized controlled trial on the effect of a silver carboxymethylcellulose dressing on surgical site infections after breast cancer surgery. PLoS One. 2018,13(5):e0195715.

39. Nagata T, Miura K, Homma Y, Fukamizu H. Comparison between negative-pressure fixation and film dressing in wound management after tissue expansion: a randomized controlled trial. Plast Reconstr Surg. 2018,142(1):37–41.

40. Gabriel A, Sigalove SR, Maxwell GP. Initial experience using closed incision negative pressure therapy after immediate Postmastectomy breast reconstruction. Plast Reconstr Surg Glob Open. 2016,4(7):e819.

41. Barr SP, Topps AR, Barnes NL, Henderson J, Hignett S, Teasdale RL, et al. Infection prevention in breast implant surgery-a review of the surgical evidence, guidelines and a checklist. Eur J Surg Oncol. 2016,42(5):591–603.

42. Tasoulis MK, Hughes T, Babiera G, Chagpar AB. Sentinel lymph node biopsy in low risk settings. Am J Surg. 2017,214(3):489–94.

43. Ahmed M, Purushotham AD, Horgan K, Klaase JM, Douek M. Meta-analysis of superficial versus deep injection of radioactive tracer and blue dye for lymphatic mapping and detection of sentinel lymph nodes in breast cancer. Br J Surg. 2015,102(3):169–81.

44. Sadeghi R, Asadi M, Treglia G, Zakavi SR, Fattahi A, Krag DN. Axillary concordance between superficial and deep sentinel node mapping material injections in breast cancer patients: systematic review and meta-analysis of the literature. Breast Cancer Res Treat. 2014,144(2):213–22.

45. Boughey JC, Suman VJ, Mittendorf EA, Ahrendt GM, Wilke LG, Taback B, et al. Sentinel lymph node surgery after neoadjuvant chemotherapy in patients with node-positive breast cancer: the ACOSOG Z1071 (Alliance) clinical trial. JAMA. 2013,310(14):1455–61.

46. Kuehn T, Bauerfeind I, Fehm T, Fleige B, Hausschild M, Helms G, et al. Sentinel-lymph-node biopsy in patients with breast cancer before and after neoadjuvant chemotherapy (SENTINA): a prospective, multicentre cohort study. Lancet Oncol. 2013,14(7):609–18.

47. Caudle AS, Yang WT, Krishnamurthy S, Mittendorf EA, Black DM, Gilcrease MZ, et al. Improved axillary evaluation following neoadjuvant therapy for patients with node-positive breast cancer using selective evaluation of clipped nodes: implementation of targeted axillary dissection. J Clin Oncol. 2016,34(10):1072–8.

48. Boughey JC, Alvarado MD, Lancaster RB, Fraser Symmans W, Mukhtar R, Wong JM, et al. Surgical standards for Management of the Axilla in breast cancer clinical trials with pathological complete response endpoint. NPJ Breast Cancer. 2018,4(1):26.

49. Woods RW, Camp MS, Durr NJ, Harvey SC. A review of options for localization of axillary lymph nodes in the treatment of invasive breast cancer. Acad Radiol. 2019,26(6):805–19.

50. Balasubramanian R, Morgan C, Shaari E, Kovacs T, Pinder SE, Hamed H, et al. Wire guided localisation for targeted axillary node dissection is accurate in axillary staging in node positive breast cancer following neoadjuvant chemotherapy. Eur J Surg Oncol. 2020,46(6):1028–33.

51. Simons JM, Scoggins ME, Kuerer HM, Krishnamurthy S, Yang WT, Sahin AA, et al. Prospective registry trial assessing the use of magnetic seeds to locate clipped nodes after neoadjuvant chemotherapy for breast cancer patients. Ann Surg Oncol. 2021,28:4277.

52. Sun J, Henry DA, Carr MJ, Yazdankhahkenary A, Laronga C, Lee MC, et al. Feasibility of axillary lymph node localization and excision using radar reflector localization. Clin Breast Cancer. 2021; https://doi.org/10.1016/j.clbc.2020.08.001.

53. Laws A, Dillon K, Kelly BN, Kantor O, Hughes KS, Gadd MA, et al. Node-positive patients treated with neoadjuvant chemotherapy can be spared axillary lymph node dissection with wireless non-radioactive localizers. Ann Surg Oncol. 2020,27(12):4819–27.

54. Kedrzycki MS, Leiloglou M, Ashrafian H, Jiwa N, Thiruchelvam PTR, Elson DS, et al. Meta-analysis comparing fluorescence imaging with radioisotope and blue dye-guided sentinel node identification for breast cancer surgery. Ann Surg Oncol. 2021; https://doi.org/10.1245/s10434–020–09288–7.

55. Valente SA, Al-Hilli Z, Radford DM, Yanda C, Tu C, Grobmyer SR. Near infrared fluorescent lymph node mapping with Indocyanine green in breast cancer patients: a prospective trial. J Am Coll Surg. 2019,228(4):672–8.

56. Ahmed M, Purushotham AD, Douek M. Novel techniques for sentinel lymph node biopsy in breast cancer: a systematic review. Lancet Oncol. 2014,15(8):e351–62.

57. Alvarado MD, Mittendorf EA, Teshome M, Thompson AM, Bold RJ, Gittleman MA, et al. SentimagIC: a non-inferiority trial comparing superparamagnetic iron oxide versus technetium-99m and blue dye in the detection of axillary sentinel nodes in patients with early-stage breast cancer. Ann Surg Oncol. 2019,26(11):3510–6.

58. Karakatsanis A, Daskalakis K, Stålberg P, Olofsson H, Andersson Y, Eriksson S, et al. Superparamagnetic iron oxide nanoparticles as the sole method for sentinel node biopsy detection in patients with breast cancer. Br J Surg. 2017,104(12):1675–85.

59. Karakatsanis A, Christiansen PM, Fischer L, Hedin C, Pistioli L, Sund M, et al. The Nordic SentiMag trial: a comparison of super paramagnetic iron oxide (SPIO) nanoparticles versus Tc(99) and patent blue in the detection of sentinel node (SN) in patients with breast cancer and a meta-analysis of earlier studies. Breast Cancer Res Treat. 2016,157(2):281–94.

7 组织灌注的重要性与乳房切除皮瓣的评估

编者：Marios-Konstantinos Tasoulis, Gerald Gui
译者：田照坤

7.1 背景

乳房切除皮瓣质量是决定异体材料乳房重建成败的核心因素。目前已证实乳房切除术后缺血性并发症的诸多内、外源性风险因素，但即使对风险最低的理想重建病例，低灌注皮瓣亦可致重建失败。

皮瓣质量对胸肌前假体重建的影响更为显著。胸肌前假体置入术作为一种新的重建技术，可最大限度降低胸肌剥离相关并发症（如活动畸形[1]），近年再度兴起。皮瓣质量不仅显著影响胸肌前假体的功能及美学效果，更决定了该术式的可行性。

假体与皮瓣间缺乏胸肌血管层，加剧了皮肤包膜发生缺血的潜在风险。全层创面或切口愈合不良可快速进展为假体外露并需要取出。过度减薄的术后皮瓣易导致假体可见/可触及的轮廓畸形和褶皱等美学缺陷。

乳房切除皮瓣质量是一个综合指标体系，取决于多种因素，包括相对皮瓣厚度、浅层腺体结构的保留程度以及皮瓣处理的规范程度。客观评估术区皮瓣质量存在挑战性，但对术中决策具有重要指导价值。科学规范的评估可有效预防缺血性并发症，并为实现最佳手术效果提供保障。

优化乳房切除皮瓣质量的目标是在满足肿瘤学标准的前提下，通过解剖学分离及根据乳房切除情况量身定制的重建方案，实现修复与美学效果的最大化。这要求肿瘤专科与整形外科医师构建多学科协作机制，在患者全诊疗周期中通力合作[2]。

7.2 解剖学

在乳腺癌根治术中，深刻理解乳腺解

N. S. Karp (✉)
Hansjörg Wyss Department of Plastic Surgery, NYU Langone Health, New York, NY, USA
e-mail: Nolan.Karp@nyumc.org

A. A. Salibian
Division of Plastic and Reconstructive Surgery,
University of California, Davis,
Sacramento, CA, USA

© The Author(s), under exclusive license to Springer Nature Switzerland AG 2023
R. Vidya, H. Becker (eds.), *Prepectoral Breast Reconstruction*,
https://doi.org/10.1007/978-3-031-15590-1_7

剖结构及皮肤软组织血供，对于维持术后组织灌注状态及保证肿瘤根治效果至关重要[3]。乳房脂肪组织皮下层被浅层筋膜分为较薄的表层与较厚的深层[4]，完整的皮下组织通过乳房（假性）包膜与腺体分隔，此包膜即代表乳房切除术中的解剖剥离层面（图7.1）。该包膜在乳房各部位的深度并不均一，故皮下层厚度存在差异。

乳房及乳头-乳晕复合体的浅层血供系统至关重要，因为这是乳房切除术后残留组织的唯一供养来源。保护胸廓内动脉穿支（尤其是优势第二穿支）对维持皮肤软组织灌注具有决定性作用。这些血管主要走行于乳房皮下脂肪层中，若解剖剥离过程保持在乳房包膜层面即可得到有效保护[5]。

7.3 术前规划

7.3.1 患者特异性因素

术前需系统评估患者体质形态学特征及其对灌注状态的影响，特别应注意乳房下垂[6]与切除体积较大[7]均与乳房切除术后皮肤软组织缺血性并发症发生率升高密切相关。专项研究发现，在保留乳头和乳晕的乳房切除术中，切除组织400~800g患者的并发症风险增加2.6倍，≥800g者则风险攀升至5.1倍[7]。乳房体积增大与下垂程度加重可能导致需灌注皮肤表面积增大，同时伴血管源至皮瓣边缘的灌注距离增加，从而进一步损害灌注效能。

对于合并乳房下垂及巨乳症的患者，必须于术前详尽告知其皮肤软组织缺血性并发症风险上升的相关性。此类病例可考虑采用倒T形切口实施皮肤缩减手术[8,9]，但当乳房切除皮瓣血运受损或出现乳头-乳晕复合体失活时，需警惕该切口T形交汇点皮肤坏死的高风险性。另外，分期实施乳房缩小成形术可有效调控皮肤张力、优化乳房形态与乳头位置，并可能诱导血管延迟效应[10]。

术前对乳房皮下层厚度进行评估很重要。其本身乳房皮下层厚度存在显著的个体间差异，肥胖（高体重指数）者常明显增厚[11]。若患者因肿瘤评估已行MRI检查，可通过该技术测量皮下层厚度（图7.2），亦可采用床旁超声实时检测。术前精确测定皮下层厚度并与肿瘤外科医师充分讨论，有助于制订规范化乳房切除方案并预估皮瓣厚度，进而指导术中根据剩余组织厚度进行动态决策。

乳房切除术后缺血性并发症存在多种潜在高危因素，需在术前系统评估。特定合并症（如糖尿病）将导致术后缺血性

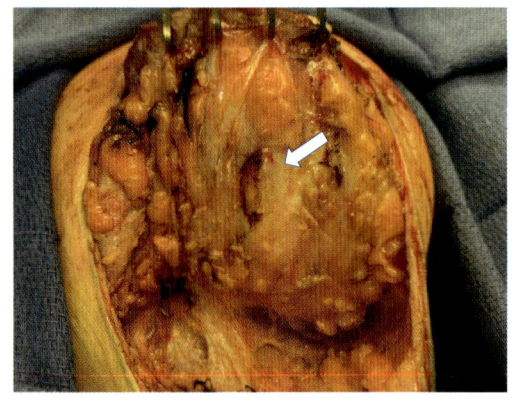

图7.1 在缩乳术中可见乳腺包膜（白箭头），分隔皮下脂肪与腺体

7 组织灌注的重要性与乳房切除皮瓣的评估

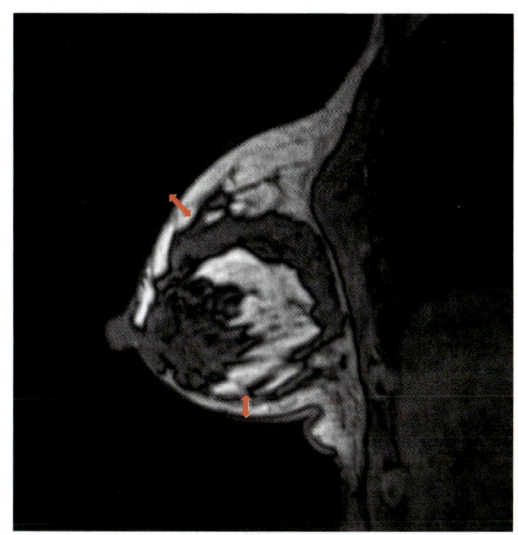

图 7.2 MRI 可评估乳房皮肤及皮下组织的厚度（红箭头），为乳房切除提供参考

发症发生率明显提高[12]。外部因素如放疗史[13]、吸烟史[14]亦需重点评估，因其已被证实对灌注功能具有不良影响并与缺血性并发症风险升高相关。

7.3.2 保留乳头和乳晕的乳房切除术

保留乳头和乳晕的乳房切除术可显著优化术后美学效果，并且已被证实与患者治疗满意度及生存质量改善存在相关性[15]。该术式因完全保留皮肤软组织覆盖，须特别关注皮瓣灌注状态，可能因手术操作空间受限、皮瓣牵拉张力增强、无法切除血运受损区等而增加技术难度。因此，此类手术（尤其是胸肌前间隙置入式重建）的成功实施有赖于精准的患者筛选与规范的术中操作。

乳房体积过大或下垂严重等形态学特征需与其他风险因素结合起来进行评估，因严重病例可能被视为该术式的相对禁忌

证。系统评估所有相关风险因素，对确定手术方案及可接受的并发症风险至关重要。我们既往建立的风险评估模型综合了12 项风险因素的加权效应，可辅助预测保留乳头和乳晕的乳房切除术联合即刻重建术的术后总体并发症风险[16]。针对每位患者开展个体化风险评估有助于术前充分沟通，从而制订最优手术方案并合理设定患者预期。

7.3.3 切口设计

切口选择对术区显露范围、乳房切除术后皮肤软组织灌注状态及美学效果具有显著影响。针对皮肤血供评估，需要了解的是，切口位置距供养血管的距离越远，切口边缘形成的"分水岭"区域范围越大。因此，在设计切口时应优先保障灌注效能（同时兼顾其他关键因素）。

保留皮肤的乳房切除联合假体重建手术通常优选椭圆形切口。该切口理想定位应距离乳房四个边缘的等距中心，以优化所有四个象限的灌注效果（图 7.3）。保留乳头和乳晕术式因需维持乳头－乳晕复合体血供，切口定位有更多选择，并且每种选择对临床转归影响更显著。

已证实乳房下皱襞切口与较低缺血性并发症发生率相关[17]，现已成为保留乳头和乳晕的乳房切除术最广泛使用的切口（图 7.4）[18]，优势包括瘢痕隐蔽、为肿瘤切除提供良好术野显露且对软组织灌注影响最小[19]。需要注意的是，对于乳腺体积较大病例，可能增加上极区域解剖操作的难度，进而导致皮瓣牵拉张力增高。

对此类病例，可考虑采用辅助切口处理乳腺尾部区域[20]。外侧缘切口与垂直放射状切口同样能有效保护乳头-乳晕复合体血供，但外侧切口可能引起乳头外移[21]。倒T形切口可为肿瘤切除提供理想术野，同时实现皮肤缩减与乳头高度调整，但与较高缺血性并发症发生率相关[17,22]。最后，因明确增加乳头-乳晕复合体坏死风险，通常不推荐使用乳晕周切口[17]。

切口选择最终应由医患共同决定，综

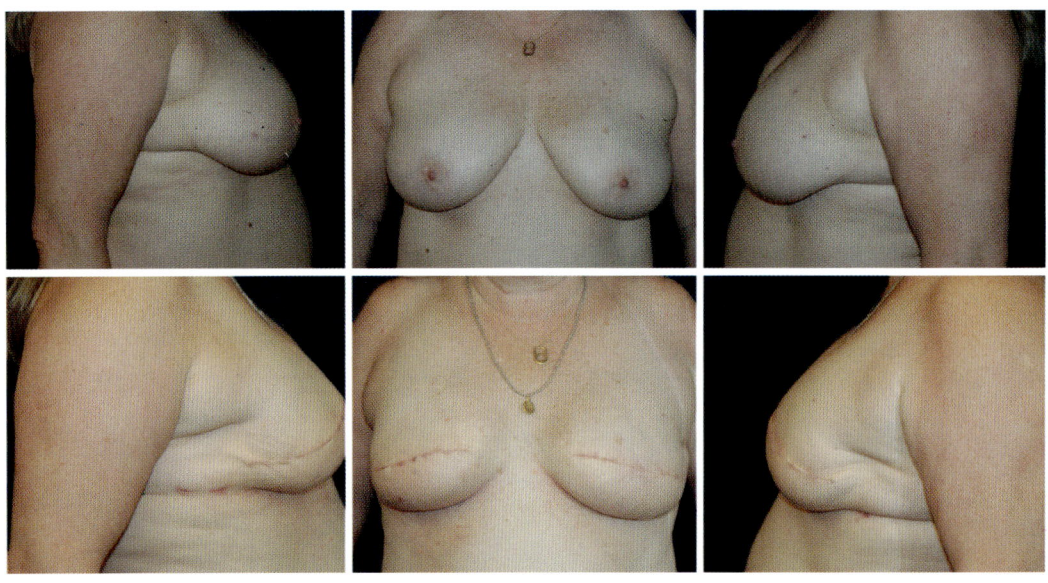

图 7.3　保留皮肤的乳房切除术后，采用中心椭圆形切口进行前胸肌重建

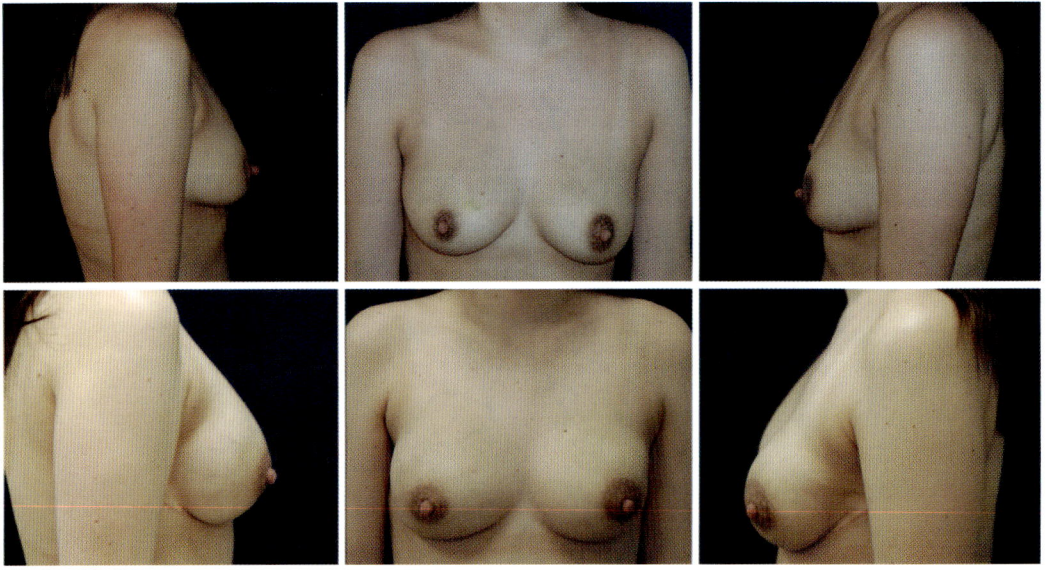

图 7.4　保留乳头和乳晕的皮下腺体切除术后，采用乳房下皱襞切口进行胸肌前重建手术

合考量患者主观诉求、肿瘤外科技术要求，以及切口对灌注效果与美学结局的影响。无论最终选择何种切口，均应向患者详细阐释各种切口方案的优劣及所有术式决策的内在风险，尤其应强调不存在普适性完美方案。建议采用多学科协作模式，结合患者个体化需求权衡不同技术方案的临床收益与潜在风险，确定最优手术计划。

7.4 术中注意事项

7.4.1 乳房切除皮瓣剥离

皮瓣质量的优劣取决于术区剥离层次的选择。尽管存在多种剥离技术规范，确立正确的剥离层面应作为各术式的不变核心要素。此层面应以乳腺包膜结构为解剖基准，确保皮瓣保留小叶状皮下组织（图7.5）。

需特别注意，皮下层厚度不仅存在显著的个体差异，同一乳房的各区域也不均一。影像学研究证实，该层次厚度具有由乳头-乳晕复合体向周边逐渐增厚的分布特征[23]，并且在解剖平面内存在多发变异。因此，实际操作中不应机械维持特定厚度，而应遵循包膜形态动态调整剥离深度，在确保切除包膜下层腺体的同时合理保留皮下脂肪层完整性。术前影像学评估可辅助预测各区域组织厚度，指导乳腺不同位点的切除深度。

穿行于皮下组织的皮肤软组织节段性灌注系需要重点保护，尤其保留乳头和乳晕的术式，胸廓内动脉第2肋间穿支的

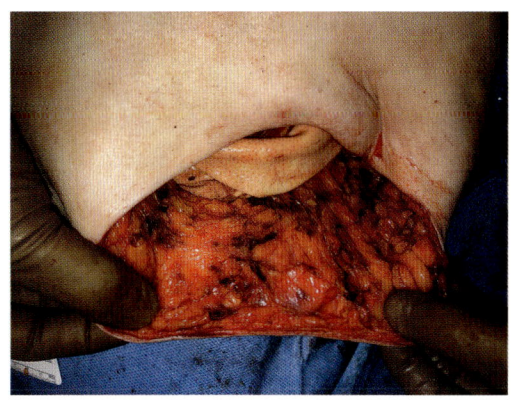

图7.5 乳房切除术应沿乳腺包膜平面切除乳腺，并尽可能保留乳房切除腺体表面皮肤的皮下脂肪

保留具有决定性意义。此外，由于乳头、乳晕后方缺乏皮下组织支持，剥离层面需转移至复合体下方的乳晕下平面。

术中的其他操作细节亦对皮瓣存活会产生显著影响。应尽量减少皮瓣牵拉，仅维持满足肿瘤切除所需的最小显露范围。推荐使用低剂量稀释肾上腺素溶液以减少出血并实现锐性剥离。值得注意的是，近期关于肿胀技术的大样本荟萃分析表明，该技术可能增加术后皮肤坏死风险[24]。术中可酌情采用精准电凝止血以减轻皮瓣热损伤。建议在切除肿瘤阶段即邀请整形外科医师协同操作，以提升整体手术质量。

7.4.2 乳房切除皮瓣质量评估

乳房切除术皮瓣质量的评估需要乳腺外科与整形外科医师对多项变量进行综合分析，重点包括皮瓣厚度参数。多项研究证实，皮瓣过薄与缺血性并发症风险升高存在显著关联性[6, 14, 23]。尤其需要指出，MRI显示术后皮瓣平均厚度<8.0mm是缺血性并发症的独立预测因子[23]。术前和术

中超声检查可作为经济高效的客观评估工具，精准测量乳腺皮下组织厚度及残余皮瓣厚度。由于皮下层本身存在厚度差异，皮瓣相对厚度参数的临床意义更突出。既往研究显示，行保留乳头和乳晕的乳房切除术后，缺血性并发症组患者的术后-术前皮瓣厚度百分比（50%厚度）显著低于无并发症组（74%厚度）[23]。尽管量化评估很重要，但根本原则是无论厚薄，在乳房切除术中保留完整皮下脂肪层并维持皮肤浅层灌注是核心目标。

皮瓣厚度不足并非等同于质量低劣。部分患者可能自身皮下层较薄，但术中若通过乳腺包膜层面的规范性解剖剥离保留该薄层，则软组织活力及质量仍可得到保障。因此，可以术前影像学皮下组织厚度测定结果为基础来评估术后厚度改变。但需要注意的是，皮瓣过薄可能对美学效果造成负面影响，尤其在胸肌前假体重建术中，可导致假体触感明显、轮廓可见度增加，甚至上极轮廓阶梯感加重。因此，术中应同步评估皮瓣厚度的缺血风险与美学效应，综合判断最优假体置入平面，以及是否需联合辅助技术以实现最佳美学效果。

除厚度参数外，存在多种其他评估皮瓣质量的方法，主要聚焦于灌注状态。我们发现，临床观察是可靠且经济的评估方式。除相对厚度外，亦应需检测皮瓣保留皮下脂肪情况、裸露真皮区域及电凝操作导致的皮肤损伤程度。其他临床参数包括切口缘出血情况、皮瓣微循环充盈状态和皮肤瘀斑，但需考虑含肾上腺素灌注液的影响。既往研究证实，即刻乳房重建术后缺血性并发症与术中医师对皮瓣质量的目测评估高度相关[25]。具体评估指标包括皮斑花斑现象、真皮暴露范围、毛细血管再充盈时间、亚甲蓝浸润效应、皮瓣边缘渗血情况及厚度预估值，验证了临床评估的实用价值。

多项辅助性灌注评估技术亦可用于术中皮瓣质量监测。此类方法主要借助吲哚菁绿血管造影系统识别局部或整体缺血区域。与单纯临床评估相比，吲哚菁绿血管造影可有效减少保皮乳房切除术后的皮瓣坏死发生率[26,27]，但判定低灌注程度及后续确定应切除组织范围的决策仍具有挑战性。系统性综述指出，吲哚菁绿或荧光素血管造影未能有效降低皮肤坏死风险，甚至可能导致错误切除健康组织[28]。其他技术如光学光谱分析及近红外组织氧饱和监测在皮瓣灌注评估中的应用尚缺乏充分循证依据。需要明确的是，组织灌注评估技术仅作为质量分析工具之一，应与临床体征检测联合应用以制定精准的术中干预策略。

7.5 受损皮瓣处理规范

7.5.1 术中处理策略

术中若发现组织灌注受限，需根据组织损伤程度及重建方案的影响因素来确定对应决策。对于保经皮肤乳房切除术或全乳切除术，血运明显受损的皮肤组织应予以切除，闭合切口时避免产生过度张力。

在保留乳头、乳晕的术式中，因为需要保持完整软组织覆盖而不能切除大面积皮肤，缺血性皮瓣处理更具挑战性。此时需调整重建方案。研究表明，与Ⅱ期组织扩张术相比，保留乳头和乳晕的手术后即刻假体重建因增加了皮瓣压力而导致更高的缺血性并发症发生率[29]。若计划行即刻假体重建但皮瓣灌注存疑，建议Ⅰ期手术优先放置组织扩张器。

存在灌注障碍时，组织扩张器应选择欠量填充（或完全不予填充）。扩张器类型亦可影响皮瓣压力：与外接式注射阀或可调节假体相比，解剖式一体化注射阀扩张器更为臃肿[30, 31]。采用空气欠量填充可降低皮肤压力（尤其对下部皮瓣）。最不利情况下应延迟重建时，以规避全层组织损伤和假体暴露导致的继发并发症。

假体置入平面亦为关键因素。灌注不良的皮瓣组织不能支持胸肌前置入式重建。因缺乏胸肌血供层的保护作用，创面愈合不良或大面积坏死将导致假体直接外露。因此，需预先告知患者可能需采用全肌肉下假体置入方案，或在软组织受损情况下选择Ⅱ期重建。需要明确的是，脱细胞真皮基质等支撑材料在此类病例中无法产生疗效。该材料需与血运充沛组织紧密接触方能整合，而在灌注不良皮瓣下放置非血管化异体真皮等同于在缺血区域置入异物。

7.5.2　术后处理要点

胸肌前乳房重建术后的皮肤软组织缺血属于严重并发症，需采取积极措施并密切随访，以最大限度降低假体外露、感染及重建失败的风险。术后皮瓣缺血需实施全面防御性干预策略，力求将组织损伤最小化。在保留乳头和乳晕的术式中，既往放疗史、即刻假体置入、脱细胞真皮基质应用、重度感染及高体重指数，已被证实为大面积缺血并发症后重建失败的独立危险因素。胸肌前间隙重建的术后管理目标为：精细处理部分厚度坏死以阻止其进展，并及时识别与处置全层损伤。

部分厚度缺血处理的要点在于密切随访配合严格的伤口护理。治疗策略需聚焦于控制感染风险并预防二次组织损伤，同时动态监测是否进展为全层坏死。推荐使用凡士林纱布辅以抗生素软膏的异物隔绝换药方案。局部应用硝酸甘油软膏与高压氧治疗可作为辅助干预手段[32, 33]。

对于全层坏死病例，必须充分强调早期主动治疗的重要性。由于假体与软组织间缺乏血管化肌肉屏障，所有创面均具有严重隐患。早期清创对促进创面闭合及减少假体囊腔污染具有决定性作用。若出现大面积坏死或创缘存在张力，取出假体并延期重建通常可实现更佳的组织愈合环境。

7.6　小结

乳房切除术皮瓣质量这一概念涵盖多元化变量指标，可归纳为皮肤软组织的相对厚度与灌注效能的综合体现。"高质量"的乳房切除术皮瓣应满足以下条件：在乳腺包膜解剖平面实施规范性剥离以完整切除腺体组织的同时，保留皮下层的全层结构从而维持关键的浅层灌注系统功能。这需要肿瘤外科与整形外科医师协力合作，在整个围术期实施多学科协作管理模式。术前影像学评估可指导制订精准的术中解剖方案，而术中对皮瓣质量的临床及辅助性评估结果应作为重建术式选择的核心依据，以最大限度降低并发症风险并优化重建与美学双重结局。

参考文献

1. Salibian AA, Frey JD, Choi M, Karp NS. Subcutaneous implant-based breast reconstruction with acellular dermal matrix/mesh: a systematic review. Plast Reconstr Surg Glob Open. 2016,4: e1139.
2. Storm-Dickerson T, Sigalove N. Prepectoral breast reconstruction: the breast Surgeon's perspective. Plast Reconstr Surg. 2017,140:43S–8S.
3. Vidya R, Iqbal FM. Breast anatomy: time to classify the subpectoral and prepectoral spaces. Clin Anat. 2017,30:434–5.
4. Rehnke RD, Groening RM, Van Buskirk ER, Clarke JM. Anatomy of the superficial fascia system of the breast: a comprehensive theory of breast fascial anatomy. Plast Reconstr Surg. 2018,142:1135–44.
5. Frey JD, Salibian AA, Choi M, Karp NS. The importance of tissue perfusion in reconstructive breast surgery. Plast Reconstr Surg. 2019,144: 21S–9S.
6. De Vita R, Zoccali G, Buccheri EM, et al. Outcome evaluation after 2023 nipple-sparing mastectomies: our experience. Plast Reconstr Surg. 2017,139:335e–47e.
7. Frey JD, Salibian AA, Karp NS, Choi M. The impact of mastectomy weight on reconstructive trends and outcomes in nipple-sparing mastectomy: progressively greater complications with larger breast size. Plast Reconstr Surg. 2018,141: 795e–804e.
8. Caputo GG, Marchetti A, Dalla Pozza E, et al. Skin-reduction breast reconstructions with prepectoral implant. Plast Reconstr Surg. 2016,137: 1702–5.
9. Rusby JE, Gui GP. Nipple-sparing mastectomy in women with large or ptotic breasts. J Plast Reconstr Aesthet Surg. 2010,63:e754–5.
10. Spear SL, Rottman SJ, Seiboth LA, Hannan CM. Breast reconstruction using a staged nipple-sparing mastectomy following mastopexy or reduction. Plast Reconstr Surg. 2012,129:572–81.
11. Frey JD, Salibian AA, Choi M, Karp NS. Optimizing outcomes in nipple-sparing mastectomy: mastectomy flap thickness is not one size fits all. Plast Reconstr Surg Glob Open. 2019,7:e2103.
12. Matsen CB, Mehrara B, Eaton A, et al. Skin flap necrosis after mastectomy with reconstruction: a prospective study. Ann Surg Oncol. 2016,23: 257–64.
13. Colwell AS, Tessler O, Lin AM, et al. Breast reconstruction following nipple-sparing mastectomy: predictors of complications, reconstruction outcomes, and 5-year trends. Plast Reconstr Surg. 2014,133:496–506.
14. Algaithy ZK, Petit JY, Lohsiriwat V, et al. Nipple sparing mastectomy: can we predict the factors predisposing to necrosis? Eur J Surg Oncol. 2012,38:125–9.
15. Didier F, Radice D, Gandini S, et al. Does nipple preservation in mastectomy improve satisfaction with cosmetic results, psychological adjustment, body image and sexuality? Breast Cancer Res Treat. 2009,118:623–33.
16. Frey JD, Salibian AA, Choi M, Karp NS. Putting together the pieces: development and validation of a risk-assessment model for nipple-sparing mastectomy. Plast Reconstr Surg. 2020,145: 273e–83e.
17. Frey JD, Salibian AA, Levine JP, Karp NS, Choi M. Incision choices in nipple-sparing mastectomy: a comparative analysis of outcomes and

evolution of a clinical algorithm. Plast Reconstr Surg. 2018,142:826e–35e.
18. Daar DA, Abdou SA, Rosario L, et al. Is there a preferred incision location for nipple-sparing mastectomy? A systematic review and meta-analysis. Plast Reconstr Surg. 2019,143:906e–19e.
19. Wagner JL, Fearmonti R, Hunt KK, et al. Prospective evaluation of the nipple-areola complex sparing mastectomy for risk reduction and for early-stage breast cancer. Ann Surg Oncol. 2012,19:1137–44.
20. Salibian AH, Harness JK, Mowlds DS. Inframammary approach to nipple-areola-sparing mastectomy. Plast Reconstr Surg. 2013,132:700e–8e.
21. Mori H, Uemura N, Okazaki M, Nakagawa T, Sato T. Nipple malposition after nipple-sparing mastectomy and expander-implant reconstruction. Breast Cancer. 2016,23:740–4.
22. Munhoz AM, Aldrighi CM, Montag E, et al. Clinical outcomes following nipple-areola-sparing mastectomy with immediate implant-based breast reconstruction: a 12-year experience with an analysis of patient and breast-related factors for complications. Breast Cancer Res Treat. 2013,140:545–55.
23. Frey JD, Salibian AA, Choi M, Karp NS. Mastectomy flap thickness and complications in nipple-sparing mastectomy: objective evaluation using magnetic resonance imaging. Plast Reconstr Surg Glob Open. 2017,5:e1439.
24. Siotos C, Aston JW, Euhus DM, et al. The use of tumescent technique in mastectomy and related complications: a meta-analysis. Plast Reconstr Surg. 2019,143:39–48.
25. Frey JD, Salibian AA, Bekisz JM, et al. What is in a number? Evaluating a risk assessment tool in immediate breast reconstruction. Plast Reconstr Surg Glob Open. 2019,7:e2585.
26. Rinker B. A comparison of methods to assess mastectomy flap viability in skin-sparing mastectomy and immediate reconstruction: a prospective cohort study. Plast Reconstr Surg. 2016,137:395–401.
27. Liu EH, Zhu SL, Hu J, et al. Intraoperative SPY reduces post-mastectomy skin flap complications: a systematic review and meta-analysis. Plast Reconstr Surg Glob Open. 2019,7:e2060.
28. Khavanin N, Qiu C, Darrach H, et al. Intraoperative perfusion assessment in mastectomy skin flaps: how close are we to preventing complications? J Reconstr Microsurg. 2019,35:471–8.
29. Frey JD, Choi M, Salibian AA, Karp NS. Comparison of outcomes with tissue expander, immediate implant, and autologous breast reconstruction in greater than 1000 nipple-sparing mastectomies. Plast Reconstr Surg. 2017,139:1300–10.
30. Becker H, Zhadan O. Filling the Spectrum expander with air-a new alternative. Plast Reconstr Surg Glob Open. 2017,5:e1541.
31. Becker H, Mathew PJ. Immediate Prepectoral breast reconstruction in suboptimal patients using an air-filled spacer. Plast Reconstr Surg Glob Open. 2019,7:e2470.
32. Turin SY, Li DD, Vaca EE, Fine N. Nitroglycerin ointment for reducing the rate of mastectomy flap necrosis in immediate implant-based breast reconstruction. Plast Reconstr Surg. 2018,142:264e–70e.
33. Alperovich M, Harmaty M, Chiu ES. Treatment of nipple-sparing mastectomy necrosis using hyperbaric oxygen therapy. Plast Reconstr Surg. 2015,135:1071e–2e.

8 胸肌前乳房重建术的补片与内置物选择

编者：Kylie M. Edinger, Ahmed M. Afifi
译者：冯志浩　刘文涛

8.1 引言

乳房重建技术正持续发展与革新，这些变革主要由假体设计与补片技术的进步驱动。20世纪70年代，乳房重建手术多采用胸肌前假体置入式，因肌下技术尚未被充分描述与认知[1]。1981年，Gruber等发表肌下与胸肌前乳房重建技术的比较研究后，业界开始从胸肌前转向肌下重建[2]。该研究通过对文献的系统回顾，揭示了与肌下重建相比，胸肌前重建的包膜挛缩、感染、假体移位和假体丢失发生率更高。然而，该研究的所有研究对象均采用直接假体置入（无须组织扩张），未使用补片产品，突显了假体选择和补片应用对实施胸肌前重建成功的重要性。即便以当今技术标准来衡量，未能正确选择假体或支撑补片的胸肌前乳房重建同样可能失败。简而言之，胸肌前乳房重建的实现依赖正确的假体与补片应用。

脱细胞真皮基质（ADM）的问世重新燃起了人们对胸肌前重建技术的关注，使其成为肌下重建的良好替代方案[3]。如ADM等生物补片与合成补片可优化假体置入与囊袋控制，增强软组织覆盖效果，减少皱褶形成，并可能降低包膜挛缩发生率。补片技术支持使用更大规格假体并获得更高的初始扩张容积[4-6]。目前，美国超过50%的乳房重建手术采用了ADM[7]。

在胸肌前乳房重建中，选择合理假体与补片是实现手术成功的关键。尽管不同外形假体对于肌下重建影响甚微，但在胸肌前重建中此类决策会显著影响手术效果，对此应持审慎态度。通过规范操作与适宜材料的选择应用，胸肌前重建可获得优异效果，这也是该技术迅速获得医患双方认可的重要原因（图8.1）。Marks等2019年的研究表明，胸肌前重建的普及度

K. M. Edinger
Division of Plastic Surgery, University of Wisconsin, Madison, WI, USA

A. M. Afifi (✉)
Division of Plastic Surgery, University of Wisconsin, Madison, WI, USA

Division of Plastic Surgery, Cairo University, Cairo, Egypt

© The Author(s), under exclusive license to Springer Nature Switzerland AG 2023
R. Vidya, H. Becker (eds.), *Prepectoral Breast Reconstruction*,
https://doi.org/10.1007/978-3-031-15590-1_8

8 胸肌前乳房重建术的补片与内置物选择

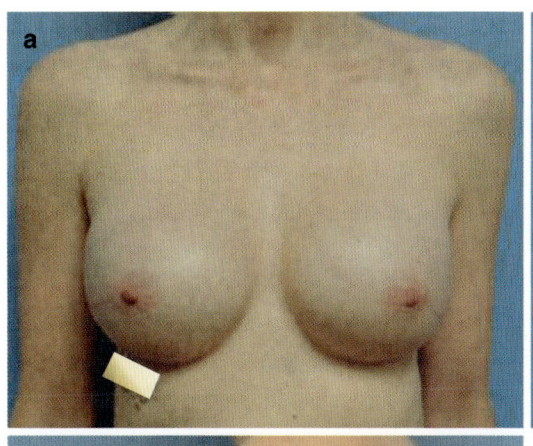
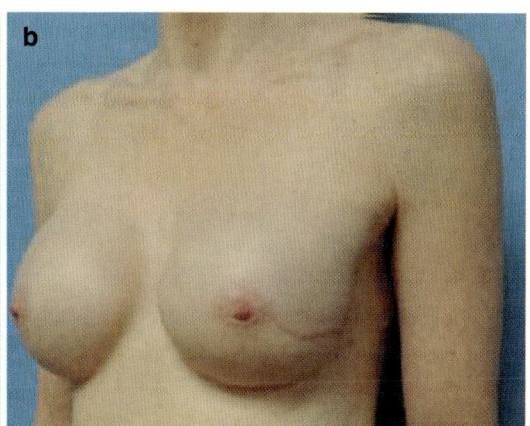
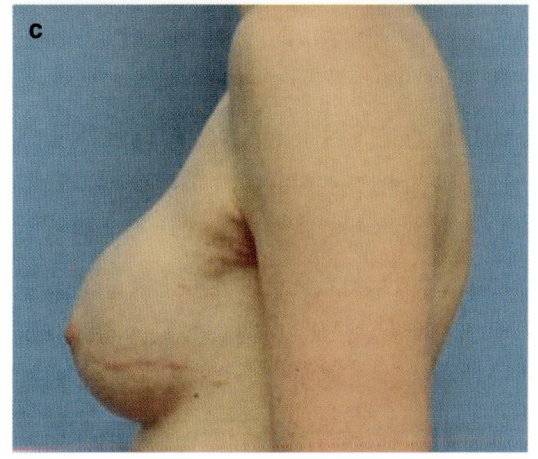

图 8.1 胸肌前假体重建理想病例，展示术后自然外形，含正（a）、斜位（b）及侧位（c）观

已超过肌下重建[8]。随着外科领域经验的积累及假体与补片技术的持续改进，我们预计这一趋势仍将延续。

8.2 假体选择

选择适宜的乳房假体是成功开展胸肌前乳房重建的核心要素之一。选择假体时需综合考量容积、外形、凝聚度、表面质地、基底宽度及凸度等多重因素。乳房假体通常根据三大制造参数分类：硅胶与盐水，毛面与光面，圆形与解剖型。

8.2.1 硅胶与盐水假体

硅胶与盐水乳房假体外壳均由硅胶弹性体制成。盐水假体内部填充无菌盐水，而硅胶假体则填充不同凝聚度的硅凝胶。硅凝胶交联化程度越高，其凝聚性及坚实度越高。高凝聚性假体皱褶发生率低于低凝聚性假体，但下垂感较弱，呈现更趋圆润的非自然外观。

在美国，多数乳房重建术使用硅胶假体。2019 年，异质材料乳房重建手术中硅胶假体占比超 95%，盐水假体仅占 5%[9]。硅胶假体因比盐水假体更具自然触感与外观特征，通常作为重建首选。全球范围内

85

硅胶假体在乳房重建术与隆乳术中的普及率均高于盐水假体。欧洲、拉丁美洲及亚洲的隆乳术数据显示，硅胶假体在全球市场中占主导地位[10]。

研究证实，盐水假体与硅胶假体使用寿命相近：盐水假体平均失效时间为 8.4 年，硅胶假体为 8.1 年[11]。关键差异使硅胶假体成为胸肌前重建优选：硅胶假体除具皱褶更少、外观触感更自然等优势外，其单位容积重量更低。400mL 盐水假体仅比同容积硅胶假体重 25g，但即便轻微重量差异也可增加切口张力，切口裂开及假体外露的风险增加[12]。本章后续内容将聚焦硅胶假体重建，因其为目前广泛应用的首选方案，亦为本机构临床实践所用。

8.2.2 毛面与光面假体

毛面处理是通过机械或化学方法改变假体表面，形成粗糙抓持纹理的技术。毛面处理可降低假体移位与包膜挛缩发生率，是胸肌前重建假体最具优势的特性之一。该特性在肌下重建中的重要性不高，但对胸肌前重建成功则至关重要。各厂商的毛面处理工艺迥异，通常通过化学或机械处理使硅胶表面变粗糙。大孔毛面技术较之微孔毛面技术可生成更宽大深陷的微孔结构，研究证实其组织黏附性更优，假体移位率更低[13]。

Allergan 曾采用失盐技术（lost-salt technique），即在未固化的湿润硅胶外壳浸渍盐颗粒混合物，来制成颗粒状毛面[1]。此法因与假体相关间变性大细胞淋巴瘤（BI-ALCL）有关而在多个国家被禁用并最终停产。目前，Allergan 全线产品为光面假体。Mentor 通过微孔毛面工艺，采用聚氨酯模具在未固化硅胶表面机械压印纹理[14]。Sientra 未公开其微孔毛面工艺细节。Mentor 与 Sientra 所用毛面技术尚未发现与 Allergan 既往大孔毛面假体同等强度的 ALCL 关联性，但所有毛面假体均存在 BI-ALCL 潜在风险，需经充分医患沟通后方可使用。

近年来，美国市场因 BI-ALCL 相关性，毛面假体接受度显著下降，但其仍为胸肌前重建最优假体选择。FDA 虽未正式禁止毛面假体使用，但多数厂商已遵循建议主动停产。尽管毛面假体在全球仍有应用，多国已着手禁止大孔毛面产品。法国于 2019 年基于 BI-ALCL 数据，同时禁止了大孔毛面与聚氨酯毛面假体。Surgitek 曾在美国推出聚氨酯毛面假体，后因聚氨酯分解产物 2,4-甲苯二胺（2,4-TDA）潜在致癌风险退市[15]。即使 2,4-TDA 仅在动物模型中显示致癌性，聚氨酯假体仍与 BI-ALCL 相关。该类型假体在欧洲仍被广泛使用。

8.2.3 圆形与解剖型假体

圆形假体具有球状圆周轮廓，而解剖型假体为水滴形态，旨在营造更自然的下垂外观。圆形假体可为光面或毛面，填充材料可选硅胶或盐水。解剖型假体亦可填充硅胶或盐水，但多数采用毛面设计以降低在胸壁发生旋转与移位的风险。目前仅 Motiva 公司生产光面解剖型假体，其设计通过定位卡扣保证假体在胸壁的稳定性[16]。

该产品尚未获批进入美国市场,但在美国已启动临床试验,有望近期于北美上市。

解剖型假体在胸肌前重建中尤具优势,与传统圆形假体相比,其能形成更自然的下垂形态及平缓的乳房上极过渡。虽然其为胸肌前重建的重要工具,但因美国市场缺乏光面解剖型假体,其应用率较低。若光面解剖形假体进入美国市场,预计其将提升在胸肌前重建中的普及度。尽管毛面解剖型假体在拉美应用较少,但在欧亚地区仍广泛使用[10]。

本机构因收治多例 ALCL 患者,现已禁用毛面装置并全面转用光面假体及扩张器,临床常采用解剖型扩张器配合圆形假体。期望未来能深化对 ALCL 的认知,推动假体技术创新,开发更安全的解剖形产品,当前本机构认为其风险代价过高。

8.2.4 凝聚度

凝聚度是胸肌前重建的重要考量因素,高凝聚度假体皱褶更少。根据乳房切除皮瓣厚度选择适宜凝聚度至关重要:薄皮瓣宜选高凝聚度假体以减少皱褶,厚皮瓣可选用低凝聚度假体以实现自然外观并减轻上极充盈感[4]。高凝聚度假体隆突感明显,乳房上极与胸壁过渡陡峭。若需渐变过渡,可采用脂肪移植修饰。皮瓣脂肪移植亦有助于减轻皱褶,但需医患对改善程度保持客观预期。观察性研究显示,使用高凝聚度假体进行胸肌前重建更易发生假体翻转(即前后移位,假体后表面对向皮肤及乳头)[17]。本机构优选中度凝聚度假体,可在减少皱褶与保持自然形态、降低翻转率间取得良好平衡(图 8.2,图 8.3)。

8.2.5 基底宽度

因需实现假体与组织囊袋的严密切合以预防皱褶、假体移位及错位,正确选择假体基底宽度与凸度对胸肌前乳房重建至关重要。由于厂商不同,硅胶假体通常具备多种凸度选项(低、中、高)。针对具

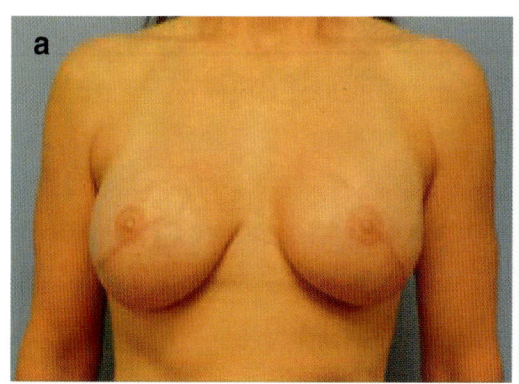 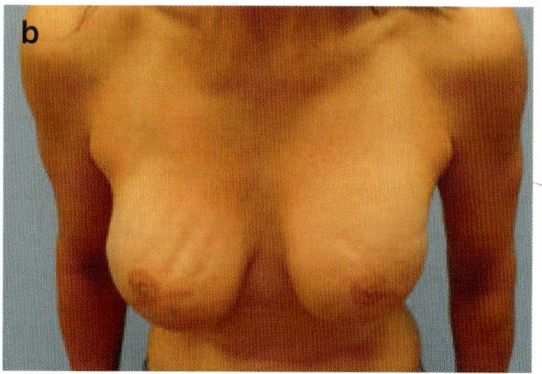

图 8.2 乳房重建患者影像对照:右侧使用普通假体,左侧应用高内聚假体(右侧假体因意外破裂紧急置换为普通假体)。(a)直立位双侧重建效果近似;(b)右侧普通假体下极明显皱褶,凸显高内聚假体在胸肌前间隙重建中的优势

胸肌前乳房重建

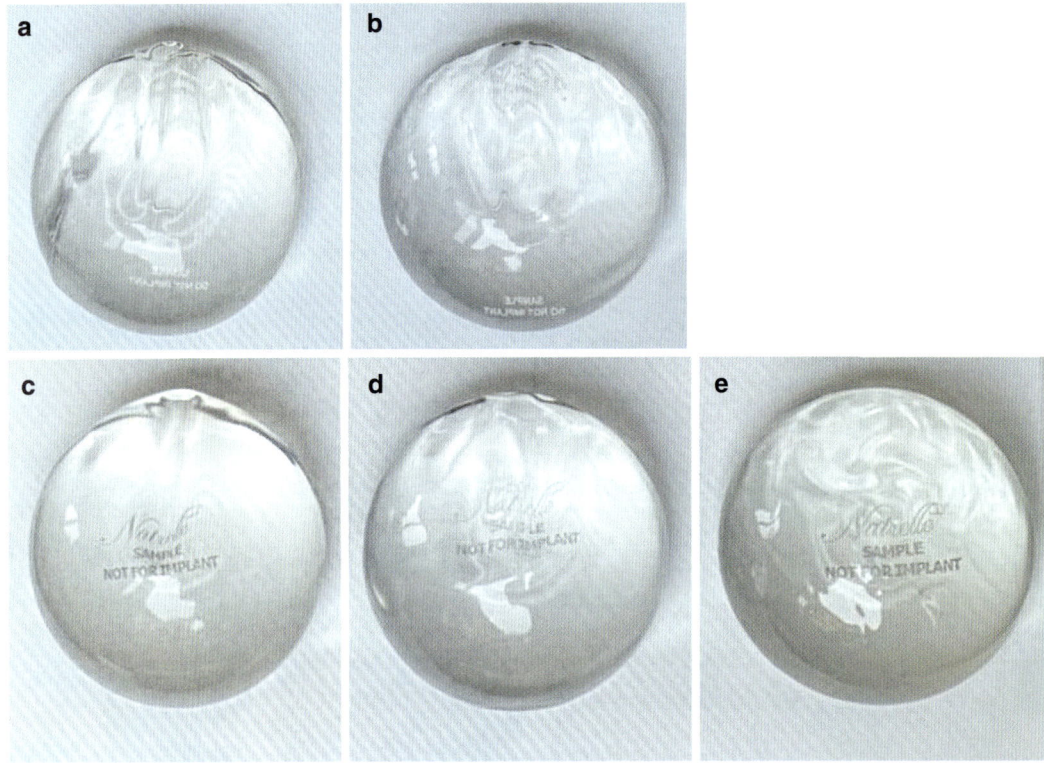

图 8.3　不同内聚性假体表面皱褶程度对比：Sientra 高内聚假体 HSC+ 型（a）、Sientra 低内聚假体 HSC 型（b）、Allergan 极高内聚假体 SCX 型（c）、Allergan 中内聚假体 SSX 型（d）、Allergan 低内聚假体 SRX 型（e）

体病例选择假体时，需由术者与患者共同确定期望凸度、基底宽度及容积三要素，其中任两项指标组合即可确定最适配假体。基底宽度是保障囊袋内假体紧密性的首要考量因素，亦为选择扩张器或假体的初始依据。

乳房基底宽度应自腋前线至乳房内侧测量，据此选择对应基底宽度假体以达到严密切合效果。圆形假体基底宽度与高度相等。胸腔横向宽度较大及肩部宽阔患者宜选大基底宽度假体，但需确保不牺牲凸度。胸壁凹陷患者选择高凸度假体有助于实现充分凸度[18]。

8.2.6　假体容积

随着假体容量增加，对乳腺组织及皮肤覆膜的要求相应提高。Vidya 等指出乳房（容积）超过 500g 者应行分阶段重建以降低手术失败风险[19]。Choi 等的大型多中心回顾性研究表明，400g 以上假体可增加感染及乳房切除术后皮瓣坏死的风险[20]。假体容量选择主要取决于乳房切除术皮瓣健康状况及患者体型特征。若切除皮瓣厚实健康且患者 BMI 较高，在胸肌前重建中使用大容量假体仍为安全的（图 8.4）。若切除皮瓣条件欠佳（薄或血供不足）或

8 胸肌前乳房重建术的补片与内置物选择

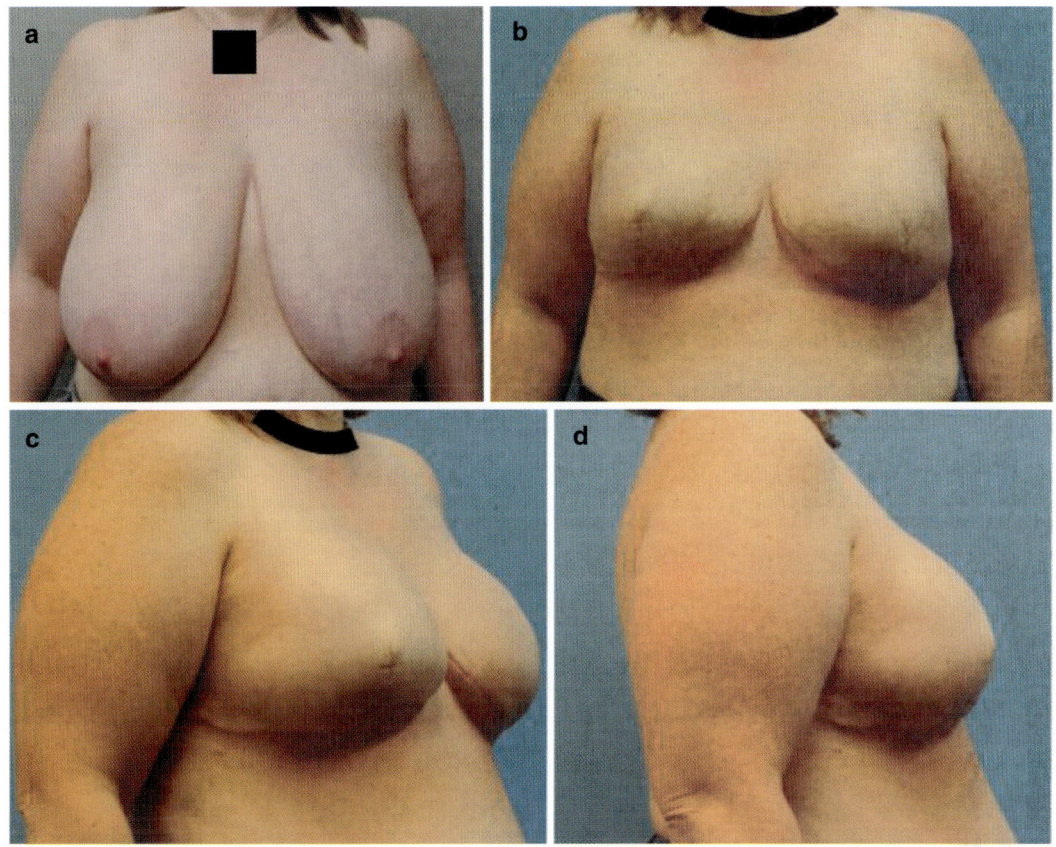

图 8.4 高体重指数（BMI）患者接受胸肌前大容量假体重建安全性验证：术前影像（a），术后正位（b）、斜位（c）、侧位（d）观；使用曼托光滑圆形超高凸度 790mL 硅胶假体

患者 BMI 较低，宜选择较小假体。胸肌前重建假体容量选择虽无绝对界限，但需综合评估皮瓣厚度及患者 BMI 确定容量。

8.3 假体制造商

经系统性调研已发表文献、社交媒体互助组、专业博客及区域外科医疗机构官方网站，现梳理当前主流应用的假体产品如下。全球乳房假体制造商众多，本节所列清单并不具备排他性。亦存在本章未述及的其他可用优质假体，临床实践中可根据需求合理选用。

8.3.1 Allergan

Allergan 为全球知名假体制造商，生产不同凝聚度的 Natrelle 系列盐水与硅胶假体。其前身为 McGhan，后更名为 Inamed，现归属 Allergan 旗下。产品（NuSil 硅胶假体）产地为哥斯达黎加。因证实与大孔毛面假体存在 BI-ALCL 相关性，该企业已全面退市相关产品。现为美国市场四大获批假体企业之一[21]。

8.3.2 Sientra

Sientra 是专供美国市场的假体供应

商。该公司原为巴西 Silimed 假体的北美代理商，但 2014 年 Silimed 巴西生产基地发现产品污染问题后终止合作，并将生产总部迁至美国威斯康星州富兰克林市。Sientra 现仅提供硅凝胶假体（圆形 / 解剖型、光面 / 毛面），未涉足盐水假体领域[22]。

8.3.3　Mentor

Mentor 为美国加利福尼亚州企业，专注美国本土假体供应，隶属强生公司旗下。产品线涵盖硅胶与盐水假体，其硅胶原料产自哥斯达黎加并进口至美国完成手工组装。该企业独家提供可调节容积的 Spectrum 盐水假体，术者可通过留置式注水管在术后 6 个月内调整假体容量[23]。

8.3.4　Silimed

Silimed 系巴西厂商，为拉美地区规模最大的假体供应商。产品线包含多种规格硅胶假体（圆形 / 解剖型、光面 / 毛面）。该公司曾为美国 Sientra 生产假体，后因 2014 年合作终止，现 Sientra 已在美国威斯康星州建立自主生产基地[24]。

8.3.5　Polytech

Polytech 为全球领先硅胶假体制造商之一，主要覆盖欧洲及中东市场。其产品包括光面与毛面假体，毛面处理采用聚氨酯工艺（该工艺在美国被列为禁用材料）[25]。

8.3.6　Ideal Implant

Ideal Implant 为专注美国市场的另一假体品牌。其硅胶原料源自哥斯达黎加，假体组装于威斯康星州维斯塔市。该企业仅生产盐水假体，采用双硅胶外壳设计以减少皱褶，旨在模拟硅胶假体的外观触感，同时避免硅胶破裂风险[26]。

8.3.7　GC Aesthetics

GC Aesthetics 公司通过旗下分支企业 Nagor（英国 / 苏格兰）与 Eurosilicone（法国）生产乳房假体。其硅胶假体覆盖全球 70 多个国家，但未进入美国市场[27]。

8.3.8　Laboratories Arion

Laboratories Arion 向南美洲、欧洲、北非、中东部分区域及越南供应假体。除单囊硅胶假体系列外，该公司还提供独特的生物相容性可降解水凝胶假体。该假体于 X 线检查下完全透明，破裂后可自行坍缩，无须 MRI 监测即可通过体检即时发现。美国市场未引入该企业产品[28]。

8.3.9　韩世生物

韩世生物（Hans Biomed）是亚洲本土企业，生产首款亚洲产硅胶假体 BellaGel（贝拉凝胶）。该产品已获欧洲认证，并计划扩展至中国及美国市场[29]。

8.3.10　Ceraplas

法国 Ceraplas 公司生产 Cereform 硅凝胶假体，涵盖圆形 / 解剖型、光面 / 毛面规格。主要销售区域为欧洲、中东及南美洲[30]。

8.3.11 Establishment 公司

Establishment 公司生产的 Motiva 硅胶假体覆盖欧洲、日本、澳大利亚及韩国等市场。目前正在美国进行临床试验，预计近期将进军北美市场。其为全球唯一生产配备胸壁固定卡扣结构的光面解剖型假体企业[31]。

8.3.12 Sebbin

法国 Sebbin 公司采用全手工生产硅胶假体，产品覆盖欧洲、非洲、南美洲、澳大利亚及印度市场[32]。

8.3.13 广州万和

广州万和塑胶材料公司系中国本土企业，专业研发生产硅胶乳房假体产品。

8.3.14 CollPlant

以色列 CollPlant 公司致力于开发基于 3D 生物打印技术制作的乳房假体。目前相关产品尚未上市[33]。

8.4 组织扩张器

对于接受乳房切除术的患者而言，即刻乳房重建仍是全球应用最广泛的术式。即刻重建可通过Ⅰ期手术直接置入假体，或采用分期术式：初始置入组织扩张器再行假体置换。多数术者更倾向于Ⅱ期手术重建，因扩张器可作为初始模板，同时可确保保险覆盖后续置换费用，借此实现囊袋精确塑形及效果优化。此外，扩张器亦适用于计划行放疗、乳房切除术皮瓣血供欠佳（可行空载扩张或注气维持容积），以及要求术后罩杯尺寸大于术前的患者[34, 35]。美国约80%异质材料重建采用分期手术方式进行。

尽管即刻重建被视为标准方案，仍有部分患者选择延迟重建，原因包括患者个人倾向、计划术后行放疗或基础病情不允许同期重建。延迟重建必须使用组织扩张器。Zenn 于 2015 年提出的分阶段即刻重建技术，既规避了即刻重建中皮肤及乳头坏死风险，又解决了因扩张导致的乳头错位问题[35]。其团队对高危或薄皮瓣患者建议在乳房切除术后 2 周再行重建，使皮瓣血供得以改善，避免因扩张导致的继发乳头移位（图 8.5）。

胸肌前重建中组织扩张器的选择需确保构建精确可控的囊袋以紧密容受最终假体。过度扩张将导致假体与囊袋贴合不良，增加皱褶、移位及翻转风险。建议先低容量填充扩张器，以保证假体置入后与囊袋紧密契合，避免皮肤松弛。此为胸肌前与肌下重建的重要区别。圆形假体常选中低高度扩张器，解剖型假体则多采用全高型[4]。通常选择基底宽度较目标假体小 0.5~1.0cm 的扩张器，以防止过度扩张[18]。最终高度选择需综合考量患者体型、测量参数、患者意愿及术者偏好等因素。Ⅰ期手术目标在于建立标准化的乳腺解剖形态基础，确保Ⅱ期修整操作最小化。

与假体类似，组织扩张器亦分毛面与光面两类。随着对 BI-ALCL 与毛面假体相关性认知的深入，近年来对毛面产

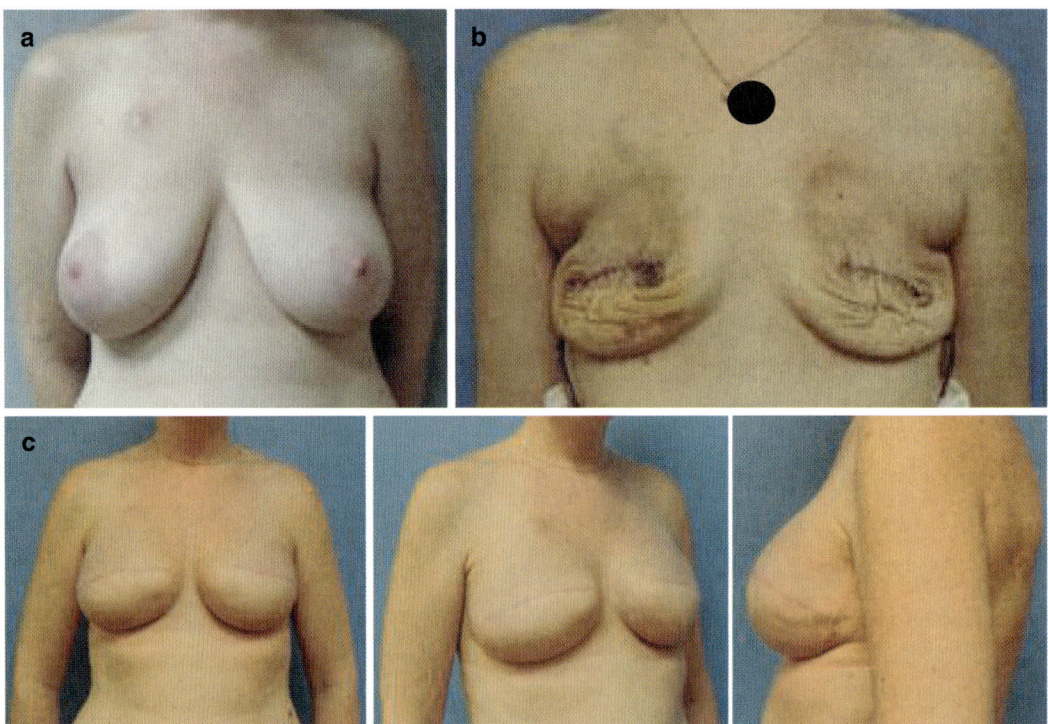

图 8.5　分期即刻假体置入重建病例影像序列：术前乳房状态（a）；乳房切除术后 1 周显示愈合中的皮瓣（b）；延期 2 周后置入 Mentor 光滑高凸度 Xtra MemoryGel 圆形 700mL 双侧重建假体，术后 3 个月随访影像（c）

品的应用更为审慎。Mentor、Allergan 及 Sientra 均在美国市场投放光面扩张器。Mentor 的 Artoura 扩张器采用动态控制技术，通过内部结构设计仅扩张下极区域，实现精准囊袋塑造[36]。Sientra 新近推出的双端口光面扩张器配备注水口与浆液引流口，理论上可避免术后留置引流管[37]。该特性对胸肌前重建尤为重要，因胸肌前假体置入血清肿发生率高于肌下置入。PMT 与 GC Aesthetics 在欧洲供应光面扩张器，但多数海外厂商仍仅提供毛面产品。双侧置入 Mentor 高凸圆形 Xtra MemoryGel 700mL 光面假体完成重建。本病例于乳房切除术后 2 周实施重建，确保皮瓣充分愈合（图 8.5）。

8.5　补片选择

近年来补片技术的突破显著推动了胸肌前乳房重建的成功率与普及度的提升。额外覆盖层可减轻皱褶，保障假体胸壁定位，减少移位及旋转异常，塑形强化乳房下皱襞，潜在抑制炎症反应，并降低皮瓣受压点风险[38, 39]。补片技术革新了胸肌前重建体系，对其成功实施具有决定性作用。

脱细胞真皮基质（ADM）于 2006 年首次引入并迅速应用于乳房重建[3]。最初 ADM 用于补充肌下重建中预计术后接受放疗患者的胸肌后缘覆盖[40]。随着其对包膜挛缩及囊袋控制的改善，ADM 应用拓展至胸肌前重建领域。研究表明，与未使用 ADM 相比，使用 ADM 可减少假体皱褶，支持薄皮瓣患者直接行即刻重建（否则需延迟重建），并允许多种大容量假体及高初始填充量的组织扩张器应用[4-6]。ADM 问世后，生物补片与合成补片市场持续扩展，胸肌前重建适应证范围亦同步拓宽。

可采取两种方式使用生物与合成补片时，覆盖假体强化皮瓣薄弱区域，或环形包裹假体。美国将 ADM 包裹假体归类为超说明书使用（off-label use）。此外，生物补片置入体内后需与组织充分接触，以促进整合。

8.6 生物补片

生物补片是由胎牛、猪及人类尸体皮肤成分配制的脱细胞真皮基质。其弊端在于成本高且存在血清肿与感染率升高的潜在风险。价格平均为每平方厘米 20~30 美元，单侧乳房重建费用为 5 000~20 000 美元[39, 41]。Chun 的研究比较了应用 ADM 与未应用 ADM 的肌下假体重建，显示使用 ADM 组感染及血清肿发生率显著增高[42]。尽管此研究聚焦肌下重建，但可推想此差异在需使用大面积补片的胸肌前重建中更为明显。Ho 等的系统综述纳入 16 篇文献，对 ADM 辅助与非 ADM 辅助重建进行了比较[43]，发现应用 ADM 使血清肿风险增加近 4 倍，感染风险增加近 3 倍，重建失败率增加近 3 倍。Marks 等对美国整形外科学会会员的调查数据亦支持此结论[8]。但研究同时指出，ADM 可提高术中初始扩张容积，可预防包膜挛缩。

人源性真皮基质制造商包括 Alloderm、Cortiva、Dermamatrix、FlexHD 与 Dermacell 等。

8.6.1 Alloderm

Alloderm 系无菌处理并冻干的人类尸体分层厚皮移植片（STSG），需冷藏保存（保质期 2 年），复水后须在 4 小时内使用。置入时基底膜面应朝向假体（因此面抗血液吸附），真皮面朝向组织以促进整合。产品提供多样厚度（0.23~3.30mm）和不同尺寸[44]。

8.6.2 Cortiva

Cortiva 前身为 AlloMax/NeoForm，是唯一通过终端灭菌工艺的人类真皮移植物。其置入体内无面性要求，仅提供单层厚度（0.8~1.8mm）多规格片型[45]。

8.6.3 Dermamatrix

Dermamatrix 为表皮经化学剥离的人源性脱细胞真皮，无须冷藏（保质期 3 年）但需复水处理。产品厚度多样（0.2~4mm、0.4~0.8mm、0.8~1.7mm 及 1.71mm）但存在特定朝向要求。禁用于自身免疫性结缔组织病患者[46]。

8.6.4 FlexHD

FlexHD 为乙醇保存的人源脱细胞异体移植物,无须复水。厚度分三种规格(常规 0.4~0.8mm,加厚 0.8~1.7mm,超厚 1.8mm),并提供多尺寸片型。与 Dermamatrix 相似,自身免疫性结缔组织病为禁忌证[47]。

8.6.5 Dermacell

Dermacell 是一种经万古霉素和庆大霉素处理的脱细胞真皮基质。该产品可室温保存,无须水化,提供三种厚度(0.2~1.0mm、0.75~1.5mm 和 1.25~2.0mm)及不同尺寸[48]。

除人类尸体来源的生物基质外,生物补片也可由动物源性产品制备。牛源性和猪源性补片是最常见的。

8.6.6 SurgiMend

SurgiMend 是唯一的胎牛真皮胶原基质产品,据称其胶原含量是其他皮肤替代品的 3 倍。该产品在波士顿生产,于美国、英国及部分英格兰地区销售,为预制孔隙的脂肪膜片材料,无须特定方向置入,厚度规格为 1.0~4.0mm。产品需室温保存且使用前需水化[41, 49]。

8.6.7 Strattice

Strattice 是主流猪真皮基质产品之一,产自新泽西州,于美国、英国及部分欧洲地区销售。该产品为经终端灭菌处理的猪真皮组织,含稳定剂以减少组织粘连[19],原设计用于减少疝修补术中的组织粘连,理论上可降低乳房重建术后包膜挛缩率。产品提供柔软型和硬挺型两种选择,需水化使用,仅有单层厚度规格(1.5~2.0mm),有不同尺寸[50]。

8.6.8 Braxon

Braxon 是另一主流猪真皮基质产品,系目前唯一预制形状的脱细胞真皮基质,产自意大利,主要在欧洲市场使用。该产品设计用于完全包裹 500mL 容量以下的假体,仅有 0.6mm 单层厚度规格,是目前最薄的生物源性猪补片产品,制造商宣称其设计旨在加速组织整合。产品采用干燥保存,使用前需水化复张[19, 51]。

除真皮基质外,其他生物补片亦有供应。Meso Biomatrix 为猪腹膜基质,厚度规格为 0.3mm 并有多种尺寸[52]。Biodesign(曾用名 Surgisis)是由牛小肠黏膜下层制成的基质产品[53]。Tutopatch 和 Veritas 则为牛心包基质制品[54]。尽管应用较少,文献中均有报道这些基质被用于乳房重建的案例。

8.7 合成补片

合成补片是较生物补片更经济的替代选择,技术难点在于在增强强度的同时需保持弹性并避免过度炎症反应[55, 56]。这类产品通常分为针织型与编织型,兼具可吸收与不可吸收两种特性。针织补片通常较编织型具有更高的多孔性和柔韧性,而后者的强度更高[56]。可吸收补片的设计原理近似生物补片，可随时间推移逐渐与组织整合，但无法达到生物补片所具备的组织长入及新生血管化程度。其劣势在于仍会增加感染与血清肿风险（但程度低于生物补片），尚不明确远期是否能持续提供支撑力[57-59]。不可吸收补片不会降解并永久留存体内，使用时应考虑其应用于胸肌前乳房重建术时可能造成的终生可触及异物感，以及未来修复手术的操作难度。

8.7.1 可吸收补片

常见可吸收补片包括 TIGR 基质、SERI 外科支架和 Galatea 支架。

8.7.2 Galatea 支架

Galatea 支架为经三羧酸循环代谢的聚合物，18~24 个月内可完全吸收（Levy）。该产品 16 周时可保留 50% 强度，降解过程中允许组织长入与新生血管形成[60]。

8.7.3 TIGR 基质

TIGR 基质为长效可吸收补片，由快吸收纤维（6 个月）与慢吸收纤维（3 年）构成[61]。

8.7.4 SERI 外科支架

SERI 外科支架采用类似设计理念，通过缓慢吸收维持降解过程中的力学强度。显微镜下观察显示 12 个月时大部分被吸收，24 个月时仅残留微量纤维[62]。

8.7.5 不可吸收补片

不可吸收补片不会随时间降解。聚丙烯补片是乳房重建领域唯一应用的不可吸收补片，代表产品包括 TriLoop Bra、ULTRAPRO 和 SERAGYN BR。

8.7.6 TriLoop Bra

TriLoop Bra 为单丝聚丙烯补片经气态钛处理以减轻炎症反应，专为胸肌前乳房重建术中包裹假体设计，存在肉芽肿形成的潜在风险[63]。

8.7.7 ULTRAPRO

ULTRAPRO 由等量可吸收单乔缝线（聚卡普隆）与不可吸收聚丙烯单丝复合构成，其中可吸收组分设计为 84 天内完全吸收[64]。

8.7.8 SERAGYN

SERAGYN 为部分可吸收补片，其硬度高于 TriLoop Bra，可吸收组分设计为 90~120 天内完全降解[65]。

虽然补片的应用推动了胸肌前乳房重建的技术革新，但其并非必需选择。Becker 等对 25 例条件欠佳患者进行了回顾性分析，这些病例均接受了 I 期手术直接置入乳房重建术（使用 Mentor Spectrum 假体且未应用脱细胞真皮基质或补片）[66]。该研究纳入的肥胖、有胸壁放疗史、显著乳房下垂/肥大的患者群体，传统上被认为不适宜胸肌前重建。作者对高风险患者采用 Spacer 理念，即通过充气暂时扩张非适应证应用 Spectrum 假体，随后换注生理盐水。1 例放疗史患者出现假体外露需取出；5 例发生乳房切除皮瓣皮肤边缘坏死，需清创处理，但无须进一步干预。该研究结果证实，高风险患者可不使用脱细胞真皮基质安全进行Ⅰ期手术重建，有助于降低费用和总体并发症发生率，缩短手术时间。

同样，Manrique通过研究对比了应用与未应用脱细胞真皮基质患者的并发症发生率及美学效果，结果显示两组在血清肿、血肿等并发症发生率及美学效果方面无显著差异，再次证明胸肌前乳房重建术无须依赖脱细胞真皮基质即可成功实施[67]。

8.8 手术技术

尽管相关证据不断增加，目前仍无适用于所有患者和外科医师的特定推荐方案。遗憾的是，胸肌前重建中不同假体与补片的使用都存在学习曲线，每位术者需要根据自身临床环境选择最优方案。

使用脱细胞真皮基质（ADM）的重建效果通常优于不使用补片或使用合成补片，因为ADM可为乳房切除术后皮瓣提供长期支撑及额外厚度，并可能降低包膜挛缩风险，但需综合考量增加并发症风险（主要为血清肿、感染及假体丢失）及高昂成本。若重建术区皮瓣肥厚、血供良好且所在机构感染率低，ADM可能是最佳选择。然而此类理想条件并不常见，常需考虑替代方案。主要依据乳房切除皮瓣厚度：皮瓣肥厚时，我们倾向于不使用补片并放置扩张器，待包膜形成后再置入假体；皮瓣菲薄时，可吸收补片是首选。ADM可按需后期添加，但此类情况罕见。

选择扩张器的适宜尺寸比品牌更为关键。在胸肌前重建中置入扩张器时，需关注以下异于胸肌后重建的要点：首先，最高点的固定片（12点方向固定片）与胸壁缝合尤为重要。胸肌后重建时，胸大肌可为扩张器上缘提供胸壁支撑，其固定片缝合重要性较低；而胸肌前重建中，若未固定该处，扩张器上缘易前移，严重时甚至呈水平卧位，需再次手术纠正。其次，需采用不可吸收缝线多点牢固固定扩张器，确保包括足够厚的胸壁组织，否则极易发生扩张器旋转或移位。再次，与胸肌后重建相比，选择适当宽度与高度的扩张器更为重要，尺寸匹配良好的扩张器不仅利于局部麻醉下轻松更换假体，更能减少包膜切开需求，便于术区全面实施脂肪移植。第四，扩张器过度充填效果不一，部分病例会出现囊袋解剖形态破坏，继而影响美学效果。最终，假体选择亦可显著影响疗效。波纹现象仍是胸肌前重建的重要缺陷[8]。脂肪移植无法改善症状性波纹，但使用较高内聚性假体对减轻波纹有效，故当前仍作为所有胸肌前重建首选方案。我们强调假体尺寸与患者BMI的比值比绝对容积更重要：高BMI患者仍可使用最大型号假体，但对消瘦患者应更谨慎。

尽管胸肌前乳房重建现已成为多机构的标准术式，我们预期在材料与技术层面可获重大改进，以期未来能找到并发症率可接受、成本合理且适用于绝大多数患者的补片及假体。

参考文献

1. Schlenker JD, Bueno RA, Ricketson G, Lynch JB. Loss of silicone implants after subcutaneous mastectomy and reconstruction. Plast Reconstr Surg. 1978,62(6):853–61.
2. Gruber RP, Kahn RA, Lash H, Maser MR, Apfelberg DB, Laub DR. Breast reconstruction following mastectomy: a comparison of submuscular and subcutaneous techniques. Plast Reconstr Surg. 1981,67(3):312–7.
3. Salzberg CA. Nonexpansive immediate breast reconstruction using human acellular tissue matrix graft (AlloDerm). Ann Plast Surg. 2006,57(1):1–5.
4. Kim SE. Prepectoral breast reconstruction. Yeungnam Univ J Med. 2019,36(3):201–7.
5. Jones G, Antony AK. Single stage, direct to implant pre-pectoral breast reconstruction. Gland Surg. 2019,8(1):53–60.
6. Preminger BA, McCarthy CM, Hu QY, Mehrara BJ, Disa JJ. The influence of AlloDerm on expander dynamics and complications in the setting of immediate tissue expander/implant reconstruction: a matched-cohort study. Ann Plast Surg. 2008,60(5):510–3.
7. Nguyen J, Carey J, Wong A. Use of human acellular dermal matrix in implant- based breast reconstruction: evaluating the evidence. J Plast Reconstr Aesthet Surg. 2011,64(12):1553–61.
8. Marks JM, Farmer RL, Afifi AM. Current trends in prepectoral breast reconstruction: a survey of american society of plastic surgeons members. Plast Reconstr Surg Glob Open. 2020,8(8):e3060.
9. Surgeons ASoP. Plastic Surgery Statistics Report. 2019. Available from: https://www.plasticsurgery.org/documents/News/Statistics/2019/reconstructive-breast-procedures-age-2019.pdf.
10. Heidekrueger PI, Sinno S, Hidalgo DA, Colombo M, Broer PN. Current trends in breast augmentation: an international analysis. Aesthet Surg J. 2018,38(2):133–48.
11. Van Slyke AC, Carr M, Carr NJ. Not all breast implants are equal: a 13-year review of implant longevity and reasons for explantation. Plast Reconstr Surg. 2018,142(3):281e–9e.
12. Spies RJ, Robert J. SPIES, MD, FACS BOARD CERTIFIED IN PLASTIC AND RECONSTRUCTIVE SURGERY [updated May 16, 2012]. Available from: https://www.azplasticsurgerycenter.com/blog/which-breast-implant-weighs-more-silicone-or-saline/#:~:text=A%20400cc%20saline%20implant%20weighs,%2F20%20of%20a%20pound).&text=Silicone%20implants%20are%20more%20similar,breast%20tissue%20than%20saline%20impla.
13. Maxwell GP, Scheflan M, Spear S, Nava MB, Heden P. Benefits and limitations of macrotextured breast implants and consensus recommendations for optimizing their effectiveness. Aesthet Surg J. 2014,34(6):876–81.
14. Webb LH, Aime VL, Do A, Mossman K, Mahabir RC. Textured breast implants: a closer look at the surface debris under the microscope. Plast Surg (Oakv). 2017,25(3):179–83.
15. Castel N, Soon-Sutton T, Deptula P, Flaherty A, Parsa FD. Polyurethane-coated breast implants revisited: a 30-year follow-up. Arch Plast Surg. 2015,42(2):186–93.
16. Labs, Establishment: Motiva; [updated 2019]. Available from: https://motiva.health/patients/implants/anatomical-truefixation-breast-implant/?rtid=3b79abf43c0e4ff0a9cf11dd03296f960e29699e53e54bf0808467c32fca3285.
17. Boschert M. American Society of Plastic Surgeons 2020 [updated March 2020]. Available from: https://www1.plasticsurgery.org/members/discussions/Topic.aspx?id=3531.
18. Gabriel A, Maxwell GP. Implant selection in the setting of prepectoral breast reconstruction. Gland Surg. 2019,8(1):36–42.
19. Vidya R, Berna G, Sbitany H, Nahabedian M, Becker H, Reitsamer R, et al. Prepectoral implant-based breast reconstruction: a joint consen-

sus guide from UK, European and USA breast and plastic reconstructive surgeons. Ecancermedicalscience. 2019,13:927.
20. Choi M, Frey JD, Alperovich M, Levine JP, Karp NS. "Breast in a Day": examining single-stage immediate, permanent implant reconstruction in nipple-sparing mastectomy. Plast Reconstr Surg. 2016,138(2):184e–91e.
21. Natrelle: Allergan; [updated 2020]. Available from: https://www.natrellesurgeon.com/.
22. Sientra 2020 [updated 2020]. Available from: https://sientra.com/for-us-surgeons/.
23. Breast Implants by Mentor [updated 2020]. Available from: https://www.breastimplantsbymentor.com/Products/MENTOR-breast-implants.
24. Silimed [updated 2020]. Available from: http://silimed.com/.
25. Polytech [updated 2020]. Available from: https://polytech-health-aesthetics.com/en/products/breast-implants/.
26. Ideal Implant [updated 2020]. Available from: https://idealimplant.com/overview.
27. GC Aesthetics. Available from: https://www.gcaesthetics.com/products/surgery/breast/.
28. Laboratories Arion [updated 2020]. Available from: https://www.laboratoires-arion.fr/en/.
29. Hans Biomed [updated 2020]. Available from: https://www.hansbiomed.com/en/.
30. Cereplas [updated 2020]. Available from: https://www.cereplas.com/en/produits/implants-mammaires/rondes.html.
31. Establishment Labs [updated 2020]. Available from: https://establishmentlabs.com/our-products/.
32. Sebbin [updated 2020]. Available from: https://www.sebbin.com/en/category/mammary-implants/.
33. Collplant [updated 2020]. Available from: https://collplant.com/products/breast-implants/.
34. Becker H, Zhadan O. Filling the spectrum expander with air-a new alternative. Plast Reconstr Surg Glob Open. 2017,5(10):e1541.
35. Zenn MR. Staged immediate breast reconstruction. Plast Reconstr Surg. 2015,135(4):976–9.
36. Mentor [updated 2020]. Available from: https://www.jnjmedicaldevices.com/en-US/product/mentor-artoura-breast-tissue-expanders.
37. Sientra [updated 2020]. Available from: https://sientra.com/for-us-surgeons/breast-tissue-expanders/.
38. Rebowe RE, Allred LJ, Nahabedian MY. The evolution from subcutaneous to prepectoral prosthetic breast reconstruction. Plast Reconstr Surg Glob Open. 2018,6(6):e1797.
39. Ter Louw RP, Nahabedian MY. Prepectoral breast reconstruction. Plast Reconstr Surg. 2017,140(5S Advances in Breast Reconstruction):51S–9S.
40. Breuing KH, Warren SM. Immediate bilateral breast reconstruction with implants and inferolateral AlloDerm slings. Ann Plast Surg. 2005,55(3):232–9.
41. Cheng A, Saint-Cyr M. Comparison of different ADM materials in breast surgery. Clin Plast Surg. 2012,39(2):167–75.
42. Chun YS, Verma K, Rosen H, Lipsitz S, Morris D, Kenney P, et al. Implant-based breast reconstruction using acellular dermal matrix and the risk of postoperative complications. Plast Reconstr Surg. 2010,125(2):429–36.
43. Ho G, Nguyen TJ, Shahabi A, Hwang BH, Chan LS, Wong AK. A systematic review and meta-analysis of complications associated with acellular dermal matrix-assisted breast reconstruction. Ann Plast Surg. 2012,68(4):346–56.
44. Allergan [Available from: https://media.allergan.com/actavis/actavis/media/allergan-pdf-documents/labeling/alleoderm_rtm_ifu.pdf.
45. RTI Surgical Implants [updated 2020]. Available from: https://www.rtix.com/en_us/implants/cortiva-1mm-allograft-dermis.
46. Synthes [Available from: http://synthes.vo.llnwd.net/o16/Mobile/Synthes%20North%20America/Product%20Support%20Materials/Brochures/CMF/MXBRODermaMatrixAcellular-J7237D.

pdf.
47. MTF Biologics [updated 2020]. Available from: https://www.mtfbiologics.org/our-products/detail/flexhd-structural.
48. Stryker [updated 2020]. Available from: https://www.stryker.com/us/en/endoscopy/products/dermacell.html.
49. Surgimend. Available from: https://www.surgimend.com/products/by-brand/surgimend.
50. Strattice [updated 2020]. Available from: http://hcp.stratticetissuematrix.com/en/products.
51. Raise Healthcare [updated 2020]. Available from: https://www.raisehealthcare.co.uk/products/breast-reconstruction/braxon/.
52. MTF Biologics [updated 2020]. Available from: https://www.mtfbiologics.org/our-products/detail/mesobiomatrix.
53. Cook Medical [updated 2020]. Available from: https://www.cookmedical.com/surgery/the-path-from-surgisis-to-biodesign.
54. rti Surgical [updated 2020]. Available from: https://www.rtix.com/en_us/implants/tuto-patch-bovine-pericardium%2D%2Dtutomesh-fenestrated-bovine-pericardium.
55. Breast Cancer and Breast Reconstruction. In: Luis Tejedor SGM, Lachezar Manchev, Arli Aditya Parikesit editor. London: IntechOpen; 2020.
56. FitzGerald JF, Kumar AS. Biologic versus synthetic mesh reinforcement: what are the pros and cons? Clin Colon Rectal Surg. 2014,27(4):140–8.
57. Potter S, Conroy EJ, Cutress RI, Williamson PR, Whisker L, Thrush S, et al. Short-term safety outcomes of mastectomy and immediate implant-based breast reconstruction with and without mesh (iBRA): a multicentre, prospective cohort study. Lancet Oncol. 2019,20(2):254–66.
58. Dieterich M, Angres J, Stachs A, Glass A, Reimer T, Gerber B, et al. Patient-report satisfaction and health-related quality of life in TiLOOP(R) bra-assisted or implant-based breast reconstruction alone. Aesthetic Plast Surg. 2015,39(4):523–33.
59. Hallberg H, Rafnsdottir S, Selvaggi G, Strandell A, Samuelsson O, Stadig I, et al. Benefits and risks with acellular dermal matrix (ADM) and mesh support in immediate breast reconstruction: a systematic review and meta-analysis. J Plast Surg Hand Surg. 2018,52(3):130–47.
60. Galatea Surgical [updated 2020]. Available from: https://www.galateasurgical.com/surgical-scaffolds/what-is-p4hb/.
61. Novus Scientific [updated 2020]. Available from: https://novusscientific.com/row/products/tigr-matrix/.
62. Seri Surgical Scaffold [updated 2020]. Available from: https://seri.com/about/product-characteristics.html.
63. PFM Medical [updated 2020]. Available from: https://www.pfmmedical.com/productcatalogue/mesh_implants_breast_surgery/tiloopr_bra/index.html.
64. Ethicon [updated 2020]. Available from: https://www.jnjmedicaldevices.com/en-US/product/ultrapro-mesh-ethicon.
65. Serag Wiessner [updated 2020]. Available from: https://www.serag-wiessner.de/en/products/textile-implants/seragyn-br/.
66. Becker H, Mathew PJ. Immediate prepectoral breast reconstruction in suboptimal patients using an air-filled spacer. Plast Reconstr Surg Glob Open. 2019,7(10):e2470.
67. Manrique OJ, Huang TC, Martinez-Jorge J, Ciudad P, Forte AJ, Bustos SS, et al. Prepectoral two-stage implant-based breast reconstruction with and without acellular dermal matrix: do we see a difference? Plast Reconstr Surg. 2020,145(2):263e–72e.

9 胸肌前假体乳房重建：预成型补片全覆盖

编者：Raghavan Vidya, Simon Cawthorn
译者：刘在波

每年乳腺癌全球年新发病例约 100 万例。在英国，每年约有 50 000 例新发乳腺癌患者，其中四成女性接受乳房切除术作为一线治疗方案[1]。在英国实施的所有乳房重建术中，40%~60% 为假体乳房重建；在美国，该比例达 75%[2, 3]。

近十年来，补片与假体的创新推动了假体乳房重建术发生变革。传统胸肌后假体乳房重建基于胸肌剥离后使用补片覆盖下方外侧象限的原则，但肌束剥离可导致动态畸形和肩关节功能损害[4]，促使术式逐渐转变为胸肌前或保留肌肉技术。与传统的胸肌后重建相比，该术式具有保留胸壁正常解剖结构，改善体像且并发症少的优势[5]。

假体重建是即刻乳房重建最常用方法：欧洲国家多采用 Ⅰ 期手术，美国则以 Ⅱ 期手术为主流：Ⅰ 期置入扩张器，Ⅱ 期更换为永久假体[6, 7]。

9.1 患者选择

胸肌前假体重建适用于所有假体重建适应证患者。术前应行常规咨询，包括讨论诊断、潜在治疗方案及相关风险与获益[8]。选择患者时应重点关注 BMI 高（>35）、糖尿病控制不良、免疫抑制及既往放疗损伤等增加围术期并发症风险的因素，应将此类情况视为相对禁忌证[9]。肿瘤学禁忌证包括局部晚期肿瘤、累及皮肤或胸壁肌肉及炎性乳腺癌[9, 10]。

术前乳房形态评估应涵盖基底轮廓、乳房体积及下垂程度。捏皮试验可预判胸肌前假体置入的皮肤厚度适宜性，亦有数字乳腺 X 线摄影或磁共振成像（MRI）预测皮肤厚度的报道[11, 12]。依据基底轮廓与乳房形态学特征，术前应详细讨论假体适用类型（圆形/解剖型），提供毛面/光面假体选择建议并基于现有证据详述利弊。

R. Vidya (✉)
The Royal Wolverhampton NHS Trust, Wolverhampton, UK
e-mail: Raghavan.Vidya@nhs.net

S. Cawthorn
The Breast Unit, Southmead Hospital, Bristol, UK

© The Author(s), under exclusive license to Springer Nature Switzerland AG 2023
R. Vidya, H. Becker (eds.), *Prepectoral Breast Reconstruction*,
https://doi.org/10.1007/978-3-031-15590-1_9

英国多采用Ⅰ期手术假体重建术；而对乳房切除皮瓣灌注不良、吸烟及预计乳房（重量）超过550mL的患者，则考虑Ⅱ期手术组织扩张器重建方案。

9.2　适应证

尽管胸肌前乳房重建主要作为乳腺癌术后Ⅰ期修复方案（图9.1），其适应证已拓展至降低风险手术及修复性手术领域[13]。

9.3　术前规划

根据肿瘤位置、乳房形态、腋窝分期需求及医患双方意愿合理规划切口尤为重要。原则上来说，切口设计应最大限度减少皮下脉管系统损伤。保留乳头或皮肤乳房切除术常用切口[14]包括乳房下皱襞切口、垂直切口、外侧"S"形切口；不保留乳头的术式则采用标准椭圆形切口。需要切除乳头时可选择保留乳晕的术式，后期利用乳晕重建乳头。术前应标记乳房基底轮廓，包括起始点、乳房下皱襞、内外侧边界，以指导精确剥离。

9.4　技术要点

胸肌前间隙是乳房切除后形成的潜在腔隙[15]，容积取决于胸壁解剖学尺度、皮肤弹性及质量，后者直接影响安全容纳假体/补片的程度。

Ⅰ期手术乳房切除术的成功高度依赖切除皮瓣质量。术中应全程维持患者体温并使用酒精基皮肤消毒剂。围术期需依据医院规范单剂量静脉预防性应用抗生素。

保留乳头乳房切除皮瓣皮下层及其穿支血管是手术成功的关键[15]。术中应于标准肿瘤学平面[16]行乳房切除术，使用低功率单极电刀以保障皮瓣血供，减少热损伤风险。必须在彻底切除乳腺组织与保护解剖平面间取得平衡，术中维护皮瓣良好血供为手术成功核心要素。多数学者通过皮瓣色泽、真皮层无暴露及电刀损伤范围在临床对血供进行评估[15, 17]。若可行，建议采用皮瓣血运评估设备（尤其血供存疑时）以提高判断准确性[17, 18]。若皮瓣血供受损，则应考虑其他重建方式。建议切除创缘（闭合伤口前）以改善皮瓣缝合线血流灌注——切除牵拉剥离所致的2mm皮肤条带后，皮瓣远端渗血增加为血供可靠征象。

用大量温生理盐水冲洗乳房切除腔，于胸肌前间隙留置1~2根闭式负压引流管。

Braxon®（意大利威尼斯Decomed公

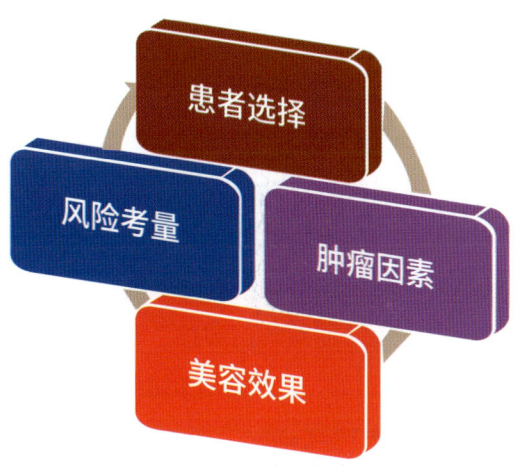

图9.1　影响乳房切除术指征的相关因素

司）为厚 0.6mm 的预成型非交联猪源脱细胞真皮基质（ADM），使用时需用生理盐水水化至少 10 分钟。该补片规格为 30cm×20cm，最大可容纳 500mL 假体（经网眼化处理可扩展至 560mL）。补片前瓣中轴含裂缝，缝合后可塑形；后瓣双窗设计可防止假体周围血清肿形成。前瓣裂隙与双翼采用 2-0 薇乔线连续缝合闭锁[19]。图 9.2 展示补片－假体包裹操作流程。

根据对称性需求选择定容硅胶/盐水、解剖型或圆形假体。若术中评估皮瓣血供存疑，可选用可调式扩张假体：初始欠量填充以避免皮瓣压力过载，确认血运稳定后延迟扩张[20]。

将选定假体置入 ADM 后，标记所需补片边缘以确保其紧密包裹假体且无冗余腔隙。塑形时补片边缘留取 2~5mm 空隙便于胸壁固定。ADM 前后缘以 2-0 薇乔线缝合形成假体囊袋。Braxon® 下缘可自然下垂，无须额外锚定；外侧间隙闭合以优化形态并减少死腔。

ADM-假体复合体置入胸肌前间隙后，以 2-0 薇乔线于 3 点、9 点、12 点位缝合固定（图 9.2）。皮肤闭合前还可于补片与皮下层间附加缝合（尤其外侧与前侧）。保留胸肌筋膜利于补片锚定，建议自腋侧闭合外侧壁并进行胸壁内加固缝合以缩小死腔。

皮下层缝合选择 2-0 薇乔线，皮内缝合采用 3-0 单乔线。常于距离假体囊袋 6~8cm 处留置 1~2 根闭式负压引流管，联合腋窝清扫时需单独引流。严格维护引流管出口位置，引流量连续 2 天（48 小时）低于 20mL 后拔除。围术期预防性使用（口服）抗生素，用药时长可依据风险分层调整[21, 22]。

术后疼痛轻微，患者可当日出院，佩戴支撑型运动文胸（图 9.3a）。作者建议对 BMI>35、合并糖尿病、有新辅助化疗史、同期行腋窝清扫或既往放疗患者预防性应用负压敷料[23]（图 9.3b）。超声影像学及组织学检查证实 ADM 整合良好[24]，详见 Marucci 等[25]编写的后续章节。图 9.4、图 9.5 展示了术前、术后效果对比。

胸肌前假体重建术患者报告不适感轻、术后疼痛轻微、无肩功能障碍或动态畸形且恢复迅速，整体满意度高（含心理社会与性健康维度）[26, 27]。美学效果与患者自评结果积极，但仍需远期研究验证。

9.5 文献综述

该技术最初由 Berna 等于 2014 年提出[28]，作者报道的 100 例手术队列为严格筛选的低合并症患者，结果示并发症率低且效果良好（可能归因于病例选择偏倚与术者经验）[29]。

波纹现象始终与该技术相关，现有文献报道胸肌前乳房重建术发生率可达 35%[30]。所有患者术前必须被充分告知该并发症。减轻波纹的措施包括：均匀皮下层厚度、适当假体－皮肤体积比及硅胶假体应用。脂肪移植术可辅助矫正波纹，本组约 10% 患者需手术干预[31]。近期报道样本量最大的 IBAG 审计研究（纳入 1 450 例，随访 6 年）显示，假体丢失率为 6.1%，包膜挛缩率为

9 胸肌前假体乳房重建：预成型补片全覆盖

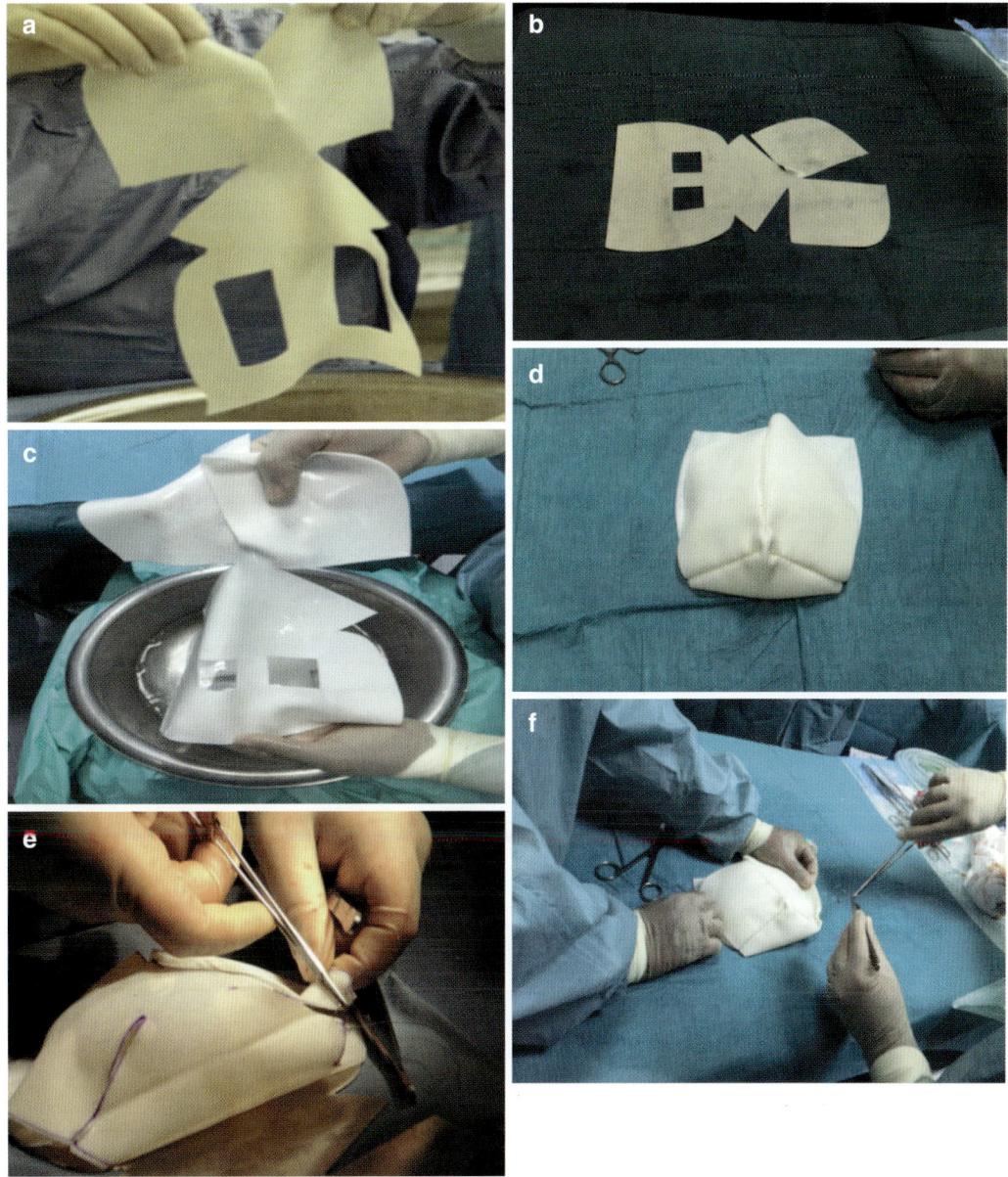

图 9.2 Braxon® 预制网片制备假体包膜技术。（a，b）Braxon® 为厚 0.6 mm、无防腐剂冻干猪源脱细胞真皮基质（ADM），基质开窗部分（后覆层）用于构成假体包膜后部以防止血清肿。（c）以常温生理盐水浸泡基质至少 5~10 分钟，使其柔润水化。（c）使用可吸收缝线（Vicryl 2/0）缝合真皮囊袋前层。（d）连接 Braxon® 前、后覆层。（e）标记并修剪多余基质，保留 2 mm 边缘以利胸壁固定。（f）可吸收缝线（Vicryl 2/0）连续缝合前、后壳形成严密假体包裹

103

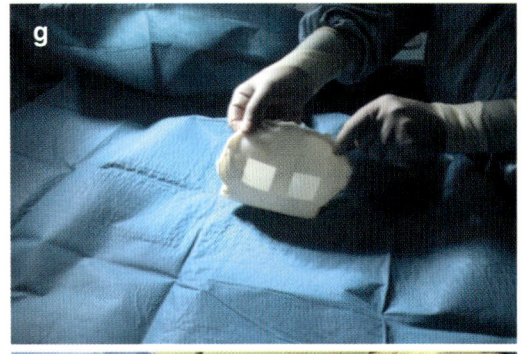
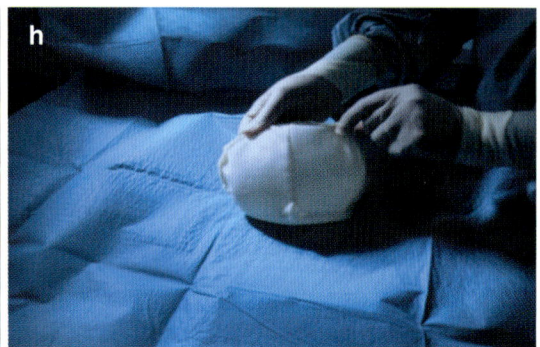
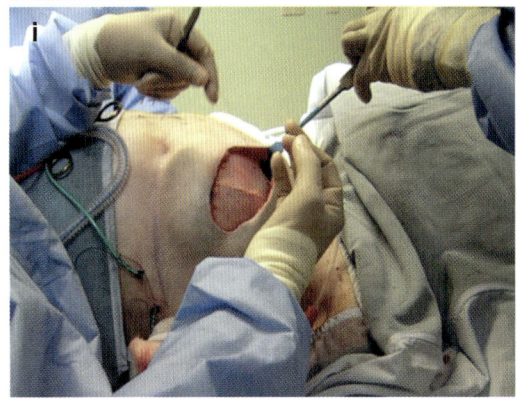

图9.2（续）（g）Braxon®后覆层开窗设计防止积液，该部分被包裹的假体置于胸肌前并固定于胸壁。（h）假体包裹前部结构。（i）假体包裹整体覆盖胸肌并固定于胸壁

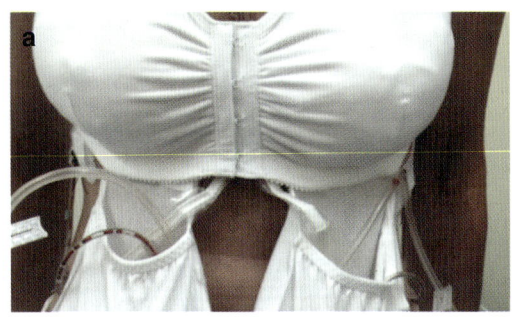
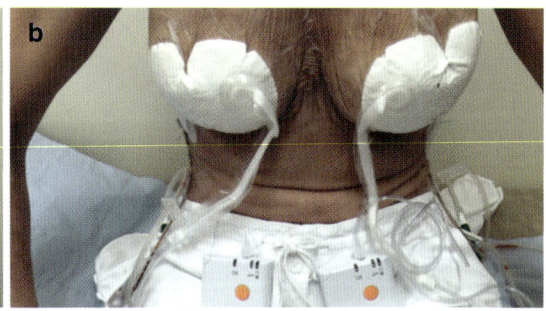

图9.3　（a）术后即刻敷料包扎与胸衣适配。（b）高危患者预防性应用负压引流等特殊包扎技术

2.1%。此为迄今最大规模胸肌前乳房重建技术研究[32]。

9.6　小结与技巧

9.6.1　预成型补片

- 补片应用推动了微创手术的临床实施。

- 胸肌前假体重建术并发症少且患者预后良好。
- Braxon®为目前唯一可体外完全包裹假体的预成型ADM补片。
- 由于学习曲线的存在，早期严格筛选病例至关重要。
- 保留乳房切除皮瓣血供是手术成功关键，保留胸肌筋膜利于补片锚定。

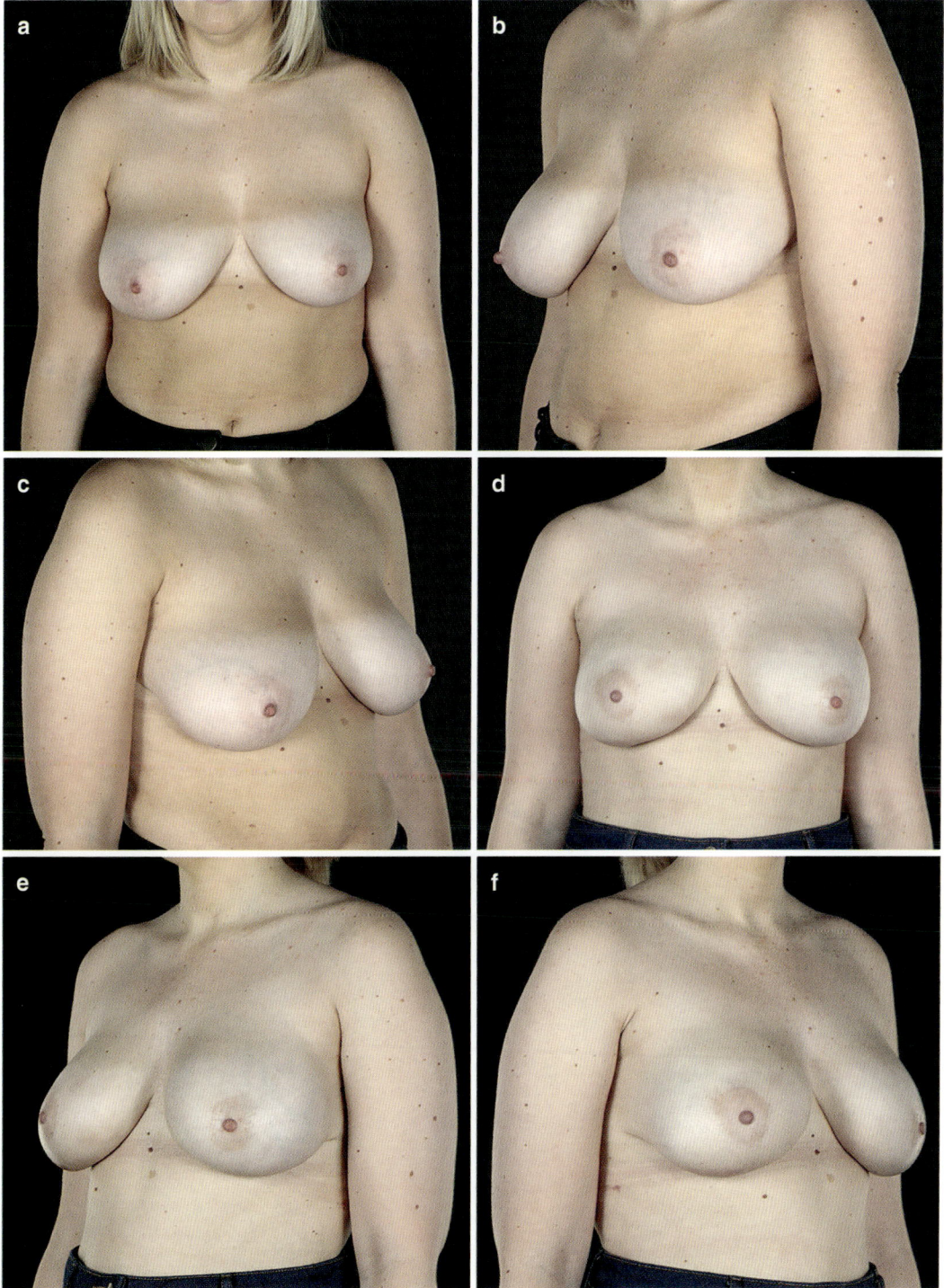

图 9.4 40 岁 BRCA 基因阳性女性患者,行双侧保留乳头和乳晕的乳房切除术联合胸肌前假体重建(560 mL 解剖型硅胶假体及 Braxon®ADM 应用)术前(上)与术后 1 年随访影像(下)

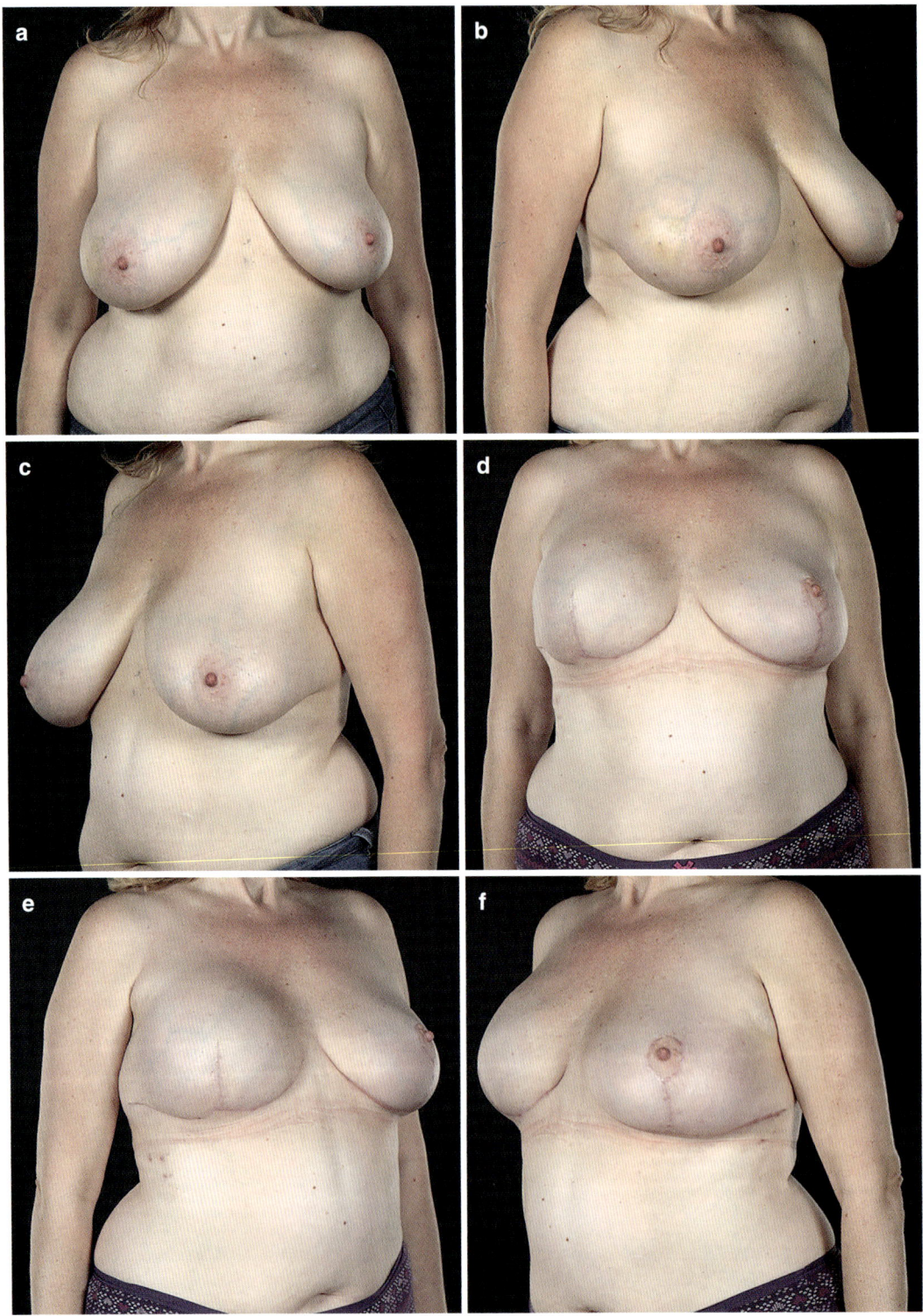

图 9.5 48 岁女性患者，因右乳浸润性导管癌行右侧不保留乳头乳房切除联合腋窝清扫及胸肌前假体重建（550 mL 假体联合真皮吊带），同期对左乳行对称性缩小术；术前（上）与术后 6 个月随访影像（下）

- 可按术者偏好选择剥离方式，但应最大限度减少皮瓣牵拉与热损伤。
- 补片－假体复合体需紧贴囊壁，以促进整合并降低血清肿风险。
- 应用大量温盐水冲洗乳房切除腔，清除游离脂肪及碎屑以减少感染风险。
- 闭合外侧间隙以优化形态并减少死腔。
- 限制手术室人员流动并缩短手术时间，双侧手术推荐双团队协作。
- 血清肿危害显著，应积极预防并立即引流（防止切口裂开）。

参考文献

1. Cancer Research UK. Breast Cancer Statistics. http://www.cancerresearchuk.org/health-professional/cancer-statistics/statistics-by-cancer-type/breast-cancer. 04/13/2016.
2. Jeevan R, Cromwell D, Browne J, Van Der Meulen J, Pereira J, Caddy C, et al. The National Mastectomy and breast reconstruction audit. A national audit of provision and outcomes of mastectomy and breast reconstruction surgery for women in England. Second Annu Rep; 2009.
3. ASoP surgeons. Plastic surgery statistics report. Am Soc Plast Surg Arlingt Height; 2012.
4. Sbitany H, Serletti JM. Acellular dermis–assisted prosthetic breast reconstruction: a systematic and critical review of efficacy and associated morbidity. Plast Reconstr Surg. 2011,128(6):1162–9.
5. Tasoulis MK, Iqbal FM, Cawthorn S, MacNeill F, Vidya R. Subcutaneous implant breast reconstruction: time to reconsider? Eur J Surg Oncol. 2017,43(9):1646–3.
6. Serletti JM, Fosnot J, Nelson JA, Disa JJ, Bucky LP. Breast reconstruction after breast cancer. Plast Reconstr Surg. 2011,127(6):124e–35e. https://doi.org/10.1097/PRS.0b013e318213a2e6.
7. Albornoz CR, Bach PB, Mehrara BJ, Disa JJ, Pusic AL, McCarthy CM, et al. A paradigm shift in U.S. breast reconstruction: increasing implant rates. Plast Reconstr Surg. 2013,131(1):15–23.
8. Vidya R, Berna G, Sbitany H, Nahabedian M, Becker H, Reitsamer R, Rancati A, Macmillan D, Cawthorn S. Prepectoral implant-based breast reconstruction: a joint consensus guide from UK, European and USA breast and plastic reconstructive surgeons. Ecancermedicalscience. 2019,13:927.
9. Sbitany H. Important considerations for performing Prepectoral breast reconstruction. Plast Reconstr Surg. 2017,140(6S):7S–13S.
10. Abbate O, Rosado N, Sobti N, Vieira BL, Liao EC. Meta-analysis of prepectoral implant-based breast reconstruction: guide to patient selection and current outcomes. Breast Cancer Res Treat. 2020,182(3):543–54.
11. Rancati AO, Angrigiani CH, Hammond DC, et al. Direct to implant reconstruction in nipple sparing mastectomy: patient selection by preoperative digital mammogram. Plast Reconstr Surg Glob Open. 2017,5(6):e1369. https://doi.org/10.1097/GOX.0000000000001369.
12. Frey JD, Salibian AA, Choi M, Karp NS. Mastectomy flap thickness and complications in nipple-sparing mastectomy: objective evaluation using magnetic resonance imaging. Plast Reconstr Surg Glob Open. 2017,5(8):e1439.
13. Vidya R, Iqbal FM. A guide to prepectoral breast reconstruction: a new dimension to implant-based breast reconstruction. Clin Breast Cancer. 2017,17(4):266–71.
14. Frey JD, Salibian AA, Levine JP, Karp NS, Choi M. Incision choices in nipple-sparing mastectomy: a comparative analysis of outcomes and evolution of a clinical algorithm. Plast Reconstr Surg. 2018,142:826e–35e.
15. Vidya R, Iqbal FM. Breast anatomy: time to classify the subpectoral and prepectoral spaces. Clin Anat. 2017,30(4):434–5.
16. Rehnke RD, Groening RM, Buskirk ERV, Clarke JM. Anatomy of the superficial fas-

16. cia system of the breast. Plast Reconstr Surg. 2018,142(5):1135–44. https://doi.org/10.1097/prs.0000000000004948.
17. Phillips BT, Lanier ST, Conkling N, et al. Intraoperative perfusion techniques can accurately predict mastectomy skin flap necrosis in breast reconstruction: results of a prospective trial. Plast Reconstr Surg. 2012,129:778e–88e.
18. Mattison GL, Lewis PG, Gupta SC, et al. SPY imaging use in postmastectomy breast reconstruction patients: preventative or overly conservative? Plast Reconstr Surg. 2016,138:15e–21e.
19. Vidya R. Prepectoral breast reconstruction or muscle-sparing technique with the Braxon porcine acellular dermal matrix. Plast Reconstr Surg Glob Open. 2017,5(6):e1364.
20. Becker H, Zhadan O. Filling the spectrum expander with air-a new alternative. Plast Reconstr Surg Glob Open. 2017,5(10):e1541. https://doi.org/10.1097/GOX.0000000000001541.
21. Vidya R. Risk assessment and antibiotic administration model. Plast Reconstr Surg. 2017,139(5): 1206e–7e.
22. Barr SP, Topps AR, Barnes NL, Henderson J, Hignett S, Teasdale RL, McKenna A, Harvey JR, Kirwan CC, Northwest Breast Surgical Research Collaborative. Infection prevention in breast implant surgery - A review of the surgical evidence, guidelines and a checklist. Eur J Surg Oncol. 2016,42(5):591–603.
23. Irwin GW, Boundouki G, Fakim B, Johnson R, Highton L, Myers D, Searle R, Murphy JA. Negative pressure wound therapy reduces wound breakdown and implant loss in prepectoral breast reconstruction. Plast Reconstr Surg Glob Open. 2020,8(2):e2667. https://doi.org/10.1097/GOX.0000000000002667.
24. Iqbal FM, Bhatnagar A, Vidya R. Host integration of an acellular dermal matrix: Braxon mesh in breast reconstruction. Clin Breast Cancer. 2016,16(6):e209–11. https://doi.org/10.1016/j.clbc.2016.06.009.
25. Onesti MG, Maruccia M, Di Taranto G, et al. Clinical, histological, and ultrasound follow-up of breast reconstruction with one-stage muscle-sparing "wrap" technique: a single-center experience. J Plast Reconstr Aesthet Surg. 2017,70(11):1527–36.
26. Walia GS, Aston J, Bello R, Mackert GA, Pedreira RA, Cho BH, et al. Prepectoral versus subpectoral tissue expander placement: a clinical and quality of life outcomes study. Plast Reconstr Surg Glob Open. 2018,6(4):e1731.
27. Vidya R, Green M. Minimal pain with prepectoral implant based breast reconstruction. Plast Reconstr Surg. 2019,143(1):236e. https://doi.org/10.1097/PRS.0000000000005135.
28. Berna G, Cawthorn SJ, Papaccio G, Balestrieri N. Evaluation of a novel breast reconstruction technique using the Braxon® acellular dermal matrix: a new muscle-sparing breast reconstruction. ANZ J Surg. 2017,87(6):493–8. Epub 2014 Sep 29
29. Vidya R, Masià J, Cawthorn S, et al. Evaluation of the effectiveness of the prepectoral breast reconstruction with Braxon dermal matrix: first multicenter European report on 100 cases. Breast J. 2017,23(6):670–6.
30. Downs RK, Hedges K. An alternative technique for immediate direct-to-implant breast reconstruction-a case series. Plast Reconstr Surg Glob Open. 2016,4:e821. https://doi.org/10.1097/GOX.0000000000000839.
31. Vidya R, Iqbal FM, Becker H, Zhadan O. Rippling associated with pre-pectoral implant based breast reconstruction: a new grading system. World J Plast Surg. 2019,8(3):311–5. https://doi.org/10.29252/wjps.8.3.311.
32. Masià J, iBAG Working Group. The largest multicentre data collection on prepectoral breast reconstruction: The iBAG study. Surg Oncol. 2020,122(5):848–60. https://doi.org/10.1002/jso.26073.

10 胸肌前内置物联合补片乳房重建术

编者：Roland Reitsamer, Andreas Sir
译者：李小磊　刘兆芸

10.1 引言

目前，保留乳头-乳晕复合体的乳房切除（NSM）术已成为需要切除乳腺且腺体表面皮肤未被肿瘤浸润患者的标准术式。NSM 术后局部复发率较低，与传统乳房切除术相当，其肿瘤学安全性已在多项研究中得到证实[1]。自体或异体乳房重建是 NSM 的重要组成部分，80% 的乳房切除术后患者选择假体置入重建，20% 选择自体组织重建。胸肌后假体重建沿用数十年，目前已成为标准术式。该术式采用胸大肌（PMM）、部分前锯肌及腹直肌筋膜来实现假体的肌肉全覆盖，有多种改良术式，但与胸肌前假体重建相比有若干缺点。胸大肌覆盖假体上极联合脱细胞真皮基质（ADM）覆盖下极的术式可改善美学效果，但仍存在破坏胸大肌的缺陷。应用 ADM 的初衷在于覆盖假体下极，稳定离断的胸大肌并形成假体悬吊结构，但该理论旋即引发争议。若假体置于类似悬吊结构的空腔中（即 ADM 覆盖假体下极），胸大肌仍可因缺少固定而收缩；若 ADM 对假体下极固定过紧，虽可稳定胸大肌，但当胸大肌收缩时仍会牵拉 ADM 及假体上移，导致美学效果欠佳及乳房不对称。由于胸大肌起点的解剖变异，其覆盖范围可从假体体积的三分之二到仅三分之一不等[2,3]，意味着可能多达三分之二的假体需要依靠基质或补片覆盖。胸肌后假体重建的缺陷如肌力减弱、术后疼痛加重、恢复期延长及乳房运动畸形持续存在。与此相比，未离断胸大肌的胸肌前假体重建具备显著优势，可规避上述不足，但需实现假体表面完全肌肉覆盖及假体固定。假体固定可用 ADM、补片或自体去上皮真皮瓣来实现。

10.2 假体直接置入 I 期手术（DTI）或两阶段重建

假体直接置入（DTI）I 期手术或两

R. Reitsamer (✉) · A. Sir
Department of Senology, Breast Center Salzburg,
Paracelsus Medical University Salzburg,
Salzburg, Austria
e-mail: r.reitsamer@salk.at; a.sir@salk.at

© The Author(s), under exclusive license to Springer Nature Switzerland AG 2023
R. Vidya, H. Becker (eds.), *Prepectoral Breast Reconstruction*,
https://doi.org/10.1007/978-3-031-15590-1_10

阶段乳房重建的问题已被反复讨论，均有理论支持。临床决策需综合考量皮肤厚度、皮肤质地、皮瓣活性、前期/辅助治疗与放疗方案及患者意愿等多种因素。

假体直接置入 I 期乳房重建手术（DTI）优势在于乳房切除与重建可一次完成。首要考量心理学因素——患者术后苏醒即见再造乳房；次要经济效益——避免二次手术可节省支出。该术式适用于希望维持原乳房体积或适度增大者，亦可应用于巨乳/下垂乳房患者的缩小性乳房切除术。

两阶段重建优势在于在第二阶段可进行调整。最终病理学报告结果明确后，可将辅助治疗计划纳入考量。可评估皮肤存活状态，对乳房体积有增大需求者可行扩张器注水。

DTI 术式弊端包括皮肤/乳头存活不良风险。罕见情况下，根据终末病理学报告可能需再次手术。

胸肌前假体置入相关文献多报道"扩张器-假体两阶段乳房重建术"[4-6]。近年来，胸肌前假体直接置入 I 期重建手术的报道逐渐增多[7-20]。

10.3　胸肌前假体置入的优缺点

与胸肌后假体置入相比，胸肌前假体置入的主要优势在于保留了胸大肌（PMM）的完整性，无须进行胸大肌剥离或抬高操作，也不会造成肌肉缺损。胸大肌剥离会影响体育活动、锻炼或重体力劳动的进行。若不剥离胸大肌，术后疼痛较轻，还可避免乳房动态畸形（即所谓"跳跃胸"）的发生。其他优势包括缩短手术时间，改善美学效果，减少包膜纤维化（尤其放疗后）等。

10.3.1　胸肌前假体置入的缺点

胸肌前假体置入的问题在于：对于纤瘦患者，假体的可显性及可触及性较为明显；患者前倾时，皱褶现象会更加突出；部分放疗后患者的皮肤会在假体上方形成紧缩，增加假体可见性和皱褶现象。

可通过脂肪移植及脂肪填充改善上述缺陷。这一简单术式是完美的辅助手段，可矫正乳房间沟区域的皱褶或微小组织缺损。

10.4　内置物的覆盖方法

自保留乳头-乳晕复合体的乳房切除术（NSM）开展以来，在假体置入乳房重建过程中如何覆盖假体始终是讨论焦点。目前的技术主要包括：使用补片或网片进行部分覆盖联合胸肌后部分置入，胸肌前假体置入联合前部覆盖/完全覆盖，以及在某些特殊病例中无须覆盖。本团队总结经验认为，补片或网片的应用不仅有助于固定假体，更可在假体与皮肤间形成再生平面，建议并倾向采用前部覆盖方式，利用富余补片或网片对假体背侧进行部分覆盖。

10.5　假体前覆盖技术

选择假体后，制备脱细胞真皮基质

（ADM）或合成网片用于假体覆盖。我们使用猪源 ADM Strattice™ 或 Artia™ 重建组织基质（LifeCell™ 公司，美国新泽西州布里奇沃特）。由于欧洲无法获得所需尺寸的 ADM，将两片 8cm×16cm 的 Strattice™ 或 Artia™ 用生理盐水彻底清洗后，采用间断 Vicryl® 3/0 缝线缝合拼接。将扩容后的 16cm×16cm ADM 于每侧纵缘各切开两处并行网化处理以增加柔顺性。此类切开可形成四片直型筋膜瓣（通过缝线固定）及四片角型筋膜瓣（包裹假体四角，图 10.1），共同构建假体前囊袋。ADM 上缘直型筋膜瓣采用三针间断缝合，固定于胸大肌筋膜与胸浅筋膜间的致密结缔组织。随后将 ADM 内侧直型筋膜瓣以三针缝线固定于筋膜。接着将尺寸适配的假体置于该 ADM 包裹下的胸肌前间隙。将角型 ADM 筋膜瓣分别向内－头端、内－尾端、外－头端及外－尾端包绕假体，确保形成完整的 ADM 囊袋来覆盖假体。之后以三针缝线固定外侧直型筋膜瓣，最后采用三针间断缝合固定尾侧直型筋膜瓣于筋膜。置入单根负压引流管并缝合双层创面，24 小时引流量低于 20mL 时拔除引流管。

若使用合成基质 TIGR™（Novus Scientific AB，瑞典乌普萨拉，10cm×15cm 或 20cm×30cm），可采用相似方式修剪并切开网片，但仅以三针缝线固定于网片上缘（图 10.1b）。用网片包绕假体，将多余网片覆盖表面及部分背面，随后将包裹后的假体置入乳房切除腔隙并通过三针留置缝线固定。TIGR™ 基质为 II 期手术降解、可完全吸收的长效合成网片，含速溶纤维与慢溶纤维。本组中 113 例（56.5%）乳房使用 ADM，87 例（43.5%）乳房使用 TIGR™ 基质。

10.6 技术与材料进展

为改善操作体验和缩短手术时间，我们将猪源性基质 Strattice® 和 Artia® 替换为牛源性 ADM Surgimend® 网化基质（图 10.1c，Integra LifeSciences 公司，美国马萨诸塞州波士顿）。该材料柔软且带网孔结构，可轻松展平覆盖假体表面而无褶皱，剩余 ADM 可在数分钟内缝至假体背面，操作便捷且节约手术时间。随后采用少量缝线将覆盖好的假体固定于腔隙内以防移位。

10.7 血清肿

关于 NSM 联合假体乳房重建术后血清肿形成的争论持续存在。ADM 及网片被视为血清肿形成诱因。由于缺乏血清肿发生率评估标准，文献中各类 ADM 或网片的相关比较研究难以开展。Glenda Caputo[21] 对 12 项单用特定 ADM 行完全胸肌前假体乳房重建的研究进行综述时，报道了血清肿发生率的巨大差异（1.4%~23.4%）。有趣的是，作者发现血清肿形成的直接诱因并非 ADM，而是与手术相关因素有关。此结论并不令人意外——我们一直主张血清肿形成源于手术导致的皮瓣内创面面积过大。所有外科医师都清楚，单纯乳房切除或改良根治术后

胸肌前乳房重建

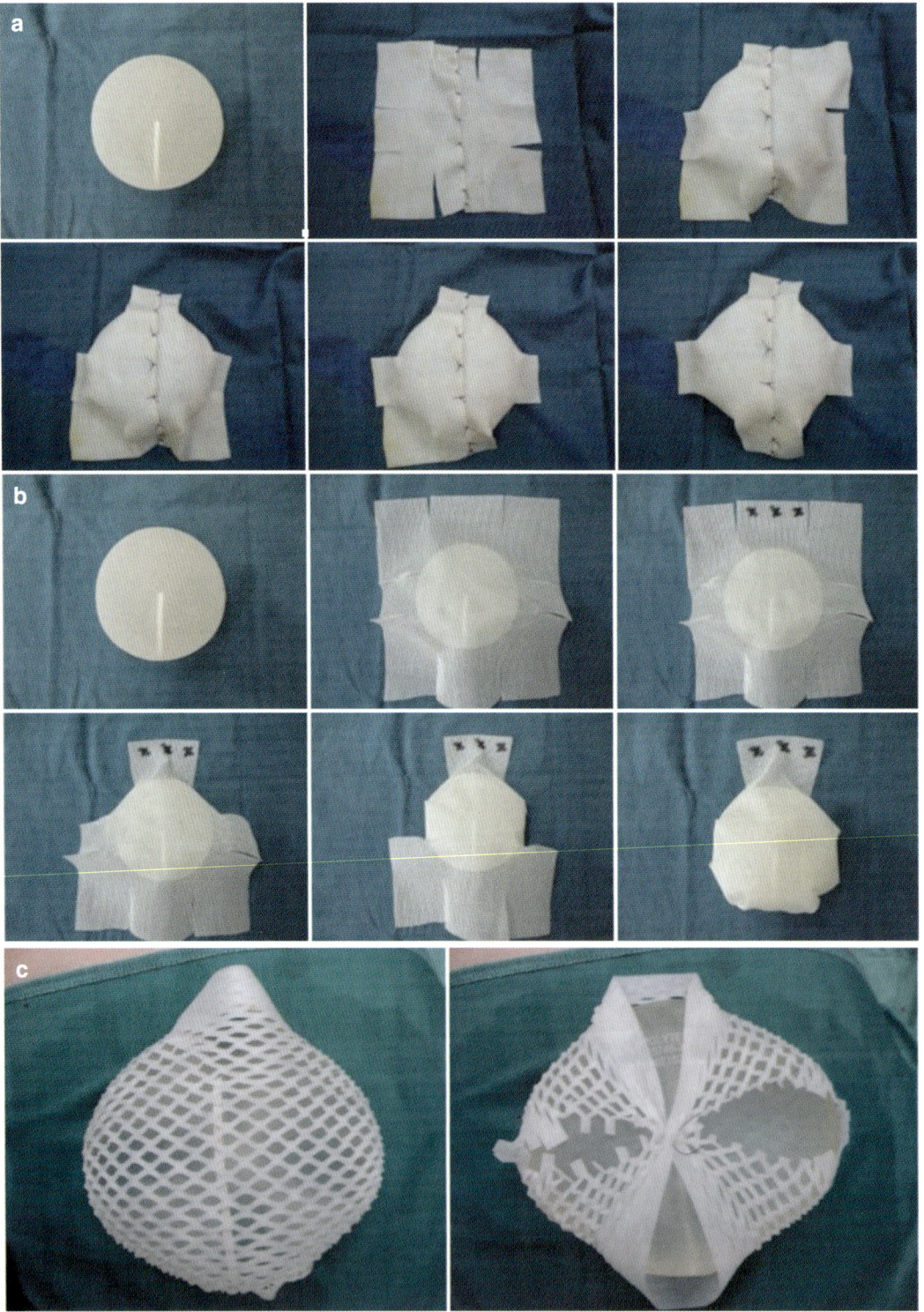

图 10.1 （a）使用猪源性 ADM（Strattice®）包裹假体。（b）使用合成补片 TIGR® 包裹假体。（c）使用牛源性 ADM（Surgimend®）网状物包裹假体

未行重建时仍可出现血清肿。这是组织对手术创伤的反应，其发生率与创伤面积、术式及操作技术相关，是淋巴引流中断的结果，而如多数文献所述，并非与某类基质的使用直接相关。

10.8 胸肌前假体直接置入（DTI）乳房重建

我们开展并报道了[22]连续200例NSM联合胸肌前假体直接置入乳房重建手术，其中假体前方均采用猪源ADM（Strattice™ 或 Artia™）或合成网片TIGR® Matrix进行完整覆盖。

现简要概述研究关键数据：134例患者（200侧乳房）接受NSM联合胸肌前假体Ⅰ期乳房重建手术（DTI）。134例患者中66例（49.3%）行双侧切除术，68例（50.7%）行单侧切除术。200侧乳房中，58侧（29.0%）接受某种形式的放疗，其中32侧（16.0%）于NSM及DTI重建术后接受放疗；26侧（13.0%）因曾行放疗且出现复发性浸润性乳腺癌或复发性导管原位癌而接受NSM联合DTI治疗。切除乳房平均体积342mL（59~1 092mL），假体平均重量340g（110~735g）。所有患者均采用了保留乳头术式，79.5%的手术选择乳房下皱襞切口。

10.9 结果

本组共200侧乳房完成重建。术后并发症包括：轻度并发症（14侧，7.0%）表现为乳头局限性坏死；重度并发症含假体取出（7侧，3.5%）及血肿二次手术清除（8侧，4.0%）。平均引流时间为5天（3~12天）。

平均随访36个月（3~68个月），美容效果评估为优（117侧，58.5%）、良（63侧，31.5%）、中（13侧，6.5%）及差（7侧，3.5%）。无假体移位出现，5例（2.5%）发生假体旋转。3例极度消瘦患者乳房上极区可见并触及假体边缘，另有2例极度消瘦者观察到波纹效应。

32例（16.0%）患者单侧乳房接受术后放疗，其中31例未出现严重放疗相关不良事件（图10.2）。1例患者因放疗后4周出现严重肿胀、水肿及感染，随后移除假体（图10.3）。未见Ⅲ级或Ⅳ级包膜挛缩，短期随访显示美容效果优良。26例

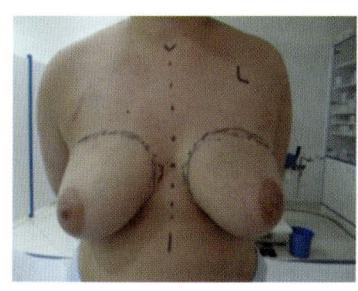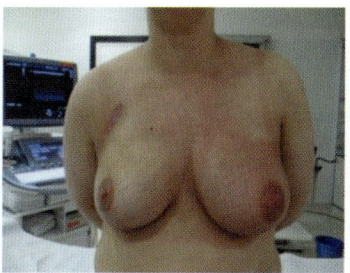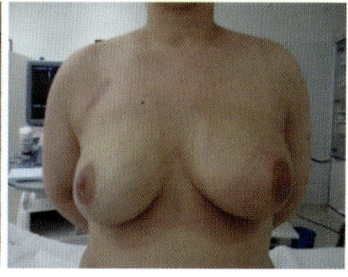

图10.2　美容效果：双侧胸肌前假体置入乳房重建后，左乳接受放疗后及放疗后1年的效果

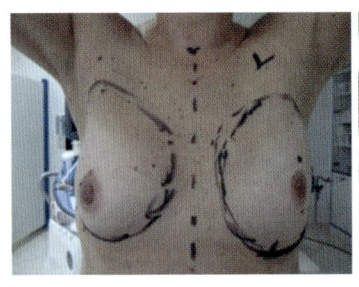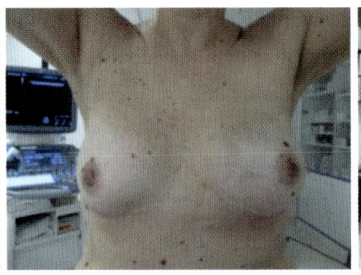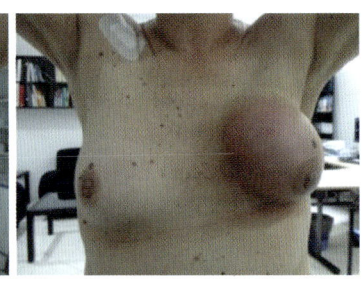

图 10.3　美容效果：左侧胸肌前假体置入乳房重建术，放疗后效果

（13.0%）患者单侧乳房既往有放疗史，其中 6 例（23.0%）乳房出现各类并发症，4 例（15.3%）发生重度并发症 [1 例取出假体，3 例因血肿行翻修手术清除，2 例（7.7%）出现乳头局限性坏死]。ADM 与合成网片在并发症发生率及美容效果方面无显著差异。

更新后的数据集涵盖 350 侧重建乳房，总体结果与前次报道一致。轻度并发症（23/350 侧，6.6%）以乳头局限性坏死为主，重度并发症包括因皮瓣坏死或感染致假体取出（14/350 侧，4.0%），以及因血肿行翻修手术（10/350 侧，2.9%）。

10.10　大而下垂乳房的胸肌前假体直接置入术

假体直接置入 I 期乳房重建术是中小乳房患者的优选方案。针对大而下垂乳房患者，常推荐采用两阶段甚至三阶段术式（先行乳房缩小悬吊术，再行保留乳头和乳晕的乳房切除术及扩张器重建术，最后置换为永久假体）。皮肤缩减保留乳头和乳晕的乳房切除术（SR-NSM）可有效缩小过剩的皮肤被覆结构，用去表皮自体真皮覆盖假体，降低胸肌前假体置入乳房重建的难度。大而下垂的乳房为采用自体真皮替代 ADM 或补片覆盖假体提供了理想条件。通过 I 期保留皮肤乳房切除术（SR-NSM）联合胸肌前假体直接置入重建术，同时采用去表皮自体真皮对假体进行全部或部分覆盖，是对全乳房切除术后大而下垂乳房重建技术的进一步发展[23-25]。本团队对 12 例（20 侧乳房）大而下垂乳房患者实施该术式。患者中位年龄 42 岁，中位体重 73kg，中位 BMI 25，胸骨切迹至乳头中位距离 27cm。所有病例均采用倒 T 形切口，术中完全去表皮处理过剩皮肤。设计上下双蒂乳头-乳晕复合体（NAC），通过带蒂 NAC 的内外侧双向入路可顺利完成全乳房切除术。对乳腺癌患者，可经同一切口行前哨淋巴结定位切除。选择合适假体于胸肌前置入，自体真皮充分覆盖固定。若自体真皮未能完全裹覆假体，可将小片 ADM 或合成补片塑形后缝合于自体真皮与胸浅筋膜之间。常规缝合皮肤覆盖假体及自体真皮，切除原 NAC 位置表皮后将其重新缝合至正确解剖位点。切除乳房中位重量 663g（最大 1 092g，最小 500g），假体中位容积 393mL（最大

495mL，最小255mL）。次要并发症包括4侧（20%）浅层乳头坏死（未经干预自愈）；主要并发症含2侧（10%）血肿需再次手术、1侧（5%）全层乳头坏死。13侧乳房（65%）术后无并发症发生。对于因乳腺癌或降低风险需行乳房切除的大而下垂乳房患者，SR-NSM联合直接假体置入重建术是合理选择。

10.11 小结

保留乳头和乳晕乳房切除（NSM）联合乳房重建术已成为传统乳房切除术的新标准治疗方案。早在20世纪70年代，术式焦点便集中于假体皮下或胸肌后置入定位及Ⅰ期手术重建[26, 27]。随着假体技术、脱细胞真皮基质（ADMs）及手术技术的进步，胸肌后假体置入的优越性正受到质疑。胸大肌（PPM）剥离术后疼痛与不适是常见的术后主诉，而PPM收缩引发的动态畸形亦很常见，胸大肌肌力显著减退及胸肌后假体重建术后肌力缺损问题也已得到充分阐述[28]。现有数据未能证实胸肌后假体置入在乳房重建效果上优于胸肌前置入。对于胸肌前置入术式，ADM通过在皮下组织与假体间构建组织再生中间层，发挥软组织支撑作用，有效防止假体移位。形态稳定的硅凝胶填充乳房假体的研发及各类脱细胞真皮基质的应用，使得胸肌前置入术式可实现假体全包裹重建，从而在不剥离PPM的条件下塑造外观自然的柔软乳房。假体置入乳房重建术后包膜挛缩是公认的难题，现有研究表明联合应用ADM可进一步降低包膜挛缩发生率[29~33]。另有研究报道ADM载体联合术后放疗可减少包膜形成[34, 35]。ADM可能通过减轻放射相关性炎症反应，减缓包膜形成、纤维化及挛缩进程[31, 32]。近期关于胸肌前假体置入联合术后放疗的研究提示预后良好[6, 35]。当前多数胸肌前置入文献聚焦于两阶段乳房重建[4~6, 35]，而Ⅰ期胸肌前置入术的相关研究较少[7~17]，各中心采用不同的假体覆盖技术，包括多类型ADM覆盖、钛化聚丙烯补片覆盖或可吸收合成补片覆盖等[10~18]。

胸肌前假体置入的并发症发生率处于合理范围，与胸肌后置入术式相当。其美学效果令人满意，但前屈体位下产生的波纹感仍较突出，可通过自体脂肪移植得到有效改善。值得注意的是，波纹感不仅见于胸肌前置入术式，胸肌后置入术式因胸大肌（PPM）萎缩亦可导致类似问题。本中心的经验显示，多数患者期望NSM术后保持原乳房体积。对于此类患者或有适度增大诉求者，Ⅰ期假体直接置入重建术可顺利实施。而对于需乳房减容的患者，假体直接置入术同样适用[23~25]。

NSM术后行胸肌前直接假体置入重建是一种前景广阔且安全可行的术式，可塑造柔软美观的乳房形态。优势包括保全胸廓肌群完整性，术后疼痛轻，无运动性形态畸形，多数患者仅需单次手术。目前针对胸肌前与胸肌后假体置入疗效的前瞻性多中心随机对照研究（OPBC-2/PREPEC）正在进行，结果备受期待[36]。

参考文献

1. Headon HL, Kasem A, Mokbel K. The oncologic safety of nipple-sparing mastectomy: a systematic review of the literature with a pooled analysis of 12,358 procedures. Arch Plast Surg. 2016,43(4): 328–38.
2. Madsen RJ Jr, Chim J, Ang B, Fisher O, Hansen J. Variance in the origin of the pectoralis major muscle: implications for implant-based breast reconstruction. Ann Plast Surg. 2015,74(1):111–3.
3. Wy B, Byun IH, Seok Kim Y, Jung BK, Yun IS, Roh TS. Variance of the pectoralis major in relation to the inframammary fold and the pectoralis minor and its application to breast surgery. Clin Anat. 2017,30(3):357–61.
4. Sbitany H, Piper M, Lentz R. Prepectoral breast reconstruction: a safe alternative to submuscular prosthetic reconstruction following nipple-sparing mastectomy. Plast Reconstr Surg. 2017,140(3): 432–43.
5. Salibian AH, Harness JK, Mowlds DS. Staged suprapectoral expander/implant reconstruction without acellular dermal matrix following nipple-sparing mastectomy. Plast Reconstr Surg. 2017,139(1):30–9.
6. Sigalove S, Maxwell GP, Sigalove NM, et al. Prepectoral implant-based breast reconstruction: rationale, indications, and preliminary results. Plast Reconstr Surg. 2017,139(2):287–94.
7. Colwell AS, Damjanovic B, Zahedi B, Medford-Davis L, Hertl C, Austen WG Jr. Retrospective review of 331 consecutive immediate single-stage implant reconstructions with acellular dermal matrix: indications, complications, trends, and costs. Plast Reconstr Surg. 2011,128(6):1170–8.
8. Reitsamer R, Peintinger F. Prepectoral implant placement and complete coverage with porcine acellular dermal matrix: a new technique for direct-to-implant breast reconstruction after nipple-sparing mastectomy. J Plast Reconstr Aesthet Surg. 2015,68(2):162–7.
9. Berna G, Cawthorn SJ, Papaccio G, Balestrieri N. Evaluation of a novel breast reconstruction technique using the Braxon® acellular dermal matrix: a new muscle-sparing breast reconstruction. ANZ J Surg. 2017,87(6):493–8.
10. Casella D, Bernini M, Bencini L, et al. Ti-Loop®bra mesh used for immediate breast reconstruction: comparison of retropectoral and subcutaneous implant placement in a prospective single-institution series. Eur J Plast Surg. 2014,37(11):599–604.
11. Casella D, Di Taranto G, Marcasciano M, et al. Evaluation of prepectoral implant placement and complete coverage with TiLoop®Bra mesh for breast reconstruction: a prospective study on long-term and patient reported BREAST-Q outcomes. Plast Reconstr Surg. 2019,142(1):1e–9e.
12. Vidya R, Masià J, Cawthorn S, et al. Evaluation of the effectiveness of the prepectoral breast reconstruction with Braxon dermal matrix: first multicenter European report on 100 cases. Breast J. 2017,23(6):670–6.
13. Onesti MG, Maruccia M, Di Taranto G, et al. Clinical, histological, and ultrasound follow-up of breast reconstruction with one-stage muscle-sparing "wrap" technique: a single-center experience. J Plast Reconstr Aesthet Surg. 2017,70(11):1527–36.
14. Bernini M, Calabrese C, Cecconi L, et al. Subcutaneous direct-to-implant breast reconstruction: surgical, functional, and aesthetic results after long-term follow-up. Plast Reconstr Surg Glob Open. 2016,3(12):e574. https://doi.org/10.1097/GOX.0000000000000533.
15. Downs RK, Hedges K. An alternative technique for immediate direct-to-implant breast reconstruction – a case series. Plast Reconstr Surg Glob Open. 2016,4(7):e821. https://doi.org/10.1097/GOX.0000000000000839.
16. Highton L, Johnson R, Kirwan C, Murphy J. Prepectoral implant-based breast reconstruction. Plast Reconstr Surg Glob Open.

17. Jones G, Yoo A, King V, et al. Prepectoral immediate direct-to-implant breast reconstruction with anterior AlloDerm coverage. Plast Reconstr Surg. 2017,140(6S Prepectoral Breast Reconstruction):31S–8S. https://doi.org/10.1097/PRS.0000000000004048.

18. Hallberg H, Lewin R, Elander A, Hansson E. TIGR® matrix surgical mesh – a two-year follow-up study and complication analysis in 65 immediate breast reconstructions. J Plast Surg Hand Surg. 2018,52(4):253–8.

19. Masià J, iBAG Working Group. The largest multicentre data collection on prepectoral breast reconstruction: the iBAG study. J Surg Oncol. 2020,122(5):848–60.

20. Khan A, Tasoulis MK, Teoh V, Tanska A, Edmonds R, Gui G. Pre-pectoral one-stage breast reconstruction with anterior biological acellular dermal matrix coverage. Gland Surg. 2021,10(3):1002–9.

21. Caputo GG, Mura S, Albanese R, Zingaretti N, Parodi PC. Seroma formation in pre-pectoral implant-based ADM assisted breast reconstruction: a comprehensive review of current literature. Chirurgia. 2021,116:16–23.

22. Reitsamer R, Peintinger F, Klaassen-Federspiel F, Sir A. Prepectoral direct-to-implant breast reconstruction with complete ADM or synthetic mesh coverage – 36-months follow-up in 200 reconstructed breasts. Breast. 2019,48:32–7.

23. Nava MB, Ottolenghi J, Pennati A, et al. Skin/nipple sparing mastectomies and implant-based breast reconstruction in patients with large and ptotic breast: oncological and reconstructive results. Breast. 2012,21(3):267–71.

24. Caputo GG, Marchetti A, Dalla Pozza E, et al. Skin-reduction breast reconstruction with prepectoral implant. Plast Reconstr Surg. 2016,137(6):1702–5.

25. Onesti MG, Di Taranto G, Ribuffo D, Scuderi N. ADM-assisted prepectoral breast reconstruction and skin reduction mastectomy: expanding the indications for subcutaneous reconstruction. J Plast Reconstr Aesthetic Surg. 2019 Nov 28. pii:S1748–6815(19)30492–9.

26. Hüter J, Clemens H, Ogbukagu A. Subcutaneous or subpectoral prosthesis positioning? Arch Gynecol. 1979,228(1–4):290.

27. Apfelberg DM, Laub DR, Maser MR, Lash H. Submuscular breast reconstruction – indications and techniques. Ann Plast Surg. 1981,7(3):213–21.

28. De Haan A, Toor A, Hage JJ, Veeger HE, Woerdeman LA. Function of the pectoralis major muscle after combined skin-sparing mastectomy and immediate reconstruction by subpectoral implantation of a prosthesis. Ann Plast Surg. 2007,59(6):605–10.

29. Stump A, Holton LH III, Connor J, Harper JR, Slezak S, Silverman RP. The use of acellular dermal matrix to prevent capsule formation around implants in a primate model. Plast Reconstr Surg. 2009,124:82–91.

30. Komorowska-Timek E, Oberg KC, Timek TA, Gridley DS, Miles DA. The effect of Alloderm envelopes on periprosthetic capsule formation with and without radiation. Plast Reconstr Surg. 2009,123:807–16.

31. Schmitz M, Bertram M, Kneser U, Keller AK, Horch RE. Experimental total wrapping of breast implants with acellular dermal matrix: a preventive tool against capsular contracture in breast surgery? J Plast Reconstr Aesthet Surg. 2013,66(10):1382–9.

32. Cheng A, Lakhiani C, Saint-Cyr M. Treatment of capsular contracture using complete implant coverage by acellular dermal matrix: a novel technique. Plast Reconstr Surg. 2013,132(3):519–29.

33. Salzberg CA, Ashikari AY, Berry C, Hunsicker LM. Acellular dermal matrix-assisted direct-to-implant breast reconstruction and capsular contracture: a 13-year experience. Plast Reconstr Surg. 2016,138(2):329–37.

34. Tang R, Coopey SB, Colwell AS, et al. Nip-

ple-sparing mastectomy in irradiated breasts: selecting patients to minimize complications. Ann Surg Oncol. 2015,22(10):3331–7.
35. Elswick SM, Harless CA, Bishop SN, et al. Prepectoral implant-based breast reconstruction with Postmastectomy radiation therapy. Plast Reconstr Surg. 2018,142(1):1–12. https://doi.org/10.1097/PRS.0000000000004453.
36. Kappos EA, Schulz A, Regan MM, et al. Prepectoral versus subpectoral implant-based breast reconstruction after skin-sparing mastectomy or nipple-sparing mastectomy (OPBC-2/PREPEC): a pragmatic, multicentre, randomized, superiority trial. BMJ Open. 2021,11(9):e045239.

11 胸肌前覆盖乳房重建术

编者：Glyn Jones
译者：刘岩青

11.1 引言

乳房为胸肌前结构，然而数十年来外科医师始终在胸肌后平面进行乳房重建。最初，假体置入乳房重建在皮下平面实施，后来随着人们认为肌层覆盖可提供更好的假体遮蔽效果、减轻皱褶形成并降低包膜挛缩率后，将假体于胸肌后置入的理念得到广泛接受[1~13]。目前的循证依据更倾向于包膜挛缩主要是由假体置入时的细菌污染引发生物膜形成引起的，而非假体位置因素[6,8,13]。生物膜抑制技术已显著降低包膜挛缩发生率，使得胸肌后置入的必要性部分丧失[14~16]。

传统乳房切除术后应用组织扩张器行Ⅱ期乳房重建是恢复缺损容积的常规手段[9]。保皮与保乳头技术已逐步取代传统乳房切除术，大幅降低了对组织扩张的需求[17,18]。为实现术中对扩张器的定位控制，全肌层覆盖理念曾被部分采用，现已被脱细胞真皮基质（ADM）及补片的下极覆盖技术所替代。ADM不仅可增强组织强度，更能实现更理想的腔隙控制与形态塑造，同时避免全肌层覆盖形成的压迫效应[19,20]。

理论上来说，该张力可能影响组织灌注并妨碍无张力缝合，而二者均是确保创面顺利愈合的必要条件。使此问题复杂化的另一因素在于，假体乳房重建初期的组织灌注评估技术目前尚不精确，外科医师仅能依赖临床评估及荧光检测。吲哚菁绿激光诱导荧光血管造影技术的问世，成为乳房切除术后皮瓣灌注评估的转折点，而新型多光谱成像技术则进一步提升了灌注评估的准确性[21]。

Ⅱ期胸肌后假体重建虽可获得合理效果，但胸肌后置入伴随显著的生理限制，多数患者活动时存在不同程度动态畸形[12,22-24]，并且功能可能受损。MRI研究证实，胸肌后隆乳术后12个月胸肌体积可减少50%[25]。此外，有文献报道胸肌后假体置入后患者肌力下降高达15%[22,26-31]。

G. Jones (✉)
University of Illinois College of Medicine at Peoria,
Peoria, IL, USA

© The Author(s), under exclusive license to Springer Nature Switzerland AG 2023
R. Vidya, H. Becker (eds.), *Prepectoral Breast Reconstruction*,
https://doi.org/10.1007/978-3-031-15590-1_11

基于上述研究结果，胸肌前假体置入乳房重建日益普及，优势在于：

1. 规避肌肉离断所致的疼痛。
2. 最大限度降低动态畸形。
3. 利于假体内侧精准放置以营造乳沟形态。
4. 未增加皮肤坏死发生风险。
5. 不诱发假体下垂风险升高。

胸肌前重建也存在若干不足之处：

1. 失去用于控制假体位置的肌肉"支撑"结构。
2. 需要外科医生[尤其是假体直接置入重建（DTI）] 精确控制假体位置。
3. 患者可能出现可见皱褶的风险可能更高。

为减小该术式固有风险与操作困难，采用生物补片或合成网片进行囊袋控制与前方覆盖具至关重要。必须承认，凸缘扩张器的使用确实解决了胸肌前扩张器位置控制的问题，若术者有意向亦可实现无网片重建。笔者认为，脱细胞真皮基质（ADM）带来的远期收益可能更多。实施Ⅰ期胸肌前假体置入手术时，使用网片控制假体位置的重要性将大幅提升。多数乳腺外科医师在剥离腋尾部时会突破乳房外侧皱襞，此举在美学层面上破坏乳房的自然标志结构，同时形成外侧潜在腔隙，因此未受限假体会很容易发生移位。假体外移不仅导致乳房形态异常，更会明显影响乳沟形成。应用脱细胞真皮基质（或合成网片）实施前方覆盖，既可实现假体精准定位与外侧皱襞控制，亦可引导假体向下方移位，进而模拟天然乳房下极的饱满形态。

11.2 前覆盖或全包裹？

对脱细胞真皮基质（ADM）或合成网片的前覆盖与全包裹技术的优劣存在诸多争议，笔者对两种ADM应用技术均具临床经验。

完全包裹假体或扩张器需消耗更多材料，显著增加治疗成本。使用单层ADM包裹去脂扩张器确实操作更便利。使用ADM时，术者可采用经ADM的间断缝合将包裹装置固定于胸壁；使用扩张器时，则通过凸缘缝合完成固定。全包裹支持者主张构建下缘套筒结构稳固装置，认为此为预防重建物下移的关键。更具决定性意义的是通过将ADM或网片与胸壁（非Scarpa筋膜）稳定缝合以精准定位乳房下皱襞（IMF）。若固定于筋膜层，假体可沿肌肉表面筋膜下隙向尾端滑动，进而导致皱襞异位。通过将材料直接缝合至皱襞水平胸壁肌层，既能可靠构建新IMF又无须刻意制造假体容纳沟槽。此操作可最大限度利用ADM塑造囊袋前部轮廓，以实现乳房最大限度下垂仿真形态，而非将其珍贵表面积浪费于装置后方。基于上述考量，笔者采用的手术策略是在胸肌前全面应用前覆盖技术来处理假体与扩张器。胸肌前假体直接置入重建术可为绝大多数患者提供可靠的Ⅰ期手术治疗解决方案（图11.1）。

11.3 材料与方法

目前，96%患者采用胸肌前Ⅰ期直接假体置入术（DTI）完成重建；Ⅱ期手术

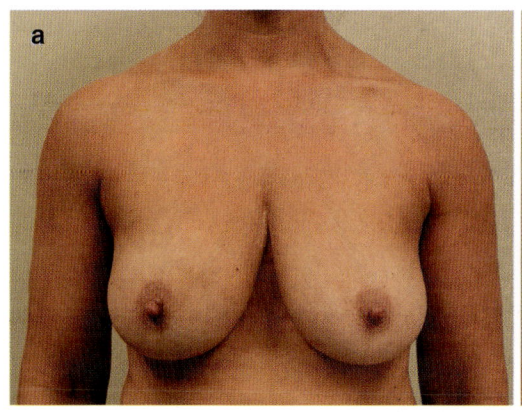 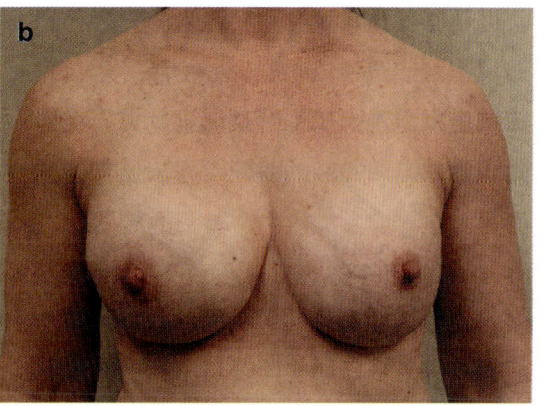

图 11.1 （a）1 例 55 岁女性 右侧乳腺癌患者术前视图；（b）双侧乳房皮下腺体切除 + Ⅰ 期胸肌前假体置入乳房重建术后 1 年

扩张器重建仅占 4%，手术平面同样位于胸肌前，适用于经 Kent Snapshot 系统（Kent 医学影像公司，卡尔加里，阿尔伯塔省）多光谱近红外成像评估存在皮肤覆盖灌注潜在风险的病例（多为重度吸烟者）。该技术因具廉价、精度高与无创等优势，在本机构已取代吲哚菁绿荧光成像技术。

在乳房切除术中，皮瓣灌注是决定是否行 Ⅰ 期重建手术的核心要素，决策取决于置入临时试模后乳房切除皮瓣的灌注充分性。在 12 年直接假体置入术实践经验的基础上，笔者发现皮瓣厚度并非核心问题，灌注质量方为关键：若存在皮肤薄弱状况，后期可通过脂肪移植予以改善；若临时试模在位时皮瓣灌注充分，则可决定行即刻重建；如灌注处于临界状态，可选择置入低充注扩张器或中止手术，并于 2 周内转行延迟 - 即刻手术。

11.4 手术操作

切除乳房后，用氯己定乙醇溶液或聚维酮碘溶液对皮肤再次消毒。置入临时试模后，用多光谱近红外成像技术评估皮瓣灌注情况（图 11.2）。该模式通过检测皮瓣氧合状态（作为灌注代用指标）实现快速评估，效果较吲哚菁绿荧光成像技术更优。多光谱成像具有无创、便携及低成本优势，单次手术中可重复多次使用。切除乳房后遗留的腔隙依次以生理盐水、原浓度聚维酮碘溶液[16, 32]行冲洗处理。

11.5 前覆盖缝合技术

取 16cm × 20cm 厚型脱细胞真皮基质（AlloDerm，艾尔建公司）按生产商规范进行冲洗。将材料覆盖于临时试模表面，用无菌标记笔对囊袋内定位进行标记后塑形修剪，通常需切除 ADM 两处小三角区域以实现囊袋上部缩窄，从而限制假体上移（图 11.3）。应在假体未就位状态下进行缝合，将 ADM 贴覆于胸大肌表面，通过定位标记确定 12 点钟位后，采用前悬吊技术[33]将其缝合固定于胸大肌前表面。

用 2-0 PDS 缝线进行连续缝合：自 12 点位至 5 点位及从 12 点位至 7 点位进行缝合后，保留下部操作窗以便假体置入（适用于乳房下皱襞切口或中央切口术式）。外侧区 ADM 缝合固定于抬高的前锯肌筋膜或肌袖（筋膜缺损时；图 11.4a）。若采用外侧切口（以右侧乳房切除术为例），则行从 12 点位至 10 点位及从 12 点经 3 点位至 7 点位的连续缝合，保留外侧假体置入通路。缝合过程中应尽可能保留 ADM 下部的冗余度，从而允许更多 ADM 膨隆覆盖假体下极以模拟乳房下极饱满形态。置入试模，复查囊袋形态与位置。移除试模后，再次以原浓度聚维酮碘溶液冲洗囊袋，术者更换手套后使用凯勒漏斗等置入假体，确保假体与皮肤无接触以降低生物膜形成风险[15, 16, 34]。随后牵拉调整 ADM 覆盖假体穹隆部，形成"戴手套"般密接状态，用 2-0 PDS 缝线将 ADM 下缘固定至胸壁（而非 Scarpa 筋膜；图 11.4b）。切忌将 ADM 与 Scarpa 筋膜缝合，否则假体可能因重力作用沿筋膜下胸壁下移，导致乳房下皱襞处于异常低位。留置双腔引流管后逐层关闭切口，创面以 Tegaderm 敷料密封固定 2 周。第 1 根引流管于术后 1 周拔除，第 2 根引流管保留至 24 小时引流量不足 20~25mL。目前研究数据提示，双管引流可有效降低术后血清肿及感染发生率。

11.6 结果

在涉及 140 例患者的 194 侧乳房的临床回顾研究中，最长随访期为 3.8 年。

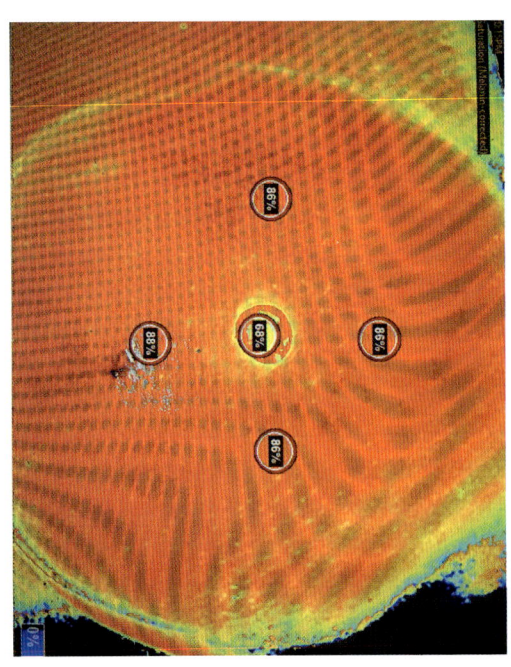

图 11.2 乳房切除术后血液灌注多光谱近红外灌注成像

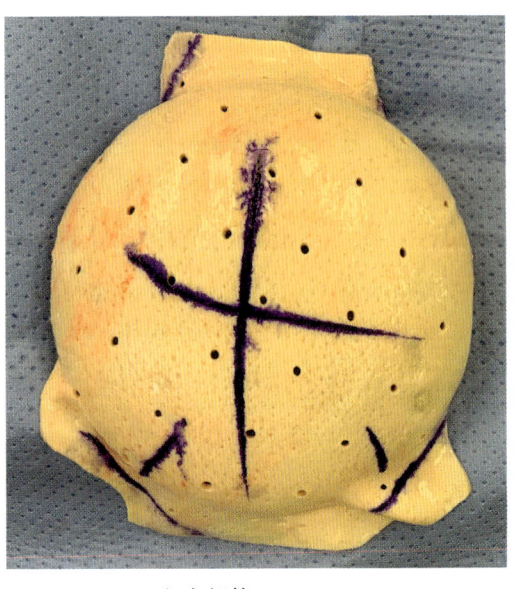

图 11.3 ADM 包裹假体

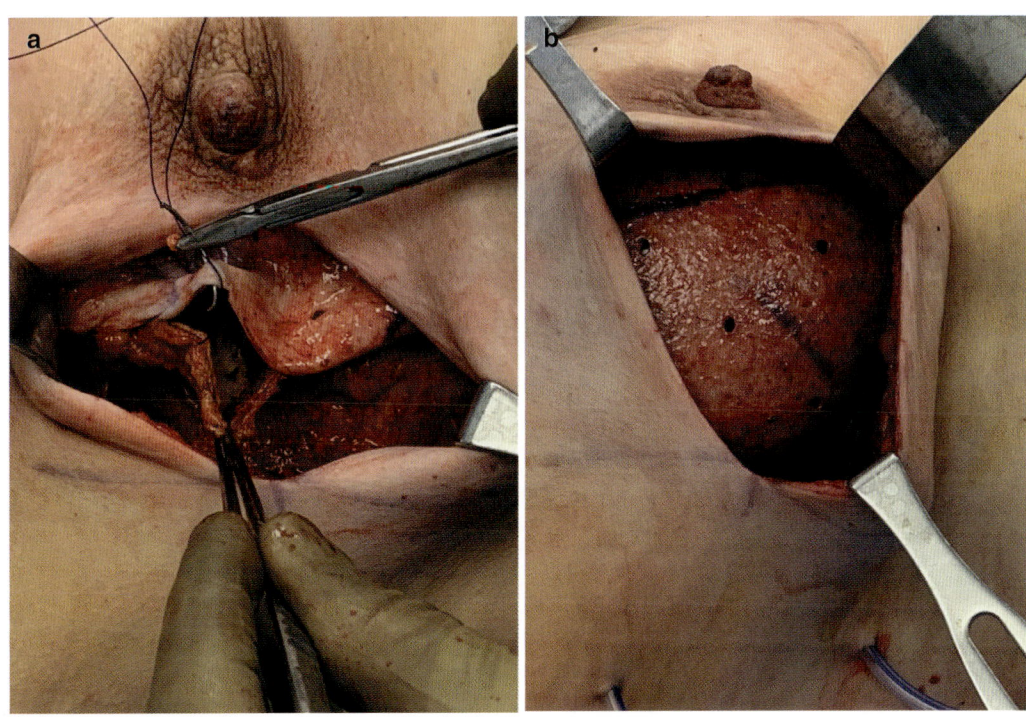

图 11.4 （a）将 ADM 的外侧缘缝合于前锯肌筋膜；（b）关闭切口前的胸肌前重建状态

目前已完成 500 余例乳房重建，长期结果相似。早期数据基于解剖型纹理面高内聚性凝胶假体（艾尔建公司，已退市）。过去 2 年，笔者已转换为仅使用全 / 中高凸度的光滑圆形中内聚性凝胶假体。初期使用高内聚性圆形光面凝胶假体（尤其超高凸度型）时，发现前后平面翻转发生率高得难以接受，故临床已弃用该类型假体，改用全高凸度中内聚性假体。目前，所有使用纹理面假体重建的病例均未发现乳房假体相关间变性大细胞淋巴瘤（BIA-ALCL），93.3% 病例获得理想效果（图 11.1）。最常见并发症包括轻度轮廓畸形（44.3%，轻微假体缘显露或凹陷）、良性血清肿（5.2%）和蜂窝织炎（5.7%）。6.7% 病例因各种原因需取出假体。无一例出现需在手术室清创缝合的全层皮肤坏死，4.1% 表浅性水疱经局部保守治疗愈合。

15% 病例存在轻度褶皱。使用解剖型高内聚性凝胶假体时，38% 病例需行脂肪移植来改善轻度轮廓畸形，该比例显著低于胸肌后重建病例的脂肪移植率。转用圆形光面假体后，为填充胸壁上极轮廓并减少低内聚性假体相关可见褶皱，脂肪移植率增至 90% 以上。非放疗患者包膜挛缩和动态畸形的发生率均为 0。将持续低发的包膜挛缩归因于生物膜减量技术及 ADM 应用。7.2% 病例实施假体更换（尺寸调整），该比例显著低于 I 期手术胸肌后重建术式。

11.7 讨论

多项研究证实了胸肌前重建术的有效性[35~44]。Gabriel 报道 39 例肥胖患者胸肌前乳房重建效果良好，仅有 1 例重建失败[35]。部分研究关注了乳房切除术后放疗（PMRT）后胸肌前重建效果[37,42,43]。Elswick 等与 Sigalove 等分别基于 93 例与 52 例短期回顾性数据发现，PMRT 后胸肌前重建患者不良结局风险无显著升高[37,42]。Sinnot 指出，胸肌后重建联合 PMRT 患者的包膜挛缩发生率高于胸肌前重建患者[43]，可能与放疗后胸肌纤维化导致的紧缩畸形及肩部僵硬相关。

自本团队前期研究发表后，多项胸肌前/后乳房重建的对比研究取得了积极结果。Cattelani 等的小样本前瞻性非随机研究发现，胸肌前重建患者术后疼痛更轻，上肢功能恢复更快，返岗时间更早[44]。Walia 报道，两阶段胸肌前重建患者术后疼痛显著减轻；BREAST-Q 量表分析结果显示，住院患者报告结局无显著差异，但胸肌前组乳头缺血发生率明显升高[39]。Baker 团队指出，胸肌前组与胸肌后组在疼痛评分、早期并发症及术后住院时长方面无统计学差异，但胸肌前组患者对假体褶皱情况的不满意度更高[41]。

尽管越来越多研究报道了直接假体置入胸肌前乳房重建的积极数据，多数外科医生仍愿意进行基于扩张器的两阶段重建手术[36,37,43,44]。鉴于目前的乳房切除术能保留更多皮肤（最高实现保留乳头乳房切除术[17,18]），这一现象似有矛盾。随着新术式的普及，通过扩张获得皮肤必要性显著下降。在乳房切除术中可通过松解筋膜使皮肤覆盖层可容纳与原体积相当甚至更大的假体。相比之下，我们常可通过 I 期手术重建增大乳房体积。两阶段扩张器-假体重建的经济补偿更高，可能影响临床决策。在全民医保体系中，I 期手术重建为乳房重建提供更实际的解决方案。

如前所述，直接置入假体进行重建主要取决于皮瓣灌注而非厚度，只要灌注评估成像显示皮瓣灌注良好，乳房切除术后皮瓣厚度本身不影响预后[13,35]。若术中临时假体试模在位时皮瓣灌注充足，胸肌前直接假体置入重建 I 期手术是安全的。手持式 Kent Snapshot 近红外多光谱成像设备（加拿大阿尔伯塔省 Kent Imaging 公司）能实现精准、简单、无创的灌注评估，本团队近期将发表的研究显示其准确性优于吲哚菁绿（ICG）荧光成像技术。

该技术的优势可分为近期与远期。近期来看，前覆盖技术的应用有助于控制乳房切除腔隙与假体位置，使手术效果更精准且可重复。远期来看，该技术显著降低了患者术后不适感，术后无须进行扩张，减轻了组织瓣水肿，对上肢功能基本无主观负面影响，动态畸形完全消除。

尽管在使用解剖型黏性凝胶假体时，胸肌前假体组需要脂肪移植的比例（38%）低于胸肌后假体组，但采用圆形假体后此差异消失，反映了圆形假体形状的固有缺陷。

与胸大肌收缩方向垂直的褶皱波纹现象已被根除，其形成主要与所选凝胶的稠度相关。由于假体在胸肌前置入，在内侧置入胸大肌限制假体而致乳沟形成受限的问题不再存在。通过前入路构建脱细胞真皮基质囊袋时，可根据需要充分向内侧延伸以获得更理想的乳沟形态。目前笔者团队已完全摒弃胸肌后假体乳房重建术式。同时，在皮瓣灌注可接受的前提下，亦基本放弃了常规两阶段重建方案，转而以Ⅰ期手术胸肌前重建作为首选。

11.8 小结

改良乳房切除术式可最大限度（或近全部）保留乳房皮肤组织。以脱细胞真皮基质/补片覆于圆形假体前进行重建，可精准实施Ⅰ期手术重建，患者不适与不便显著减少。通过前覆盖技术，Ⅰ期手术在胸肌前直接置入假体进行重建已基本替代两阶段扩张器重建。10年随访数据显示，该术式重建效果稳定可靠，包膜挛缩率与零动态畸形发生率极低，既往关于假体远期下垂、侵蚀或无法接受的波纹皱褶现象的质疑均未发生。

参考文献

1. Freeman BS. Subcutaneous mastectomy for benign breast lesions with immediate or delayed prosthetic replacement. Plast Reconstr Surg Transplant Bull. 1962,30:676–82.
2. Berens JJ, Stapley LA. Breast tumors treated by mastectomy (subcutaneous) with mammary replacement. Ariz Med. 1969,26(8):651–7.
3. Hueston J, McKenzie G. Breast reconstruction after radical mastectomy. Aust N Z J Surg. 1970,39(4):367–70.
4. Snyderman RK, Guthrie RH. Reconstruction of the female breast following radical mastectomy. Plast Reconstr Surg. 1971,47(6):565–7.
5. Guthrie RH. Breast reconstruction after radical mastectomy. Plast Reconstr Surg. 1976,57(1):14–22.
6. Schlenker JD, Bueno RA, Ricketson G, Lynch JB. Loss of silicone implants after subcutaneous mastectomy and reconstruction. Plast Reconstr Surg. 1978,62(6):853–61.
7. Blevins PK. Subcutaneous mastectomy and breast replacement: its role in the treatment of benign, premalignant, and malignant breast disease. Am Surg. 1981,47(7):281–6.
8. Gruber RP, Kahn RA, Lash H, Maser MR, Apfelberg DB, Laub DR. Breast reconstruction following mastectomy: a comparison of submuscular and subcutaneous techniques. Plast Reconstr Surg. 1981,67(3):312–7.
9. Radovan C. Breast reconstruction after mastectomy using the temporary expander. Plast Reconstr Surg. 1982,69(2):195–208.
10. Giraud B, Dauplat J, Gadonneix P, Jany M, Rodier JF, Issert B, et al. [Subcutaneous mammectomy with prosthetic inclusion. Apropos of 114 cases]. Chirurgie 1986,112(5):402–412.
11. Scarfì A, Ordemann K, Hüter J. Reconstruction of an ablated breast. Eur J Gynaecol Oncol. 1986,7(2):93–6.
12. Artz JS, Dinner MI, Sampliner J. Breast reconstruction with a subcutaneous tissue expander followed with a polyurethane-covered silicone breast implant. Ann Plast Surg. 1988,20(6):517–21.
13. Artz JS, Dinner MI, Foglietti MA, Sampliner J. Breast reconstruction utilizing subcutaneous tissue expansion followed by polyurethane-covered silicone implants: a 6-year experience. Plast Reconstr Surg. 1991,88(4):635–9. discussion640–1
14. Ajdic D, Zoghbi Y, Gerth D, Panthaki ZJ, Thaller S. The relationship of bacterial biofilms and capsular contracture in breast implants. Aes-

thet Surg J. 2016,36(3):297–309.
15. Deva AK, Adams WP Jr, Vickery K. The role of bacterial biofilms in device-associated infection. Plast Reconstr Surg. 2013,132(5):1319–28.
16. Jewell ML, Adams WP Jr. Betadine and breast implants. Aesthet Surg J. 2018,38(6):623–6.
17. Toth BA, Lappert P. Modified skin incisions for mastectomy: the need for plastic surgeons input. Plast Reconstr Surg. 1991,87(6):1048–53.
18. Bishop CC, Singh S, Nash AG. Mastectomy and breast reconstruction preserving the nipple. Ann R Coll Surg Engl. 1990,72(2):87–9.
19. Duncan DI. Correction of implant rippling using allograft dermis. Aesthet Surg J. 2001,21(1):81–4.
20. Baxter RA. Intracapsular allogenic dermal grafts for breast implant-related problems. Plast Reconstr Surg. 2003,112(6):1692–6.
21. Gurtner GC, Jones GE, Neligan PC, Newman MI, Phillips BT, Sacks JM, et al. Intraoperative laser angiography using the SPY system: review of the literature and recommendations for use. Ann Surg Innov Res. 2013,7(1):1–1.
22. Spear SL, Schwartz J, Dayan JH, Clemens MW. Outcome assessment of breast distortion following submuscular breast augmentation. Aesth Plast Surg. 2009,33(1):44–8.
23. Becker H, Fregosi N. The impact of animation deformity on quality of life in post-mastectomy reconstruction patients. Aesthet Surg J. 2017,37(5):531–6.
24. Nigro LC, Blanchet NP. Animation deformity in Postmastectomy implant-based reconstruction. Plast Reconstr Surg Glob Open. 2017,5(7):e1407–4.
25. Weck Roxo AC, Nahas FX, Salin R, de Castro CC, Aboudib JH, Marques RG. Volumetric evaluation of the mammary gland and pectoralis major muscle following subglandular and submuscular breast augmentation. Plast Reconstr Surg. 2016,137(1):62–9.
26. Banbury J, Yetman R, Lucas A, Papay F, Graves K, Zins JE. Prospective analysis of the outcome of subpectoral breast augmentation: sensory changes, muscle function, and body image. Plast Reconstr Surg. 2004,113(2):701–7.
27. Beals SP, Golden KA, Basten M, Kelly KM. Strength performance of the pectoralis major muscle after subpectoral breast augmentation surgery. Aesthet Surg J. 2003,23(2):92–7.
28. Becker H, Lind JG II, Hopkins EG. Immediate implant-based Prepectoral breast reconstruction using a vertical incision. Plast Reconstr Surg Glob Open. 2015,3(6):e412–9.
29. de Haan A, Toor A, Hage JJ, Veeger HEJ, Woerdeman LAE. Function of the pectoralis major muscle after combined skin-sparing mastectomy and immediate reconstruction by subpectoral implantation of a prosthesis. Ann Plast Surg. 2007,59(6):605–10.
30. Hage JJ, van der Heeden JF, Lankhorst KM, Romviel SMG, Vluttters ME, Woerdeman LAE, et al. Impact of combined skin sparing mastectomy and immediate subpectoral prosthetic reconstruction on the pectoralis major muscle function. Ann Plast Surg. 2014,72:631–7.
31. Sarbak J, Baker J. Effects of breast augmentation on pectoralis major muscle function in the athletic woman. Aesthet Surg J. 2004,24(3):224–8.
32. Campbell CA. The role of triple-antibiotic saline irrigation in breast implant surgery. Ann Plast Surg. 2018,80:S398–402.
33. Jones G, Yoo A, King V, Jao B, Wang H, Rammos C, et al. Prepectoral immediate direct-to-implant breast reconstruction with anterior AlloDerm coverage. Plast Reconstr Surg. 2017,140:31S–8S.
34. Flugstad NA, Pozner JN, Baxter RA, Creasman C, Egrari S, Martin S, et al. Does implant insertion with a funnel decrease capsular contracture? A Preliminary Report Aesthet Surg J. 2016,36(5): 550–6.
35. Gabriel A, Maxwell GP. Prepectoral breast reconstruction in challenging patients. Plast Reconstr Surg. 2017,140:14S–21S.
36. Jafferbhoy S, Chandarana M, Houlihan M, Par-

meshwar R, Narayanan S, Soumian S, et al. Early multicentre experience of pre-pectoral implant based immediate breast reconstruction using Braxon®. Gland Surg. 2017,6(6):682–8.
37. Sigalove S, Maxwell GP, Sigalove NM, Storm-Dickerson TL, Pope N, Rice J, et al. Prepectoral implant-based breast reconstruction and Postmastectomy radiotherapy. Plast Reconstr Surg Glob Open. 2017,5(12):e1631–7.
38. Paydar KZ, Wirth GA, Mowlds DS. Prepectoral breast reconstruction with fenestrated acellular dermal matrix. Plast Reconstr Surg Glob Open. 2018,6(4):e1712–4.
39. Walia GS, Aston J, Bello R, Mackert GA, Pedreira RA, Cho BH, et al. Prepectoral versus subpectoral tissue expander placement. Plast Reconstr Surg Glob Open. 2018,6(4):e1731–6.
40. Pittman TA, Abbate OA, Economides JM. The P1 method: Prepectoral breast reconstruction to minimize the palpable implant edge and upper pole rippling. Ann Plast Surg. 2018,80(5):487–92.
41. Baker BG, Irri R, MacCallum V, Chattopadhyay R, Murphy J, Harvey JR. A prospective comparison of short-term outcomes of subpectoral and Prepectoral Strattice-based immediate breast reconstruction. Plast Reconstr Surg. 2018,141(5):1077–84.
42. Elswick SM, Harless CA, Bishop SN, Schleck CD, Mandrekar J, Reusche RD, et al. Prepectoral implant-based breast reconstruction with Postmastectomy radiation therapy. Plast Reconstr Surg. 2018,142(1):1–12.
43. Sinnott CJ, Persing SM, Pronovost M, Hodyl C, McConnell D, Young AO. Impact of postmastectomy radiation therapy in prepectoral versus subpectoral implant-based breast reconstruction. Ann Surg Oncol. 2018:1–10. Springer International Publishing
44. Cattelani L, Polotto S, Arcuri MF, Pedrazzi G, Linguadoca C, Bonati E. One-step Prepectoral breast reconstruction with dermal matrix-covered implant compared to submuscular implantation: functional and cost evaluation. Clin Breast Cancer. 2018,18(4):e703–11. Elsevier Inc

Further Reading

Gur E, Hanna W, Andrighetti L, Semple JL. Light and electron microscopic evaluation of the pectoralis major muscle following tissue expansion for breast reconstruction. Plast Reconstr Surg. 1998,102(4):1046–51.

Maxwell GP, Tornambe R. Management of mammary subpectoral implant distortion. Clin Plast Surg. 1988,15(4):601–11.

Hammond DC, Schmitt WP, O'Connor EA. Treatment of breast animation deformity in implant-based reconstruction with pocket change to the subcutaneous position. Plast Reconstr Surg. 2015,135(6):1540–4.

Lesavoy MA, Trussler AP, Dickinson BP. Difficulties with subpectoral augmentation Mammaplasty and its correction: the role of subglandular site change in revision aesthetic breast surgery. Plast Reconstr Surg. 2010,125(1):363–71.

Gabriel A, Sigalove S, Sigalove NM, Storm-Dickerson TL, Rice J, Pope N, et al. Prepectoral revision breast reconstruction for treatment of implant-associated animation deformity: a review of 102 reconstructions. Aesthet Surg J. 2018,38(5):519–26.

Hammond DC. Commentary on: Prepectoral revision breast reconstruction for treatment of implant-associated animation deformity: a review of 102 reconstructions. Aesthet Surg J. 2018,38(5):527–8.

12 使用扩张器的胸肌前重建术

编者：Hilton Becker

译者：刘宪强　刘晓宇

随着胸肌前乳房重建术的优势逐渐被认可，该技术正获得越来越广泛的临床应用[1~7]。

很多医师称胸肌前假体置入不仅是其首选术式，部分术者甚至已完全摒弃胸肌后假体置入术[8]。

该术式不仅能有效避免动态畸形、肌肉不适、慢性疼痛及肩关节功能障碍，其美学效果亦常优于胸肌后重建术[9]。

需要特别强调的是，该技术取得理想疗效的前提是乳房切除后残留皮瓣具有足够的厚度并且血供充分。

当皮瓣条件欠佳时，临床医生应如何抉择？目前主要有三种解决方案：胸肌后假体置入术，延期乳房重建术，即刻-延期乳房重建术[10]。

近年来新兴的"扩张器"技术展现了良好的应用前景。该技术通过将未充盈（或空置）的光滑可调式假体置入胸肌前间隙，待确认血运良好后再行填充，其本质等同于延期重建术。当存在血管危象风险时，应采用最小化补片覆盖策略，以便必要时行切口清创处理。

开始时，假体部分充气可显著减轻对菲薄皮瓣（尤其是切口下方区域）的压力。与生理盐水的重力沉积效应相比，气体在假体内分布更为均匀。通过维持假体低充盈状态，可促使皮肤收缩，从而实现皮瓣增厚与上提的双重效果（图 12.1，图 12.2）。

若需进一步增加皮瓣厚度，可辅以实施脂肪移植或延期补片置入[11]。

12.1 操作步骤

包括胸肌前重建在内的所有术式选项均须在术前与患者充分沟通。

完成乳房切除后，必须认真评估组织瓣血供情况。若组织瓣质量良好，可考虑用凝胶假体直接行胸肌前重建术；若组织瓣质量欠佳或血供存疑，则需置入扩张器。

H. Becker (✉)
Department of Surgery, Charles E. Schmidt College of Medicine, Boca Raton, FL, USA

Florida Atlantic University, Boca Raton, FL, USA
e-mail: Hilton@beckermd.com

© The Author(s), under exclusive license to Springer Nature Switzerland AG 2023
R. Vidya, H. Becker (eds.), *Prepectoral Breast Reconstruction*,
https://doi.org/10.1007/978-3-031-15590-1_12

12 使用扩张器的胸肌前重建术

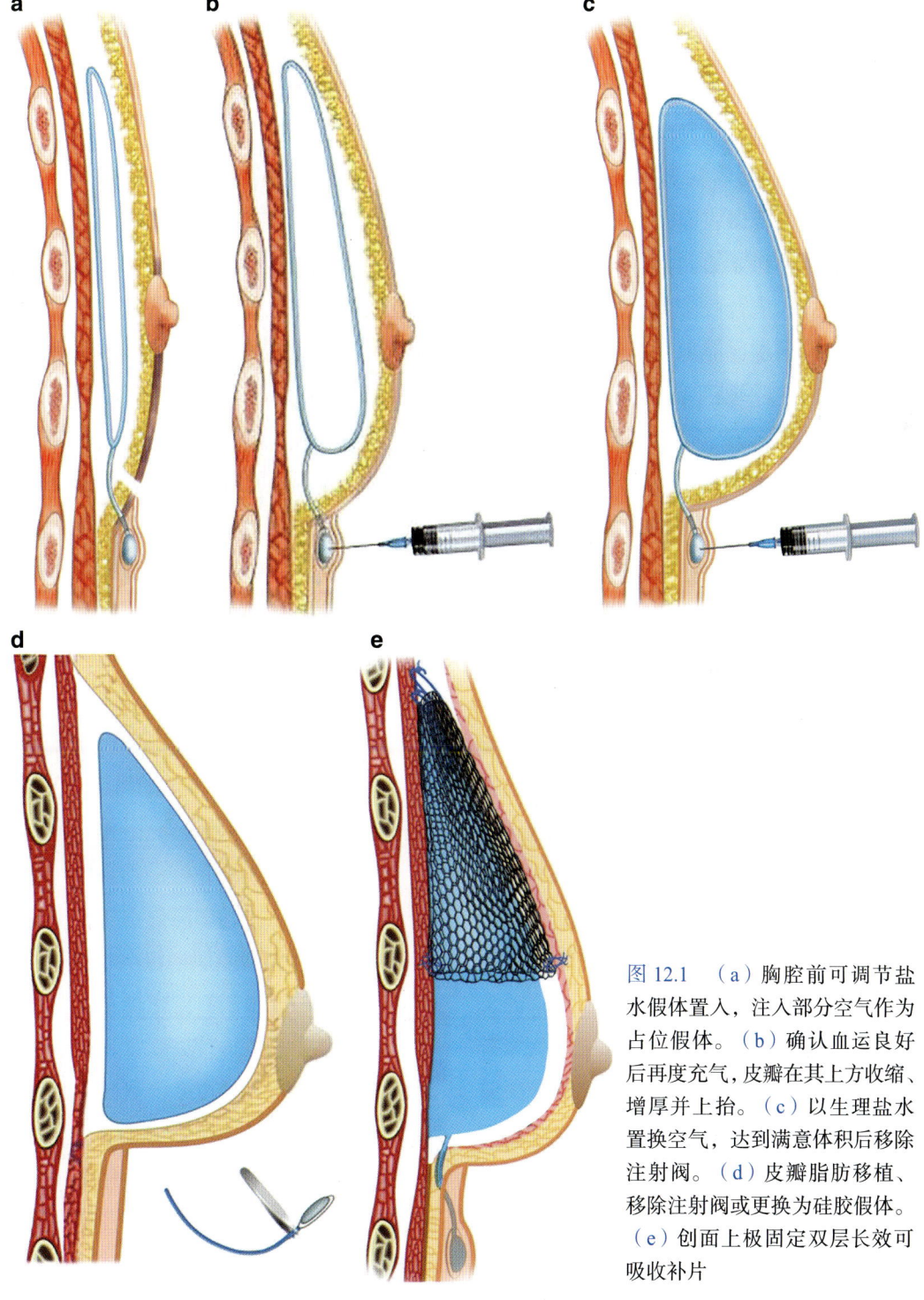

图 12.1 （a）胸腔前可调节盐水假体置入，注入部分空气作为占位假体。（b）确认血运良好后再度充气，皮瓣在其上方收缩、增厚并上抬。（c）以生理盐水置换空气，达到满意体积后移除注射阀。（d）皮瓣脂肪移植、移除注射阀或更换为硅胶假体。（e）创面上极固定双层长效可吸收补片

胸肌前乳房重建

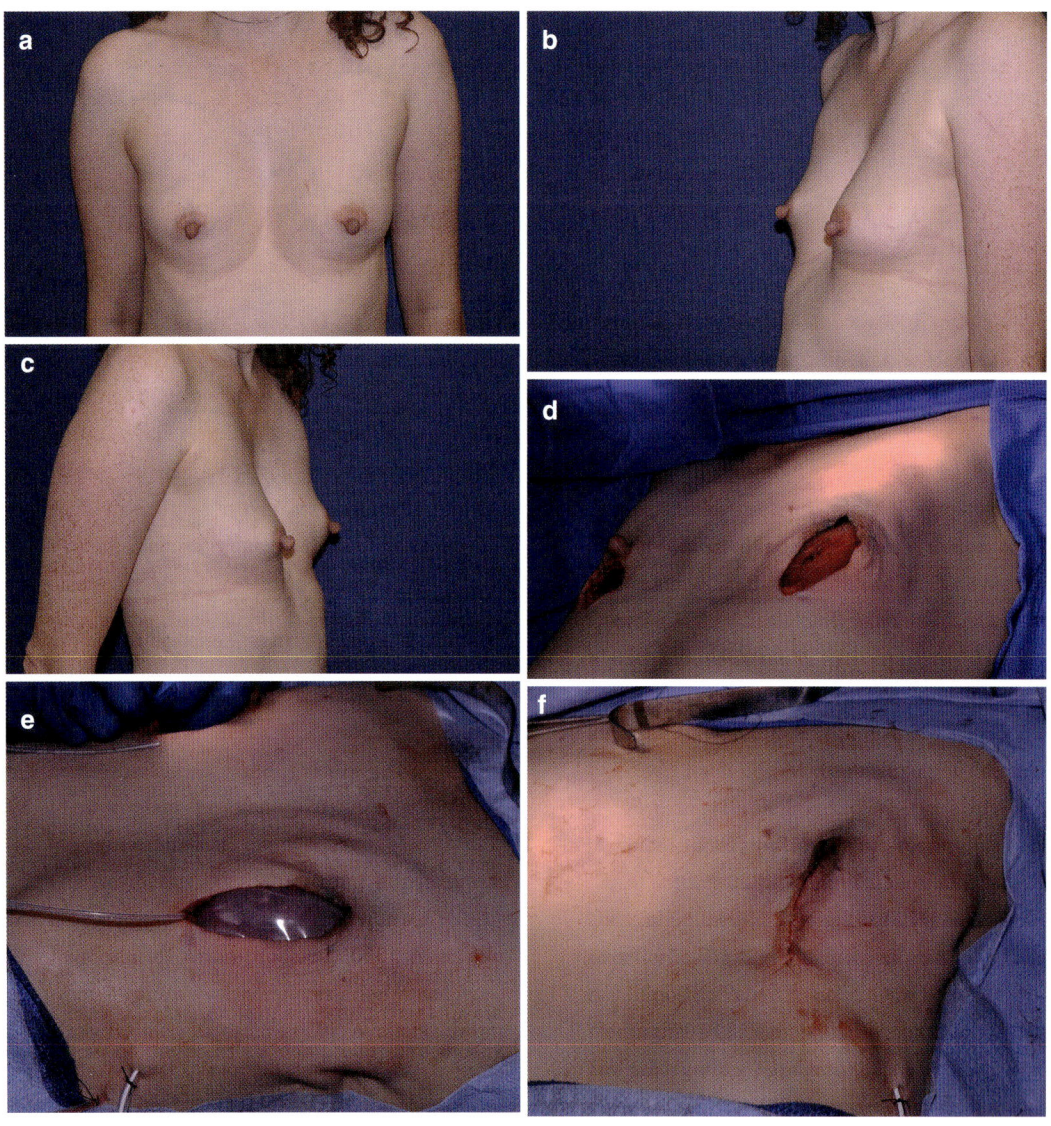

图12.2 （a~c）左乳癌患者拟行双乳切除术。（d）左侧保皮与右侧保乳手术实施后。（e）置入可调节临时占位器并记录皮瓣张力。（f）安放占位假体（基本排空）

不使用SPY（吲哚菁绿）成像技术。适度延迟皮瓣复位可为组织循环恢复创造机会，从而保留可能因循环不良而被迫切除的皮瓣。

使用2-0Vicryl缝线关闭外侧腔隙及腋窝入口，以重建乳房外侧皱襞。

经长的皮下隧道放置2根引流管，并与皮肤固定缝合。

确切止血后，用三联抗生素溶液冲洗腔隙。

最后准备光面可调节假体。可将该假体直接置入腔隙，无须ADM或补片支撑。

必要时使用单丝可完全吸收网状前片如DuraSorb（SIA）。实验表明，双层补片

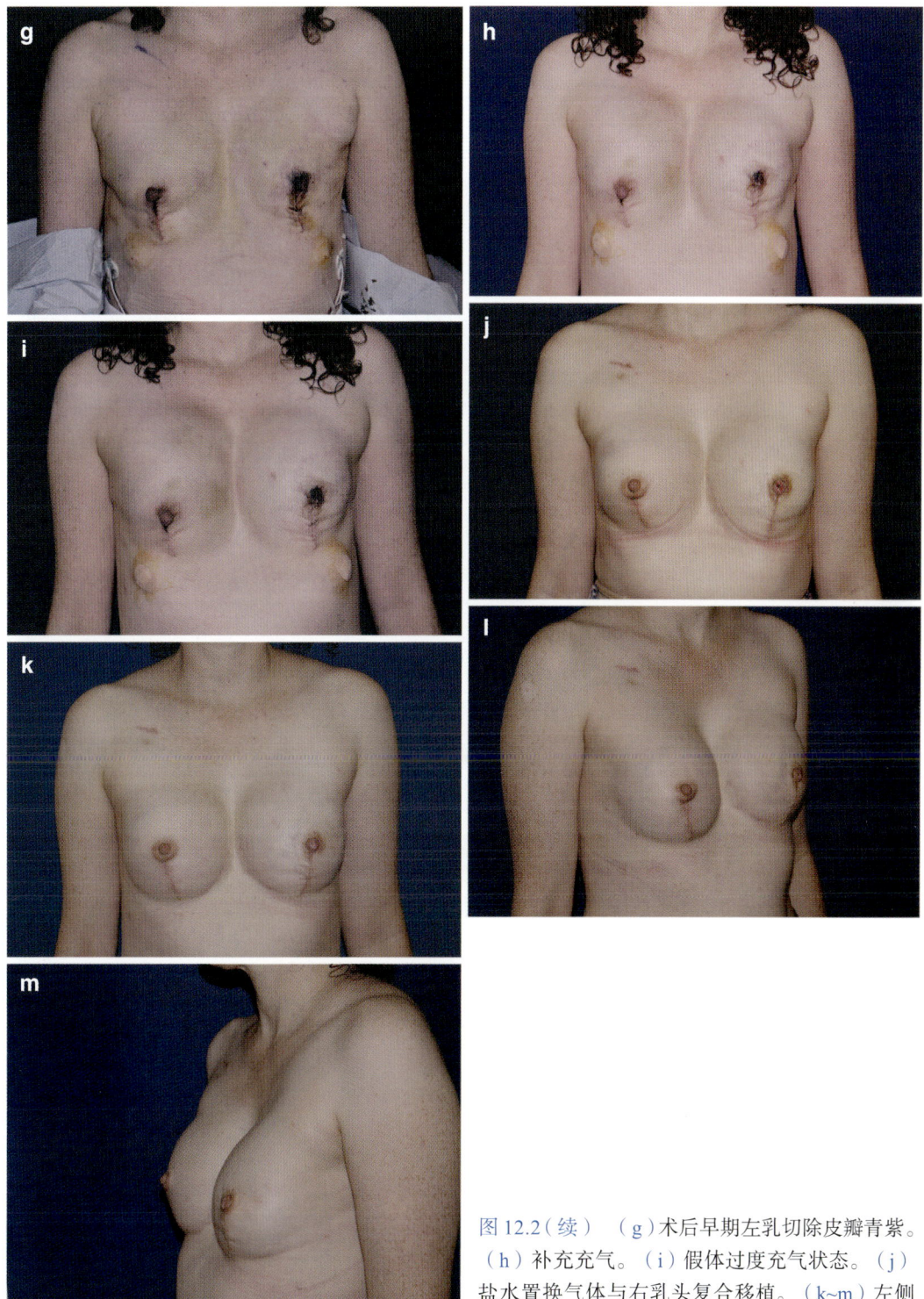

图12.2(续) (g)术后早期左乳切除皮瓣青紫。(h)补充充气。(i)假体过度充气状态。(j)盐水置换气体与右乳头复合移植。(k~m)左侧可调节盐水假体更换为光滑硅胶假体

可形成与使用 ADM 等效的三维包膜厚度效果[12]。

目前采用富血小板血浆（PRP）及脂肪浸润的双层补片，用脂肪来源血管基质成分（SVF）来模拟生物补片（图 12.3）。

因假体预充空气，使用时按需抽出部分气体形成欠充盈状态后置入腔隙。将充盈管修剪至合适长度后连接注射阀。用 Stratafx（Ethicon）缝线将补片固定于胸肌上缘（图 12.3e）。注射阀埋置于切口外侧皮下，用 1~2 针 Vicryl 线固定（图 12.4）。随后行多层缝合：真皮层用 3/0Vicryl 线，表皮层行两列 4-0Monocryl（Ethicon）缝合。

引流管外覆盖 Biopatch（Ethicon）及 Tegaderm（3M）敷料。

皮瓣表面覆以大面积 Tegaderm 敷料及轻质棉纱敷料。

术后次日评估皮瓣血供，通过 23G 蝶形针经注射阀补充假体气体。使用 $0.2\mu m$ 滤菌注射器进行注射。

出现切口边缘坏死者，需排空扩张器并行清创。皮瓣张力消除后，Ⅱ期缝合多可成功（图 12.3）。

乳房形态大小满意后择期取出注射阀。在局部麻醉下沿原切口分离至注射阀，部分游离后退出连接管。于连接器远端夹持充盈管，经假体自密封阀完整取出。

需放疗患者建议保留注射阀至治疗结束，可调节假体体积适配放疗方案，放疗结束后超量扩张数周以减轻包膜挛缩。

必要时行脂肪移植增厚组织瓣（图 12.5）。

若褶皱持续存在，可更换为光面硅胶假体。此时亦可联合补片修补和/或脂肪移植。

12.2 讨论

目前胸肌前乳房重建已成为即刻乳房重建的首选术式。当组织瓣质量欠佳时，多数术者会采用吲哚菁绿成像评估血供。若发现循环障碍，可选择清创或改行胸肌后假体置入，亦可通过延迟即刻重建促进循环恢复，避免不必要的皮肤切除。

同理，术中置入组织扩张器（可调节假体）可产生延迟皮瓣效应，为循环恢复创造治疗窗口，降低组织瓣废弃风险。

即刻乳房重建术风险较高，尤其是在组织瓣条件不佳者时行胸肌前假体置入重建时，故需实施全面风险控制措施：

1. 最小化组织瓣刺激。受损皮瓣不做额外切口，首期手术不游离乳头-乳晕复合体。

2. 置入欠充注光面扩张器。光面假体较毛面假体可减少血清肿、感染等早期并发症。通过排空气囊或降低预充注量，使假体呈现均匀表面形态且避免底部积液[13, 14]。

3. 血供稳定后续行容积调节。

4. 细单丝长效可吸收（1 年内）补片具有显著优势，几乎无感染风险。双层补片可构建三维支撑框架，联合脂肪/富血小板血浆（PRP）可增效。

5. 实现无张力组织瓣闭合。

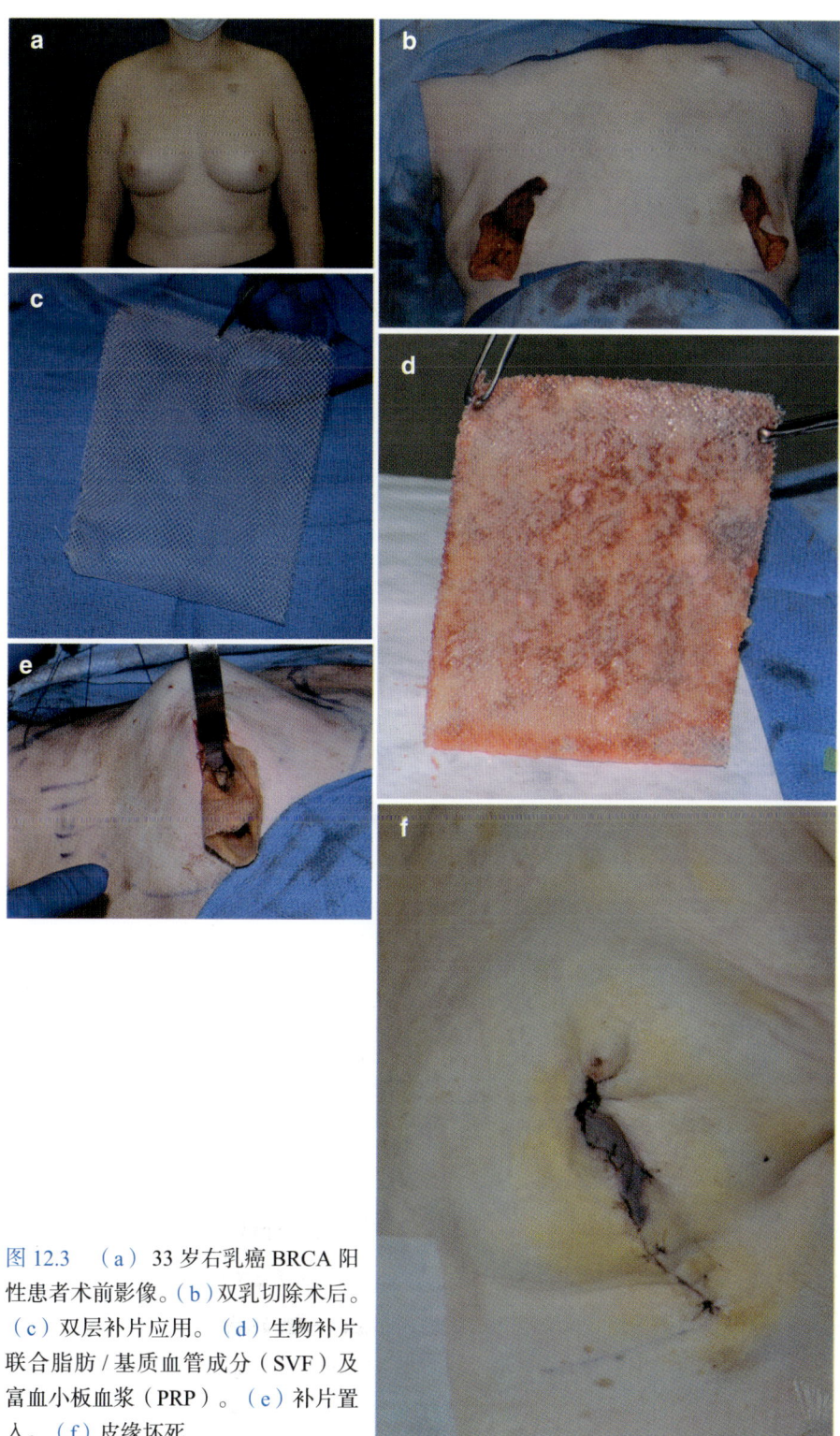

图 12.3 （a）33 岁右乳癌 BRCA 阳性患者术前影像。（b）双乳切除术后。（c）双层补片应用。（d）生物补片联合脂肪/基质血管成分（SVF）及富血小板血浆（PRP）。（e）补片置入。（f）皮缘坏死

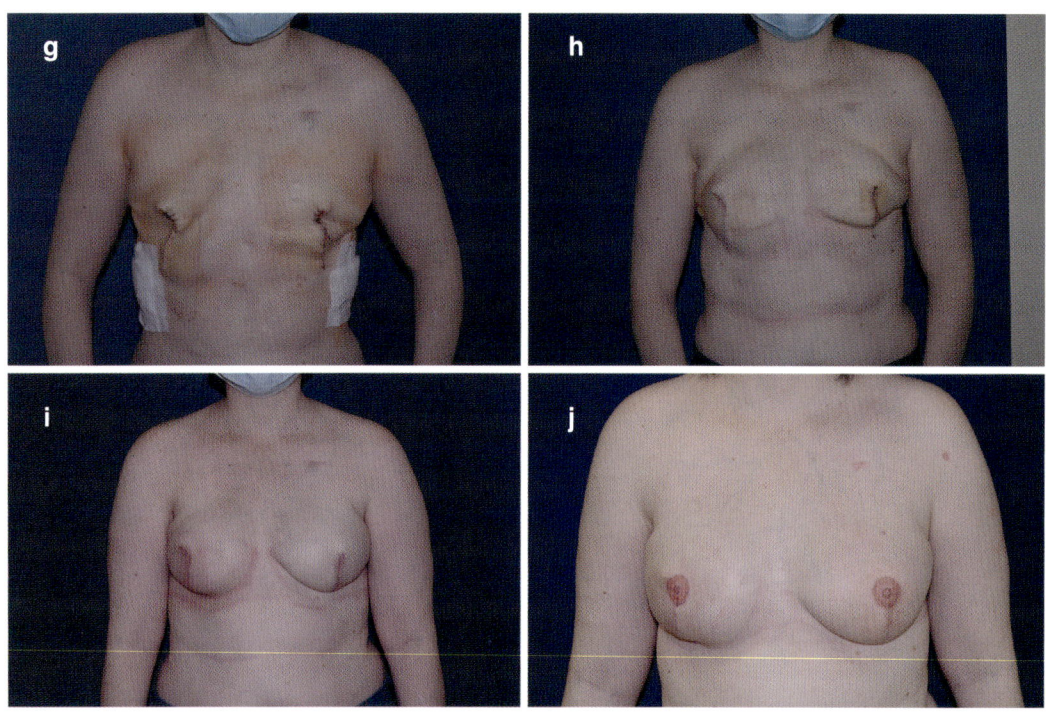

图 12.3（续） （g）清创后Ⅱ期缝合。（h）血运改善后补气。（i）气体置换为盐水。（j）假体更换及乳晕纹饰

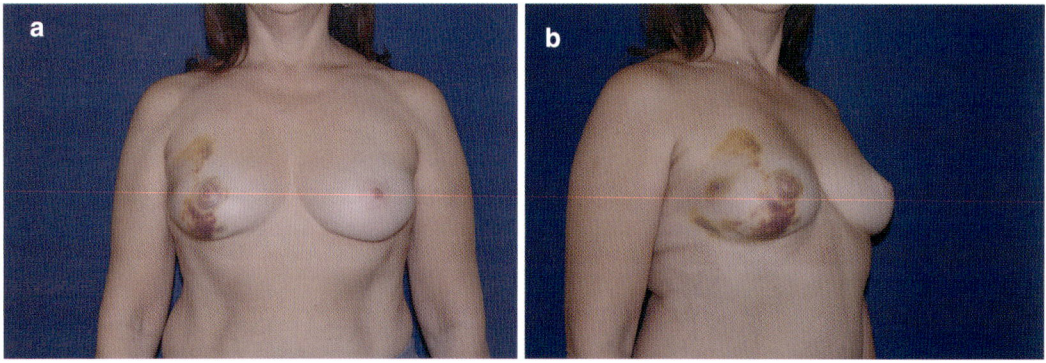

图 12.4 （a，b）右乳癌患者。（c）气体填充占位假体。（d）皮下置入占位假体。（e）注射阀置于切口外侧。（f）术后假体部分充气。（g）盐水置换气体。（h，i）更换为硅胶假体

12 使用扩张器的胸肌前重建术

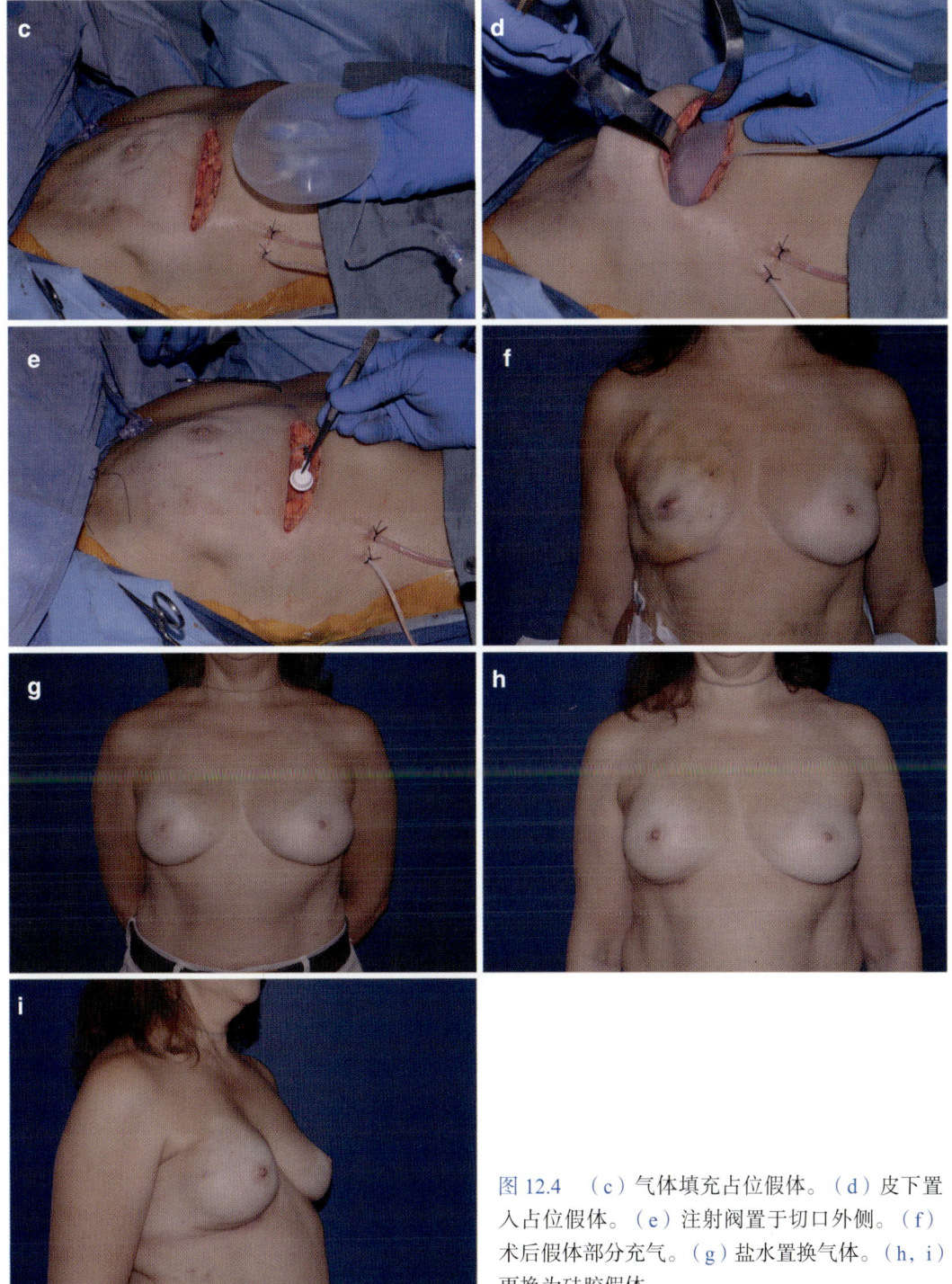

图12.4 （c）气体填充占位假体。（d）皮下置入占位假体。（e）注射阀置于切口外侧。（f）术后假体部分充气。（g）盐水置换气体。（h，i）更换为硅胶假体

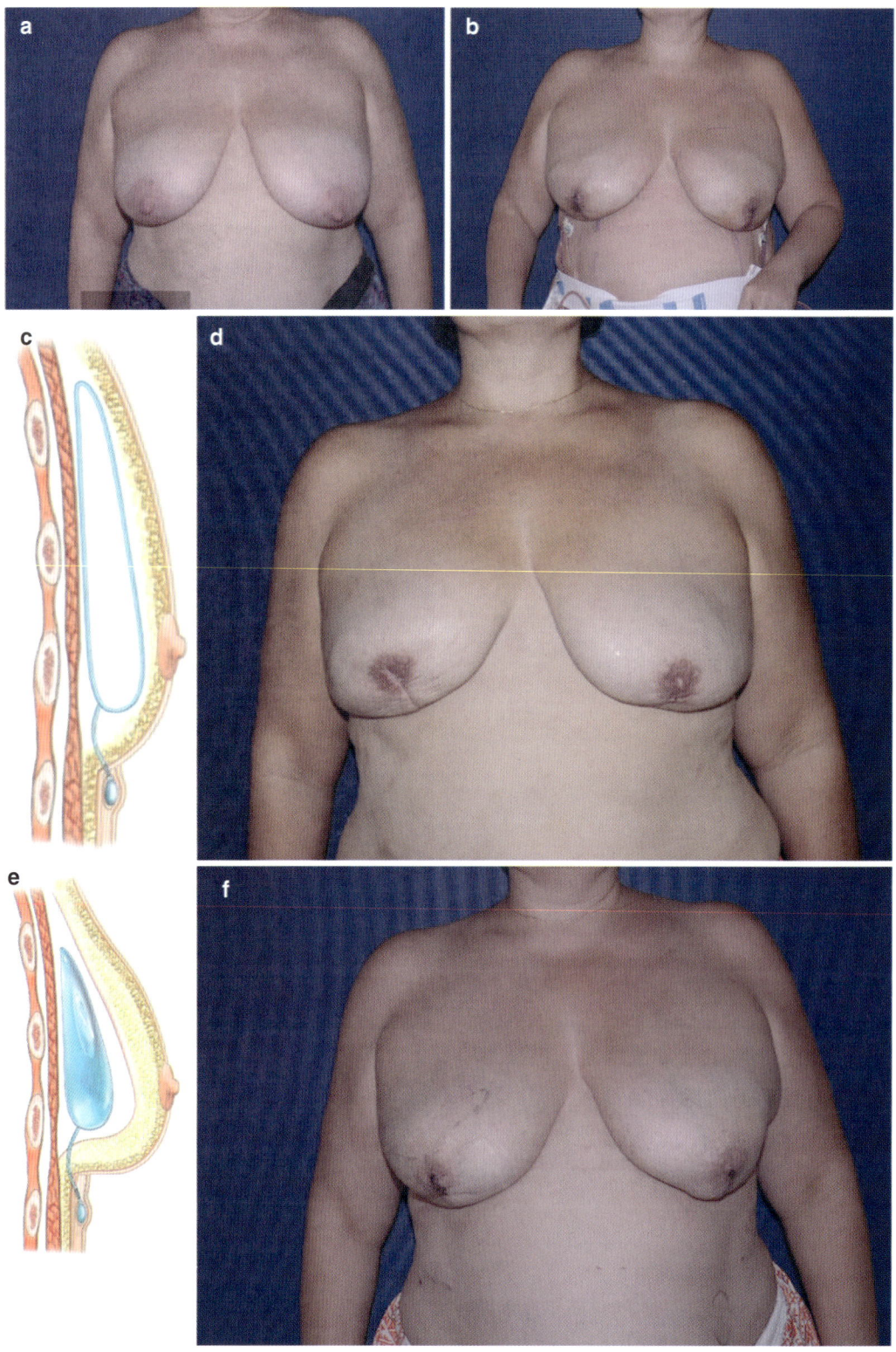

图 12.5 （a）右乳癌 BRCA 阳性患者。（b，c）双乳保皮切除术后胸肌前置入部分充气占位假体。（d，e）盐水置换后实施皮瓣脂肪移植。（f~h）体量调整并追加脂肪移植

12 使用扩张器的胸肌前重建术

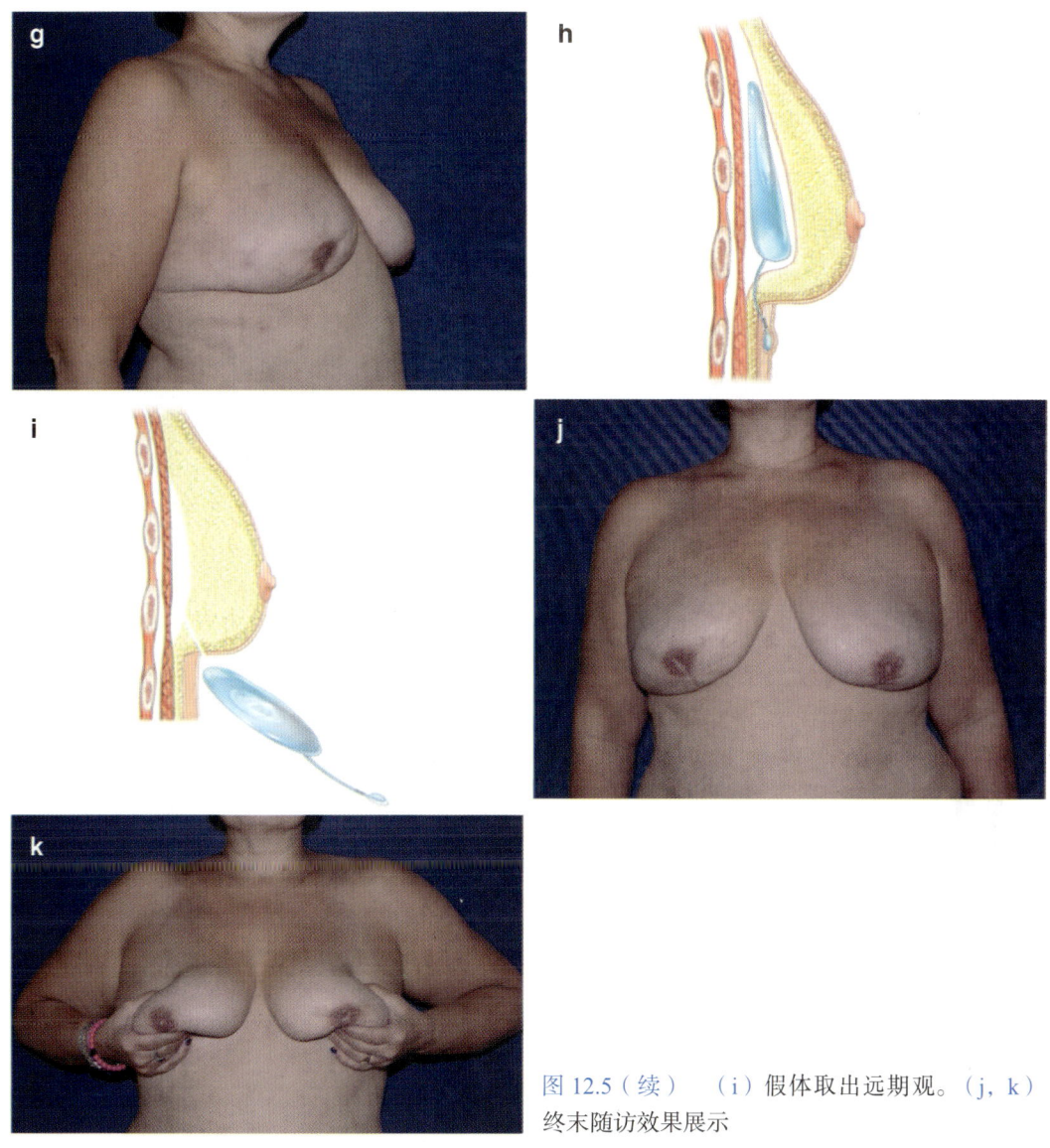

图 12.5（续） （i）假体取出远期观。（j，k）终末随访效果展示

12.3 乳房切除术中未切除的皮瓣血运较差区域

切口采用无张力缝合关闭，为皮瓣恢复创造条件。若需行创缘清创，可将假体排空后完成切口Ⅱ期无张力闭合。

通过保持假体空气未完全充盈，可使囊腔收缩，从而实现皮瓣抬升与增厚[15]。

胸肌前假体重建面临的主要问题之一是因胸肌缺失导致的乳房上极轮廓欠饱满。将多层浸渍脂肪/血管基质组分（SVF）与富血小板血浆（PRP）的 DuraSorb（SIA）补片（生物补片）缝合固定于胸大肌上部并延伸至乳晕上缘，可有效改善上极组织容量不足（图 12.3）。

12.4 小结

胸肌前重建通常需具备足够厚实的皮瓣以获得最佳疗效。若乳房切除术后皮瓣条件欠佳，应考虑使用"扩张器"。

通过促进皮肤自然收缩、延期脂肪移植及置入多层长效可吸收单丝补片等方式，可进一步增加皮瓣厚度。

参考文献

1. Sbitany H, Piper M, Lentz R. Prepectoral breast reconstruction: a safe alternative to submuscular prosthetic reconstruction following nipple-sparing mastectomy. Plast Reconstr Surg. 2017,140(3):432–43.
2. Vidya R, Iqbal FM. A guide to prepectoral breast reconstruction: a new dimension to implant-based breast reconstruction. Clin Breast Cancer. 2017,17(4):266–71.
3. Becker H, Lind JG 2nd, Hopkins EG. Immediate implant-based prepectoral breast reconstruction using a vertical incision. Plast Reconstr Surg Glob Open. 2015,3(6):e412.
4. Ter Louw RP, Nahabedian MY. Prepectoral breast reconstruction. Plast Reconstr Surg. 2017,140(5 Suppl):51S–9S.
5. Eskenazi LB. New options for immediate reconstruction: achieving optimal results with adjustable implants in a single stage. Plast Reconstr Surg. 2007,119:28–37.
6. Woo A, Harless C, Jacobson SR. Revisiting an old place: single-surgeon experience on post-mastectomy subcutaneous implant-based breast reconstruction. Breast J. 2017,23:545–53.
7. The aesthetic meeting 20/20 april Aesthetic Breast Reconstruction Co-Chairs: Nolan Karp, MD and John Kim, MD: Pre-Pectoral Breast Reconstruction.
8. Hilton Becker MD. Correction of animation deformity. Plastic surgery pulse news. 2017,7(1).
9. Zenn MR. Staged immediate breast reconstruction. Plast Reconstr Surg. 2015,135(4):976–9.
10. Mayer HF, editor. Breast reconstruction: modern and promising surgical techniques. Springer Nature;2020.
11. Becker H. Breast reconstruction using an inflatable breast implant with detachable reservoir. Plast Reconstr Surg. 1984,73:678–3.
12. Becker H, Zhadan O. Filling the spectrum expander with air—a new alternative. Plast Reconstr Surg Glob Open. 2017,6:e1541.
13. Becker H, Carlisle H, Kay J. Filling of adjustable breast implants beyond the manufacturer's recommended fill volume. Aesthetic Plast Surg. 2008,32(3):432–41.
14. 15 Tissue Contraction—A New Paradigm in Breast Reconstruction Hilton Becker, MD, FACS*†‡ Olga Zhadan, MD, MS §PRS Global Open • 2018.
15. Becker H, Maraist F. Immediate breast reconstruction after mastectomy using a permanent tissue expander. South Med J. 1987,80(2):154–60.

13 合成补片在胸肌前乳房重建中的应用

编者：D. Casella, J. Kaciulytc, V. Restaino, F. Lo Torto, M. Marcasciano
译者：刘 琪

13.1 引言

胸肌前即刻乳房重建（IBR）由 Snyderman 和 Guthrie 于 1971 年首次提出[1]。与传统的胸肌后重建术相比，该技术显著缩短了恢复周期，患者满意度也较高，因此被认为是假体重建乳房领域的重大进展[2]。尽管存在明显的预期收益，但皮下异体重建很快被发现与包膜挛缩发生率升高，假体的可见、可触及性增高、波纹形成、乳房切除术后皮瓣坏死高风险及假体外露等并发症相关。合成补片（SM）与脱细胞真皮基质（ADM）的应用逐步确立了全包裹假体理念，为假体置入乳房重建手术（尤其是胸肌前重建）开辟了新方向。

2013 年，Cheng 等[3]首次报道了一种新型外科技术，在胸肌前置入用脱细胞真皮基质完整包裹的假体，用于治疗胸肌后乳房重建术后发生的包膜挛缩。

2014 年，在一组诊断为乳腺癌并接受保留皮肤和乳头乳房切除术的患者中[4]，首次将钛涂层聚丙烯补片（TCPM）完全包裹的乳房假体置入皮下腔隙。

无论是脱细胞真皮基质（ADM）还是合成补片，并在胸肌前即刻乳房重建术（IBR）中展现了良好的美学与功能效果[5]，同时其安全性也得到证明。皮下乳房重建通过避免肌肉剥离，降低了术区发病率并保留了乳房的自然解剖结构。包裹装置的支持力可实现假体完全覆盖，从而避免其与乳房切除术后皮瓣直接接触。

D. Casella (✉) · V. Restaino
Department of Breast Cancer Surgery,
UOC Chirurgia Oncologica Della Mammella,
Azienda Ospedaliero-Universitaria Senese,
University Hospital of Siena, Siena, Italy

J. Kaciulyte · F. L. Torto
Department of Surgery "P.Valdoni", Unit of Plastic and Reconstructive Surgery, Sapienza University of Rome, Policlinico Umberto I, Roma, Italy

M. Marcasciano
Experimental and Clinical Medicine Department,
Division of Plastic and Reconstructive Surgery,
"Magna Graecia" University of Catanzaro
Germaneto, Catanzaro, Italy

© The Author(s), under exclusive license to Springer Nature Switzerland AG 2023
R. Vidya, H. Becker (eds.), *Prepectoral Breast Reconstruction*,
https://doi.org/10.1007/978-3-031-15590-1_13

与传统的肌下术式相比，胸肌前术式能显著减轻术后疼痛并缩短手术时间。此外，文献显示该术式美学效果良好，并发症发生率似与胸肌后重建相当[6]。

事实上，目前还没有适用于所有患者的标准术式，胸肌后与胸肌前乳房重建均可获得理想疗效。应根据患者的生理与病史特征提供个体化最佳重建方案，必须全面理解每项技术的优势与局限性。

与其他术式相同，胸肌前乳房重建也存在局限，充足的皮瓣血供与均匀的皮下组织厚度是确保手术成功的前提条件。软组织质量欠佳（如存在皮瓣受损或微循环障碍）的患者将面临更高的假体外露与重建失败风险[7]。

术前精准规划与严格筛选患者始终是手术成功的关键，在进行胸肌前乳房重建时须遵循[8]。

自1882年Halstead根治性乳房切除术问世以来，不断发展的肿瘤外科术式趋向保守化，致力于保留皮肤与乳头-乳晕复合体。Umberto Veronesi开创性地推动微创术式的转变，提出"从最大耐受治疗转向最小有效治疗"理念[9]。在此趋势下，"美学癌症治疗"与"肿瘤整形外科"新理念应运而生，通过有效的肿瘤切除手术联合乳房美学保护或改善，形成了动态优化的患者管理模式[10]。

胸肌前乳房重建完美契合这一现代理念。得益于假体材料与合成补片（SM）等外科器械的最新进展，该术式已演变为可靠、安全且具美学可行性的重建方案，总体并发症发生率处于可接受范围[11]。

13.2 患者选择

通过对多项术前与术中变量进行全面评估，必须严格筛选患者。手术风险需通过精准化、个体化方法进行评估，文献中的多项研究报道可为此提供参考，有助外科医生决策及判定胸肌前乳房重建的可行性。2017年，Rancati等[12]提出一项算法，核心为通过数字化乳腺X线摄影评估术前皮瓣厚度，以此指导手术规划。同样，Mlodinow等[13]引入乳房重建风险评估（BRA）评分系统，用于评估自体与异体内置物即刻乳房重建术（IBR）的术后并发症风险。2019年，Vidya等[14]发布了由欧美乳腺外科与整形重建外科医生联合签署的国际共识，可为胸肌前乳房重建术提供指导，涵盖患者筛选、手术技术及疗效等。尽管上述工具颇具价值，但针对皮下乳房重建术适应患者的鉴别标准——尤其是如何精准预测直接假体置入术（DTI）或组织扩张器两阶段重建术式的最佳适用者——尚未达成共识。实施胸肌前乳房重建术前需考虑多种变量，以最终预测乳房切除术后皮瓣缺血坏死风险。必须全面评估患者全身健康状况，包括完整个人史及常规临床检查。老年患者、BMI异常、活跃吸烟者或糖尿病患者的微循环可能受损，发生皮瓣坏死、假体外露或感染的风险升高[15-17]。同理，需行缩皮乳房切除术的乳房下垂亦与乳房下皱襞区假体外露风险增高相关[18]。

必须详尽采集患者的相关病史，既往乳房手术史、既往放疗史与术后伤口裂开及感染的高风险相关[19]。术中对乳房切除术后皮瓣厚度及潜在存活能力进行评估亦至关重要，厚度合适且含血管化皮下脂肪的皮瓣是获得良好术后效果的前提[20]。吲哚菁绿荧光血管造影技术作为一种客观可靠的评估方法，被推荐用于乳房切除术后皮瓣存活能力的评估，但该技术价格昂贵，并非在所有医疗机构均可获取。此外，目前仍缺乏高质量证据证明其优于精准的术中临床评估，所以仍需更大规模研究以推动此项创新技术的普及[21]。

13.3 合成补片

随着新技术的开发、合成及生物补片装置的改进，以及自体脂肪移植技术的进步[22]，乳房重建方式逐渐从肌下转移至胸肌前平面。合成补片约20年前已引入乳房手术[23]，与脱细胞真皮基质相比，兼具良好强度与柔顺性且价格更低，但用于乳房重建存在显著的学习曲线[24]。合成补片能形成完整的内置物包膜，并作为假体与皮下组织间的附加层发挥类似"新筋膜层"的作用[25]。

合成补片具有弹性，分为可吸收型、部分可吸收型及不可吸收型，可为假体提供牵拉支持，其强度与弹性保持平衡：强度增加时弹性减弱，同时可能加剧炎症反应[26]。合成补片与周围组织的整合能力取决于其孔隙大小，孔隙直径与组织长入量及纤维组织形成呈正相关[26]；其强度与柔韧性则由经编或编织的制造工艺决定，编织补片因纤维密度高而强度更大，经编补片则具有多孔性及柔韧性特质[27]。

表13.1总结了乳房重建领域主要合成补片的特征参数[28~33]。

不同的可吸收补片的吸收时间不同，可为数个月（乙丙交酯共聚物 Vicryl）[34]，也可为2~3年（Seri Surgical Scaffold、TIGR Matrix）[35, 36]。长期吸收的理论依据在于其含有快速降解纤维以在伤口愈合阶段提供额外支撑，而慢吸收纤维可持续数年维持内置物稳定性[37]。Seri Surgical Scaffold由丝质材料制成，其特性更接近脱细胞真皮基质（ADM），因其置入后可形成新生组织并完成力学性能转移[38, 39]。

在不可吸收补片中，仅聚丙烯（PP）材质产品被应用于乳房重建（TiLOOP Bra/Pocket、TiO2Mesh BRA）[40, 41]。此外，部分补片采用混合材质并具备部分可吸收特性（ULTRAPRO、SERAGYN BR）[31, 42]。近期，Eichler 等[43]对不可吸收 TiLOOP 补片与部分可吸收 Seragyn 补片开展对比研究，发现两者并发症发生率无显著差异，总体假体损失率与价格昂贵的脱细胞真皮基质重建术相当。

数年前本团队率先将钛化聚丙烯材料补片 TiLoop® Bra（德国科隆 pfm medical 公司）应用于胸肌前乳房重建，相关经验已发表[44-47]。该即用型补片由不可吸收的1a型钛化聚丙烯制成，无须复水处理，已通过认证并获准临床应用。近期其升级版本推出，采用预成型囊袋设计以简化术中介入操作并缩短手术时间。该补片表面钛化处理，可促进细胞生长，同时降低瘢痕形成、补片皱缩、炎症反应及包膜挛缩

表 13.1　乳房重建用合成补片

吸收性聚合物		材料来源	吸收时间	最终抗拉强度（N 或 N/cm）	乳房重建参考文献
	Vicryl 补片	乙丙交酯共聚物	3 个月	–	Faulkner 等[29]
	Seargyn BR（部分可吸收）	聚乙二醇己内酯/聚丙烯	3~4 个月	41 N/cm	Machleidt 等[31]
	ULTRAPRO（部分可吸收）	聚卡环酮-25 单丝/不可吸收聚丙烯	3~4 个月	–	József 等[32]
	Seri Surgical Scaffold	蚕丝蛋白	2 年	99.7 N	van Turnhout 等[28]
	TIGR Matrix	丙交酯-乙交酯-碳酸三亚甲基酯共聚物	3 年	86.6 N/cm	Hallberg 等[33]
不可吸收的钛涂层聚合物					
	TiLOOP Bra	镀钛聚丙烯网片	–	37 N/cm	Casella 等[30]
	TiO$_2$ Mesh Bra	镀氧化钛的单丝聚丙烯	–	–	–

的发生率，此特性为所有钛涂层合成补片共有[48~50]。

13.4　手术技术

乳腺手术团队通常由普外科与整形外科医师组成，各自提供专业技术。有研究表明，兼具乳腺肿瘤学与整形外科双重资质的复合型医师可独立完成手术，凭借对乳腺癌治疗的综合理解，可提供更广泛的手术选择并提高治疗成功率[51]。本团队的所有胸肌前乳房重建术（含永久或暂时假体置入）均由此类双资质复合型医师实施，同步把控肿瘤根治与重建环节[52]。

术前必须完善患者综合评估。若预计能保留具有活力且可靠的乳房切除皮瓣，则规划胸肌前重建术，同时须于术中对皮瓣进行再评估，保留中转为胸肌后术式的可能性。于患者站立位进行术前体表标记，包括胸骨中线与旁正中线、乳房下皱襞及切口位置。根据肿瘤学特征、病灶位置、患者个体差异及乳房形态，可选择乳房下皱襞、倒 T 形、"斜 S" 形或乳晕周切口行乳房切除术。在真皮下平面进行皮瓣分离，沿 Cooper 悬韧带行解剖分离，最终置入胸肌前永久假体前必须充分评估切缘出血状况及皮瓣活力。若皮瓣菲薄或对血供存疑，则首选临时扩张器分阶段重建。

需要特别说明的是，当保留乳头和乳晕乳房切除术后皮肤覆盖层难以支撑永久假体时，则需置入组织扩张器作为临时占位器。

皮下囊腔初始注容 30% 以避免组织愈合期皮瓣张力过高。组织扩张器在保留皮肤乳房切除术后的应用策略有差异，主要通过逐步注水扩张以期形成适宜的皮肤覆盖层用于后续永久假体置入。无论采用直接假体置入（DTI）或分步重建术式，均须将补片（SM）包绕假体后通过顶部、内侧及外侧缝合固定于胸大肌筋膜。术后即刻予以适度加压包扎，并于 60 天后更换为术后专用胸罩。对于特定病例，尤其是接受缩皮式乳房切除术或存在术后并发症高风险患者，可采用负压伤口敷料（如英国施乐辉公司 PICO 负压系统）以预防切口并发症，缩短瘢痕形成时间并减少术后复诊次数[53]。

分阶段重建病例通常于出院后 3 周进行首次术后扩张。

13.5　自体脂肪移植

自 Rigotti 等[54]于 2007 年首次报道脂肪移植的临床获益以来，该技术在乳房重建领域的重要性日益凸显，现已成为胸肌前重建路径的关键环节。自体脂肪组织取材便捷，其血管基质成分中含脂肪来源干细胞（ASC）。脂肪来源干细胞（ASC）经移植后通过自组织与分化效应，具有促进新生血管生成、抗细胞凋亡及免疫调节等作用[55]。临床可利用上述特性防治乳房重建术后或放疗后相关并发症，如褶皱形成、包膜挛缩、感染、组织溃破及假体外露等[56]。基于 ASC 的肿瘤学安全性可靠且未增加肿瘤复发风险，目前在胸肌前/胸肌后重建术中均已建立自体脂肪移植规范[57]。

关于扩张器/假体乳房重建术中脂肪移植的实施时机尚存争议，目前有多种方案[58, 59]。胸肌前重建术后脂肪移植策略的相关证据仍显不足。本团队经验显示，若皮下置入合成补片包裹的组织扩张器，可于 II 期重建阶段实施单次脂肪填充，必要时重复操作。据此，传统三步法（两次扩张联合一次填充）可精简为经典 II 期流程。该方案不仅能改善覆盖永久假体的乳房切除术后皮瓣质量，亦可预防假体表浅化、包膜挛缩及轮廓显形等问题，显著提升美学与功能疗效。对于术后放疗患者，实施脂肪移植可降低局部感染/溃破、假体移位及包膜挛缩的发生率，效果与非放疗重建病例相当[60]。

13.6　并发症

胸肌前术式具有操作快捷安全、患者耐受性良好等优势，但亦存在一定缺陷。近期系统评价显示，包膜挛缩为胸肌前乳房重建术后最常见并发症，发生率可达 8.8%[61]。包膜挛缩的病理生理机制，涉及机体异物反应、生物膜激活、菌血症侵袭或硅胶暴露等，常继发于术后放疗，导致乳房外形异常、疼痛及美学缺陷[56]。如前所述，脂肪移植或有助防治早期包膜挛缩，但部分病例仍需行包膜切开、包膜切除联合假体置换等[62, 63]。Sinnott

等的研究表明，胸肌前重建+放疗后包膜挛缩的发生率仅为胸肌后术式的1/3（16.1%：52.2%）[64]。

上述差异可能与放疗后胸大肌纤维化产生的额外机械应力导致假体移位及相关包膜挛缩进展有关[65]。另一方面，因缺乏肌层覆盖，若乳房切除术后皮瓣过薄或厚度不均（尤其是上极和内侧区域），则可能引发假体显形（波纹征），发生率为12.9%~19.4%（随随访时间延长递增）[66]。脂肪移植可改善此类问题，尤其适用于内上及外侧象限。直接假体置入（DTI）重建术后常需后续脂肪填充等修整手术，术前应与患者充分沟通。

其余并发症如血清肿（5.1%）、血肿（2.4%）、皮瓣或乳头-乳晕复合体（NAC）坏死伴假体丢失（3.3%）等，虽发生率较低但后果严重[61]。

细致止血及合理安放引流管可预防上述并发症。血清肿可引发疼痛、不适，或进一步进展为感染及皮瓣坏死等严重问题，故应及时规范处理，必要时行穿刺抽吸。可在超声引导下实施细针抽吸；使用临时扩张器时可行徒手操作，利用注水阀周围安全区抽取假体与周围组织间积液，同步完成组织扩张并避免假体意外破裂[67]。

皮瓣或乳头-乳晕复合体（NAC）坏死源于肿瘤根治性切除操作所致的血管损伤，或假体过度压迫过薄或张力过高的切除后皮瓣，表覆软组织缺损将导致灾难性后果乃至重建失败。术前精准筛选患者并在术中全面评估皮瓣活力（如吲哚菁绿灌注显像）可预防或降低此类风险。如前所述，若对皮瓣可靠性存疑，建议放弃直接假体置入术（DTI）转为分阶段组织扩张器重建方案。因置入部位及适应证不同，假体周围感染率为1.1%~35%[68]。

尽管胸肌前与胸肌后重建的感染率相近[69]，但前者相关文献数据稀疏且缺乏已获共识的管理方案。常规处置策略包括抗生素治疗及修复手术（部分/全包膜切除术并移除感染假体）以清除定植组织[70]。胸肌前囊袋修复时因包膜毗邻皮肤，存在组织减薄过度及皮瓣活力受损风险。此时，脉冲灌洗技术凭借其交替喷射-抽吸无菌生理盐水的特性可实现流体动力清洁，成为有效辅助手段[71~73]。针对胸肌前假体感染，本团队于移除扩张器时应用脉冲灌洗技术，彻底清创并重建健康皮下囊腔后直接置入永久假体，省去二次手术步骤。

红色乳房综合征为特发性术后短暂性红斑，既往仅见于应用脱细胞真皮基质重建病例，据报道发生率高达7.6%[74]。该病类似蜂窝织炎并伴瘙痒、疼痛，但无感染客观证据。目前仅有一例报道描述应用合成聚乙醇酸补片行即刻胸肌前乳房重建后出现此症并自行缓解的案例[75]。

需要强调的是，基于补片的胸肌前假体乳房重建虽可取得优良效果，但严格把控适应证、全面认识潜在并发症并采取正确处置策略，是获得理想疗效的核心要素。

13.7 当前文献回顾

乳房重建术式多样，涵盖自体组织移植至假体置入。自20世纪60年代硅凝胶乳房假体问世以来，假体乳房重建术（implant-based reconstruction，IBR）已成为主流，约占目前重建病例的70%[76]。伴随重建技术进步，乳腺肿瘤外科逐步向保乳理念发展，摒弃了 Halsted 根治性术式[77]。

随着创新假体材料、覆盖装置、皮瓣灌注评估技术及成熟脂肪移植的应用，乳腺癌根治术与乳房重建术协同发展。其中，假体覆盖装置（脱细胞真皮基质 ADM 与补片 SM）于 2006 年引入临床，为胸肌前重建提供了全新视角[78]。

胸肌前重建术将假体置于正常解剖平面，美学效果佳且并发症发生率低。但因临床复兴时间较短，现有应用补片的胸肌前重建研究随访时间偏短，远期疗效资料有限[79]。首篇合成补片应用于乳房重建的文献发表于 1997 年（Rietjens 等[80]），但其研究对象为胸肌后假体重建，术中补片用于强化假体外下极支撑，与多数文献报道方案类同。

针对补片在胸肌前重建的应用，Reitsamer 等[81]报道 200 例应用 ADM 或可吸收 TIGR 补片的即刻假体重建术疗效满意，平均随访 36 个月。Casella 等[30]应用 TiLoop 补片亦获良好结局与美学效果（平均随访 38.5 个月），并发症发生率低。

已有研究比较胸肌前与胸肌后乳房重建术的术后并发症发生率，结果显示二者在感染、皮肤坏死及血清肿等方面的发生率相似[82]。其他研究报告旨在扩大胸肌前重建术的适用范围。Caputo 等[83]描述了胸肌前重建在需要显著缩小皮肤面积的病例中取得的良好效果；Marcasciano 等[84]报道了采用胸肌前假体联合下侧皮瓣与合成补片覆盖技术进行缩乳乳房重建的类似结果。

创新与持续演进是现代肿瘤乳腺外科的显著特征。Salibian 等[85]指出，保留血供良好且具有充分活力的乳房切除皮瓣，并严格保护原生乳房下皱襞，可避免使用假体覆盖装置。

随着乳房重建效果的提升及其重要性的凸显，当代乳腺外科医师应重视持续理念更新并加强跨学科协作，因为创新与进步并非源于孤立工作，而是基于多方合作及思想与知识的共享。最新文献指出，当前医疗环境正发生明显改变，患者参与度逐步提高，对重建效果及其对生活质量影响的关注度显著提升[86]，研究进展与知识共享不可或缺，乳腺外科医师须探索新的交流途径以保持技术更新与提升，从而持续为患者提供最佳治疗方案[87]。事实上，胸肌前乳房重建术的复兴印证了科学研究的进步不仅依赖新技术的发明，亦可通过对现有技术的回溯与历史术式的改良来实现。

13.8 小结

- 假体置入乳房重建是乳房切除术后最常用的重建方式。
- 传统观点认为，胸肌后重建是标准术式。
- 脱细胞真皮基质（ADM）与合成补片（SM）的应用逐步确立了全包裹假体理念，为假体置入技术开拓了新方向，并为胸肌前乳房重建术的复兴创造了条件。

- 采用 SM 的皮下乳房重建术可避免肌肉损伤，从而减轻术后疼痛并缩短手术时间。美容效果更优，并发症发生率与胸肌后重建术相似。
- 充足的皮肤血供支持与可靠的乳房切除皮瓣质量，是胸肌前乳房重建术实施的限制因素，因此详尽的术前规划与严格的病例选择至关重要。
- 自体脂肪移植应被视为胸肌前重建的重要组成部分，研究证实其可减少术后皱褶、包膜挛缩、感染、溃疡及假体外露等并发症风险。

参考文献

1. Snyderman RK, Guthrie RH. Reconstruction of the female breast following radical mastectomy. Plast Reconstr Surg. 1971,47:565–7.
2. Kobraei EM, Cauley R, Gadd M, Austen WG Jr, Liao EC. Avoiding breast animation deformity with pectoralis-sparing subcutaneous direct-to-implant breast reconstruction. Plast Reconstr Surg Glob Open. 2016,4:e708.
3. Cheng A, Lakhiani C, Saint-Cyr M. Treatment of capsular contracture using complete implant coverage by acellular dermal matrix: a novel technique. Plast Reconstr Surg. 2013,132:519–29.
4. Casella D, Bernini M, Benci ni L, Roselli J, Lacaria MT, Martellucci J, Banfi R, Calabrese C, Orzalesi L. TiLoop® bra mesh used for immediate breast reconstruction: comparison of retropectoral and subcutaneous implant placement in a prospective single institution series. Eur J Plast Surg. 2014,37:599–604.
5. Lo Torto F, Cigna E, Kaciulyte J, Casella D, Marcasciano M, Ribuffo D. National breast reconstruction utilization in the setting of postmastectomy radiotherapy: two-stage implant-based breast reconstruction. J Reconstr Microsurg. 2017,33:e3.
6. Jafferbhoy S, Chandarana M, Houlihan M, Parmeshwar R, Narayanan S, Soumian S, Harries S, Jones L, Clarke D. Early multicentre experience of pre-pectoral implant based immediate breast reconstruction using Braxon®. Gland Surg. 2017,6:682–8.
7. Cattelani L, Polotto S, Arcuri MF, Pedrazzi G, Linguadoca C, Bonati E. One-step prepectoral breast reconstruction with dermal matrix-covered implant compared to submuscular implantation: functional and cost evaluation. Clin Breast Cancer. 2018,18:e703–11.
8. Sbitany H. Important considerations for performing Prepectoral breast reconstruction. Plast Reconstr Surg. 2017,140:7S–13S.
9. Zurrida S, Veronesi U. Milestones in breast cancer treatment. Breast J. 2015,21:3–12.
10. Kaufman CS. Increasing role of oncoplastic surgery for breast cancer. Curr Oncol Rep. 2019,21:111.
11. Maxwell GP, Gabriel A. Bioengineered breast: concept, technique, and preliminary results. Plast Reconstr Surg. 2016,137:415–21.
12. Rancati AO, Angrigiani CH, Hammond DC, Nava MB, Gonzalez EG, Dorr JC, Gercovich GF, Rocco N, Rostagno RL. Direct to implant reconstruction in nipple sparing mastectomy: patient selection by preoperative digital mammogram. Plast Reconstr Surg Glob Open. 2017,5:e1369.
13. Mlodinow AS, Lanier ST, Galiano RD, Kim JYS. Using the breast reconstruction risk assessment (BRA) score: an individualized risk calculator to assist expectation management and reconstructive decision making in the mastectomy patient. In: Harness J, Willey S, editors. Operative approaches to nipple-sparing mastectomy. Springer: Cham; 2017. p. 117–26.
14. Vidya R, Berna G, Sbitany H, Nahabedian M, Becker H, Reitsamer R, Rancati A, Macmillan D, Cawthorn S. Prepectoral implant-based breast reconstruction: a joint consensus guide from UK,

European and USA breast and plastic reconstructive surgeons. Ecancermedicalscience. 2019,13: 927.
15. Srinivasa DR, Holland M, Sbitany H. Optimizing perioperative strategies to maximize success with prepectoral breast reconstruction. Gland Surg. 2019,8:19–26.
16. Gabriel A, Maxwell GP. Prepectoral breast reconstruction in challenging patients. Plast Reconstr Surg. 2017,140:14S–21S.
17. Casella D, Di Taranto G, Lo Torto F, Marcasciano M, Kaciulyte J, Greco M, Onesti MG, Ribuffo D. Body mass index can predict outcomes in DTI prepectoral breast reconstruction. Plast Reconstr Surg. 2020,145:867e–8e.
18. Komorowska-Timek E, Merrifield B, Turfe Z, Davis AT. Subcutaneous prosthetic breast reconstructions following skin reduction mastectomy. Plast Reconstr Surg Glob Open. 2019,7:e2078.
19. Spear SL, Boehmler JH, Bogue DP, Mafi AA. Options in reconstructing the irradiated breast. Plast Reconstr Surg. 2008,122:379–88.
20. Khavanin N, Qiu C, Darrach H, Kraenzlin F, Kokosis G, Han T, Sacks JM. Intraoperative perfusion assessment in mastectomy skin flaps: how close are we to preventing complications? J Reconstr Microsurg. 2019,35:471–8.
21. Pruimboom T, Schols RM, Van Kuijk SM, Van der Hulst RR, Qiu SS. Indocyanine green angiography for preventing postoperative mastectomy skin flap necrosis in immediate breast reconstruction. Cochrane Database Syst Rev. 2020,4: CD013280.
22. Lo Torto F, Relucenti M, Familiari G, Vaia N, Casella D, Matassa R, Miglietta S, Marinozzi F, Bini F, Fratoddi I, Sciubba F, Cassese R, Tombolini V, Ribuffo D. The effect of postmastectomy radiation therapy on breast implants: material analysis on silicone and polyurethane prosthesis. Ann Plast Surg. 2018,81:228–34.
23. Jacobs JM, Salzberg CA. Implant-based breast reconstruction with meshes and matrices: biological vs synthetic. Br J Hosp Med (Lond). 2015,76:211–6.
24. Rolph R, Farhadi J. The use of meshes and matrices in breast reconstruction. Br J Hosp Med (Lond). 2018,79:454–9.
25. Sigalove S, Maxwell GP, Sigalove NM, Storm-Dickerson TL, Pope N, Rice J, Gabriel A. Prepectoral implant- based breast reconstruction: rationale, indications, and preliminary results. Plast Reconstr Surg. 2017,139:287–94.
26. Gómez-Modet S, Tejedor L. Synthetic mesh in immediate breast reconstruction. Breast cancer and breast reconstruction. IntechOpen. 2020. https://doi.org/10.5772/intechopen.90884.
27. Fitzgerald JF, Kumar AS. Biologic versus synthetic mesh reinforcement: what are the pros and cons? Clin Colon Rectal Surg. 2014,27(4):140–8.
28. Van Turnhout AAWM, Franke CJJ, Vriens-Nieuwenhuis EJC, Van der Sluis WB. The use of SERI™ surgical scaffolds in direct-to-implant reconstruction after skin-sparing mastectomy: a retrospective study on surgical outcomes and a systematic review of current literature. J Plast Reconstr Aesthet Surg. 2018,71:644–50.
29. Faulkner HR, Shikowitz-Behr L, McLeod M, Wright E, Hulsen J, Austen WG Jr. The use of absorbable mesh in implant-based breast reconstruction: a 7-year review. Plast Reconstr Surg. 2020,146:731e–6e.
30. Casella D, Di Taranto G, Marcasciano M, Sordi S, Kothari A, Kovacs T, Lo Torto F, Cigna E, Calabrese C, Ribuffo D. Evaluation of prepectoral implant placement and complete coverage with TiLoop Bra mesh for breast reconstruction: a prospective study on long-term and patient-reported BREAST-Q outcomes. Plast Reconstr Surg. 2019,143:1e–9e.
31. Machleidt A, Schmidt-Feuerheerd N, Blohmer JU, Ohlinger R, Kueper J, von Waldenfels G, Dittmer S, Paepke S, Klein E. Reconstructive breast surgery with partially absorbable bi-component Seragyn® BR soft mesh: an outcome analysis. Arch Gynecol Obstet. 2018,298:755–

32. József Z, Újhelyi M, Ping O, Domján S, Fülöp R, Ivády G, Ráchel T, Rubovszky G, Mészáros N, Kenessey I, Mátrai Z. Long-term dynamic changes in cosmetic outcomes and patient satisfaction after implant-based postmastectomy breast reconstruction and contralateral mastopexy with or without an ultrapro mesh sling used for the inner bra technique. A retrospective correlational study. Cancers (Basel). 2020,13: E73.
33. Hallberg H, Lewin R, Elander A, Hansson E. TIGR® matrix surgical mesh-a two-year follow-up study and complication analysis in 65 immediate breast reconstructions. J Plast Surg Hand Surg. 2018,52:253–8.
34. Tessler O, Reish RG, Maman DY, Smith BL, Austen WG Jr. beyond biologics: absorbable mesh as a low-cost, low-complication sling for implant-based breast reconstruction. Plast Reconstr Surg. 2014,133:90–9.
35. Cuffolo G, Holford NC, Contractor K, Tenovici A. TIGR matrix for implant-based breast reconstruction-a long-term resorbable mesh. Expert Rev Med Dev. 2018,15:689–91.
36. Pompei S, Evangelidou D, Arelli F, Ferrante G. The use of TIGR matrix in breast aesthetic and reconstructive surgery: is a resorbable synthetic mesh a viable alternative to acellular dermal matrices? Clin Plast Surg. 2018,45(1):65–73.
37. Becker H, Lind JG. The use of synthetic mesh in reconstructive, revision, and cosmetic breast surgery. Aesthet Plast Surg. 2013,37:914–21.
38. Fine NA, Lehfeldt M, Gross JE, Downey S, Kind GM, Duda G, Kulber D, Horan R, Ippolito J, Jewell M. SERI surgical scaffold, prospective clinical trial of a silk-derived biological scaffold in two-stage breast reconstruction: 1-year data. Plast Reconstr Surg. 2015,135:339–51.
39. De Vita R, Buccheri EM, Pozzi M, Zoccali G. Direct to implant breast reconstruction by using SERI, preliminary report. J Exp Clin Cancer Res. 2014,33:78.
40. Dieterich M, Reimer T, Dieterich H, Stubert J, Gerber B. A short-term follow-up of implant based breast reconstruction using a titanium-coated polypropylene mesh (TiLoop(®) Bra). Eur J Surg Oncol. 2012,38:1225–30.
41. TiO2Mesh™ – Surgical Mesh Implant. Available at: http://www.biosermedikal.com/en/tio2mesh-surgical-mesh-implant. Accessed on January 2021
42. Pukancsik D, Kelemen P, Gulyás G, Újhelyi M, Kovács E, Éles K, Mészáros N, Kenessey I, Pálházi P, Kovács T, Kásler M, Mátrai Z. Clinical experiences with the use of ULTRAPRO® mesh in single-stage direct-to-implant immediate postmastectomy breast reconstruction in 102 patients: a retrospective cohort study. Eur J Surg Oncol. 2017,43:1244–51.
43. Eichler C, Schulz C, Thangarajah F, Malter W, Warm M, Brunnert K. A retrospective head-to-head comparison between TiLoop Bra/TiMesh® and Seragyn® in 320 cases of reconstructive breast surgery. Anticancer Res. 2019,39:2599–605.
44. Bernini M, Calabrese C, Cecconi L, Santi C, Gjondedaj U, Roselli J, Nori J, Fausto A, Orzalesi L, Casella D. Subcutaneous direct-to-implant breast reconstruction: surgical, functional, and aesthetic results after long-term follow-up. Plast Reconstr Surg Glob Open. 2016,3:e574.
45. Casella D, Calabrese C, Bianchi S, Meattini I, Bernini M. Subcutaneous tissue expander placement with synthetic titanium-coated mesh in breast reconstruction: long-term results. Plast Reconstr Surg Glob Open. 2016,3:e577.
46. Lo Torto F, Marcasciano M, Kaciulyte J, Redi U, Barellini L, De Luca A, Perra A, Frattaroli JM, Cavalieri E, Di Taranto G, Greco M, Casella D. Prepectoral breast reconstruction with TiLoop® bra pocket: a single center prospective study. Eur Rev Med Pharmacol Sci. 2020,24:991–9.
47. Casella D, Di Taranto G, Marcasciano M, Sordi S, Kothari A, Kovacs T, Lo Torto F, Cigna E, Ribuffo D, Calabrese C. Nipple-sparing bilateral

prophylactic mastectomy and immediate reconstruction with TiLoop® Bra Mesh in BRCA1/2 mutation carriers: a prospective study of long-term and patient reported outcomes using the BREAST-Q. Breast. 2018,39:8–13.
48. PFM Medical. TiLoop® Bra Pocket. Available at: https://www.pfmmedical.com/en/productcatalogue/mesh_implants_breast_surgery/tiloopR_bra_pocket. Accessed: December 2020
49. Mowlds DS, Salibian AA, Scholz T, Paydar KZ, Wirth GA. Capsular contracture in implant-based breast reconstruction: examining the role of acellular dermal matrix fenestrations. Plast Reconstr Surg. 2015,136:629–35.
50. Dessy LA, Corrias F, Marchetti F, Marcasciano M, Armenti AF, Mazzocchi M, Carlesimo B. Implant infection after augmentation mammaplasty: a review of the literature and report of a multidrug-resistant candida albicans infection. Aesthet Plast Surg. 2012,36:153–9.
51. Shaterian A, Saba SC, Yee B, Tokin C, Mailey B, Dobke MK, Wallace AM. Single dual-trained surgeon for breast care leads to higher reconstruction rates after mastectomy. World J Surg. 2013,37:2600–6.
52. Casella D, Di Taranto G, Marcasciano M, Lo Torto F, Barellini L, Sordi S, Gaggelli I, Roncella M, Calabrese C, Ribuffo D. Subcutaneous expanders and synthetic mesh for breast reconstruction: long-term and patient-reported BREAST-Q outcomes of a single-center prospective study. J Plast Reconstr Aesthet Surg. 2019,72:805–12.
53. Casella D, Fusario D, Cassetti D, Miccoli S, Pesce AL, Bernini A, Marcasciano M, Lo Torto F, Neri A. The patient's pathway for breast cancer in the COVID-19 era: an italian single-center experience. Breast J. 2020,26:1589–92.
54. Rigotti G, Marchi A, Galiè M, Baroni G, Benati D, Krampera M, Pasini A, Sbarbati A. Clinical treatment of radiotherapy tissue damage by lipoaspirate transplant: a healing process mediated by adipose-derived adult stem cells. Plast Reconstr Surg. 2007,119:1409–22.
55. Cigna E, Ribuffo D, Sorvillo V, Atzeni M, Piperno A, Calò PG, Scuderi N. Secondary lipofilling after breast reconstruction with implants. Eur Rev Med Pharmacol Sci. 2012 Nov;16(12):1729–34.
56. Ribuffo D, Lo Torto F, Atzeni M, Serratore F. The effects of postmastectomy adjuvant radiotherapy on immediate two-stage prosthetic breast reconstruction: a systematic review. Plast Reconstr Surg. 2015,135:445e.
57. Calabrese C, Kothari A, Badylak S, Di Taranto G, Marcasciano M, Sordi S, Barellini L, Lo Torto F, Tarallo M, Gaggelli I, D'Ermo G, Fausto A, Casella D, Ribuffo D. Oncological safety of stromal vascular fraction enriched fat grafting in two-stage breast reconstruction after nipple sparing mastectomy: long-term results of a prospective study. Eur Rev Med Pharmacol Sci. 2018,22:4768–77.
58. Ribuffo D, Atzeni M, Guerra M, Bucher S, Politi C, Deidda M, Atzori F, Dessi M, Madeddu C, Lay G. Treatment of irradiated expanders: protective lipofilling allows immediate prosthetic breast reconstruction in the setting of postoperative radiotherapy. Aesthet Plast Surg. 2013,37:1146–52.
59. Vaia N, Lo Torto F, Marcasciano M, Casella D, Cacace C, De Masi C, Ricci F, Ribuffo D. From the "Fat Capsule" to the "Fat Belt": limiting protective lipofilling on irradiated expanders for breast reconstruction to selective key areas. Aesthet Plast Surg. 2018,42:986–94.
60. Vyas KS, DeCoster RC, Burns JC, Rodgers LT, Shrout MA, Mercer JP, Coquillard C, Dugan AJ, Baratta MD, Rinker BD, Vasconez HC. Autologous fat grafting does not increase risk of oncologic recurrence in the reconstructed breast. Ann Plast Surg. 2020,84:S405–10.
61. Wagner RD, Braun TL, Zhu H, Winocour S. A systematic review of complications in prepectoral breast reconstruction. J Plast Reconstr Aesthet Surg. 2019,72:1051–9.

62. Chopra K, Gowda AU, Kwon E, Eagan M, Grant SW. Techniques to repair implant malposition after breast augmentation: a review. Aesthet Surg J. 2016,36:660–71.
63. Harris R, Raphael P, Harris SW. Thermal capsulorrhaphy: a modified technique for breast pocket revision. Aesthet Surg J. 2014,34:1041–9.
64. Sinnott CJ, Persing SM, Pronovost M, Hodyl C, McConnell D, Ott YA. Impact of postmastectomy radiation therapy in prepectoral versus subpectoral implant-based breast reconstruction. Ann Surg Oncol. 2018,25:2899–908.
65. Casella D, Di Taranto G, Onesti MG, Greco M, Ribuffo D. A retrospective comparative analysis of risk factors and outcomes in direct-to-implant and two-stages prepectoral breast reconstruction: bmi and radiotherapy as new selection criteria of patients. Eur J Surg Oncol. 2019,45:1357–63.
66. Nahabedian MY. What are the long-term aesthetic issues in prepectoral breast reconstruction? Aesthet Surg J. 2020,40:S29–37.
67. Marcasciano M, Kaciulyte J, Marcasciano F, Lo Torto F, Ribuffo D, Casella D. "No drain, no gain": simultaneous seroma drainage and tissue expansion in pre-pectoral tissue expander-based breast reconstruction. Aesthet Plast Surg. 2019,43:1118–9.
68. Washer LL, Gutowski K. Breast implant infections. Infect Dis Clin North Am. 2012,26:111–25.
69. Avila A, Bartholomew AJ, Sosin M, Deldar R, Griffith KF, Willey SC, Song DH, Fan KL, Tousimis EA. Acute postoperative complications in prepectoral versus subpectoral reconstruction following nipple-sparing mastectomy. Plast Reconstr Surg. 2020,146:715e–20e.
70. Spear SL, Howard MA, Boehmler JH, Ducic I, Low M, Abbruzzesse MR. The infected or exposed breast implant: management and treatment strategies. Plast Reconstr Surg. 2004,113:1634–44.
71. Prince MD, Suber JS, Aya-Ay ML, Cone JD Jr, Greene JN, Smith DJ Jr, Smith PD. Prosthesis salvage in breast reconstruction patients with periprosthetic infection and exposure. Plast Reconstr Surg. 2012,129:42–8.
72. De Lorenzi C. Successful treatment of acute periprosthetic breast infection with curettage, pulse lavage, and immediate device exchange. Aesthet Plast Surg. 2005,29:400–3.
73. Antoniazzi E, Villani R, Fabbri E, Vietti Michelina V, D'Angelo G, Summo V, Cipriani R, Morselli PG, Fasano D. Management of the exposed and/or infected breast prosthesis: a proposal for a standardized approach. Plast Reconstr Surg Glob Open. 2016,4:e658.
74. Ganske I, Hoyler M, Fox SE, Morris DJ, Lin SJ, Slavin SA. Delayed hypersensitivity reaction to acellular dermal matrix in breast reconstruction: the red breast syndrome? Ann Plast Surg. 2014,73:S139–43.
75. Mayer HF, Perez Colman M, Stoppani I. Red breast syndrome (RBS) associated to the use of polyglycolic mesh in breast reconstruction: a case report. Acta Chir Plast. 2020,62:50–2.
76. Vidya R, Iqbal FM. A guide to prepectoral breast reconstruction: a new dimension to implant-based breast reconstruction. Clin Breast Cancer. 2017,17:266–71.
77. Akram M, Siddiqui SA. Breast cancer management: past, present and evolving. Indian J Cancer. 2012,49:277–82.
78. Salzberg CA. Nonexpansive immediate breast reconstruction using human acellular tissue matrix graft (AlloDerm). Ann Plast Surg. 2006,57:1–5.
79. Ter Louw RP, Nahabedian MY. Prepectoral Breast reconstruction. Plast Reconstr Surg. 2017,140:51S–9S.
80. Rietjens M, Garusi C, Lanfrey E, Petit JY. La Suspension cutanée: Reconstruction Mammaire immédiate Avec Avancement cutané Abdominal à l'aide d'une Plaque Non résorbable. Résultats préliminaires à Propos de Vingt-Neuf Cas [Cutaneous suspension: immediate breast reconstruction with abdominal cutaneous advancement

using a non-resorptive mesh. preliminary results and report of 28 cases]. Ann Chir Plast Esthet. 1997,42:177–82.
81. Reitsamer R, Peintinger F, Klaassen-Federspiel F, Sir A. Prepectoral direct-to-implant breast reconstruction with complete ADM or synthetic mesh coverage - 36-months follow-up in 200 reconstructed breasts. Breast. 2019,48:32–7.
82. Zhu L, Mohan AT, Abdelsattar JM, Wang Z, Vijayasekaran A, Hwang SM, Tran NV, Saint-Cyr M. Comparison of subcutaneous versus submuscular expander placement in the first stage of immediate breast reconstruction. J Plast Reconstr Aesthet Surg. 2016,69:e77–86.
83. Caputo GG, Marchetti A, Dalla Pozza E, Vigato E, Domenici L, Cigna E, Governa M. Skin-reduction breast reconstructions with prepectoral implant. Plast Reconstr Surg. 2016,137:1702–5.
84. Marcasciano Md M, Kaciulyte J, Gentilucci M, Barellini L, Ribuffo D, Casella D. Skin-reduction breast reconstructions with prepectoral implant covered by a combined dermal flap and titanium-coated polypropylene mesh. J Plast Reconstr Aesthet Surg. 2018,71:1123–8.
85. Salibian AH, Harness JK, Mowlds DS. Staged suprapectoral expander/implant reconstruction without acellular dermal matrix following nipple-sparing mastectomy. Plast Reconstr Surg. 2017,139:30–9.
86. Marcasciano M, Frattaroli J, Mori FLR, Lo Torto F, Fioramonti P, Cavalieri E, Kaciulyte J, Greco M, Casella D, Ribuffo D. The new trend of pre-pectoral breast reconstruction: an objective evaluation of the quality of online information for patients undergoing breast reconstruction. Aesthet Plast Surg. 2019,43:593–9.
87. Marcasciano M, Kaciulyte J, FLR M, Lo Torto F, Barellini L, Loreti A, Fanelli B, De Vita R, Redi U, Marcasciano F, Di Cesare F, dal Prà G, Conversi A, Elia L, Montemari G, Vaia N, Bernini M, Sordi S, Luridiana G, D'Ermo G, Monti M, De Luca A, Ricci F, Mazzocchi M, Gentilucci M, Greco M, Losco L, Valdatta LA, Raposio E, Giudice G, Maruccia M, Di Benedetto G, Cigna E, Casella D, Ribuffo D. Breast surgeons updating on the thresholds of COVID-19 era: results of a multicenter collaborative study evaluating the role of online videos and multimedia sources on breast surgeons education and training. Eur Rev Med Pharmacol Sci. 2020,24:7845–54.

14 复合式胸肌前乳房重建：联合皮瓣与假体

编者：Arash Momeni, Anna Zhou
译者：孙芦浩

14.1 引言

自50年前首例假体置入乳房重建问世以来，乳房切除重建术式已取得巨大进展，临床疗效显著提升，由此确立了乳房重建在乳腺癌诊疗体系中的核心地位。从胸肌后术式向胸肌前假体置入乳房重建的演进，正是现代技术降低手术并发症发生率的例证。研究证实，乳房重建可显著改善患者报告的结果及健康相关生命质量[1-3]。

传统重建路径将假体置入与自体组织重建作为互斥选项，旨在实现重建乳房的"5S"目标：合适的大小（size）、形态（shape）、对称性（symmetry）、柔软度（softness）及感觉（sensation）恢复。尽管该二元选择适用于多数病例，仍有部分患者无法通过此类简化策略获得满意疗效，尤其在双侧乳房切除日益增多的背景下[5]，自体组织供区组织量不足成为主要制约因素。针对此类拟行双侧自体组织重建但供区组织量不足的病例，目前文献提出了多种解决方案，包括皮瓣移植后Ⅰ期/Ⅱ期脂肪移植、叠合皮瓣重建术，以及复合式乳房重建（即自体组织联合假体置入）[6-11]。

尽管自体脂肪移植作为门诊短程手术，能通过矫正轮廓畸形与容量不足显著改善临床疗效，提高患者满意度[12]，但其存在诸多局限，包括脂肪吸收率不稳定、脂肪坏死风险、需多次手术干预，以及重建乳房缺乏结构性支撑等[13]。此外，需要注意的是，腹部脂肪组织量不足以行双侧乳房自体重建者，其他解剖部位的脂肪储备亦可能不足，难以通过Ⅱ期脂肪移植获取理想美学效果。

叠合皮瓣重建术可实现大体积软组织单次移植，从而完成全自体乳房重建，并且移植组织不存在继发性吸收问题。然而，多供区皮瓣获取不仅延长手术时间，增加操作复杂性，亦导致患者创伤加重。尽管

A. Momeni (✉) · A. Zhou
Division of Plastic & Reconstructive Surgery,
Stanford University School of Medicine, Stanford,
CA, USA
e-mail: amomeni@stanford.edu;
Atzhou@stanford.edu

© The Author(s), under exclusive license to Springer Nature Switzerland AG 2023
R. Vidya, H. Becker (eds.), *Prepectoral Breast Reconstruction*,
https://doi.org/10.1007/978-3-031-15590-1_14

文献显示叠合皮瓣重建效果优异[9, 14]，但该术式对术者操作技术要求较高，普及度受限。

因此，对于自体供区组织不足但坚持自体重建诉求的病例，复合式重建或为理想解决方案。

复合式乳房重建术以自体组织联合假体置入为特征，主要形式为背阔肌（LD）皮瓣与假体联合应用[15, 16]。然而，此术式存在以下缺陷：LD供区损伤，术中需重置体位，术后动态畸形风险，难以构建自然乳房下垂形态，以及继发软组织萎缩致假体显形与皱褶形成[6, 17, 18]。基于此概念的拓展术式——游离腹部皮瓣移植联合同期假体置入——可有效规避上述缺陷。

腹部皮瓣获取不仅瘢痕位置隐蔽，而且可通过更大体积的软组织转移来对抗萎缩，显著降低假体显影与皱褶发生风险[11, 19]。此外，充足的腹部皮瓣体积允许使用较小假体，故游离腹部皮瓣复合重建术后乳房外观主要由皮瓣而非假体决定，此点与 LD 皮瓣重建术形成鲜明对比。需要特别注意的是，假体在腹部皮瓣重建与 LD 皮瓣重建中的功能存在不同：在前者，假体主要起凸度塑形及支撑皮瓣覆盖基底的作用，主体体积由游离腹部皮瓣提供，主导最终乳房的形态、尺寸与柔软度；同时，降低假体占乳房总体积比例有助于减少远期假体相关并发症。在 LD 皮瓣重建术中，假体为乳房体积及外观核心决定因素，LD 皮瓣仅起血管化软组织覆盖作用。

14.2 假体置入时机的选择

假体置入时机的选择，存在点关注即刻置入与延迟置入两种策略。部分学者推荐延迟置入策略，认为其更利于控制重建结局，原因包括能更精准地构建假体囊袋及确定假体尺寸[20]。但该策略存在技术难点，尤其是接受辅助放疗者囊袋分离操作难度增加[21]；此外，延迟置入常需多次修正手术，文献报道完成最终重建最多需 6 次手术[22]。

即刻假体置入则可规避二次手术。早期研究指出，假体同期置入联合腹直肌皮瓣（TRAM）移植时假体相关并发症（如感染率高达19%）风险增加，但近期研究未证实此结论[19, 23-25]。一项对 57 例双侧复合式乳房重建患者的回顾性分析显示，仅 1 例发生术后感染[26]。即刻置入优势包括：避免二次手术；更精确调控假体位置（尤其联合补片应用时）；通过初次手术同步矫正乳房皮肤包裹与容量不匹配问题，术后乳房外观更佳。对拟行术后辅助放疗者尤为重要。因乳房切除后皮瓣愈合至较小的游离皮瓣，使皮肤包裹回展至原始维度的难度增大（游离皮瓣与乳房切除皮肤包裹粘连），放疗后粘连更甚。此时延迟置入虽可增大乳房体积，但形态与轮廓很不理想[26]。

尽管即刻复合式重建存在优势，但假体选择颇具挑战性，即刻复合式重建术后因假体尺寸引发的修正率超10%[10]。应对此问题的优化方案为延迟-即刻复合式重建，即分阶段手术：Ⅰ期行即刻胸肌前组织扩张器重建术，Ⅱ期移除扩张器并行游离腹部皮瓣移植联合假体置入术[27]。该策略可依据最终扩张器容积与皮瓣重量差值精准确定假体尺寸。延迟-即刻策略的另一优势在于，Ⅰ期术后乳房切除皮肤坏死不影响最终的美学效果，可在Ⅱ期重建前代偿性修复皮肤缺损。此外，扩张期患者可参与乳房体积决策，故更易满足其对最终乳房尺寸的个性化诉求。

14.3 放疗

放疗是另一需重点考量的因素，因为据报道，放疗后腹壁下动脉穿支（DIEP）皮瓣移植的乳房切除皮肤坏死率、包膜挛缩率及脂肪坏死率增高[28]。胸肌前假体重建术后乳房切除皮肤坏死可能危及整体重建效果，但复合式重建术中假体由血供良好的腹部皮瓣与坏死区域隔离，故无须强制性手术干预。尽管放射野内假体相关并发症风险升高，但自体组织的加入可减少放疗相关假体隐患[29]。

拟行放疗的偏瘦患者具有特殊挑战，因该人群假体重建失败率高且美学效果欠佳[30, 31]。虽然胸肌前假体置入可通过规避胸肌后重建术后放疗所致肌肉纤维化与挛缩来改善预后[32]，但薄弱的软组织覆盖问题仍然存在。消瘦患者的自体重建同样困难，因皮瓣体积不足难以获得满意乳房形态。对此类患者，复合式重建为优选方案。

14.4 假体置入平面

与假体置入乳房重建术的演进同步，复合式重建术的假体置入平面及肌肉覆盖程度亦在不断改变。早期的自体组织联合假体置入术主张假体完全被肌肉覆盖，由胸大肌（偶联合前锯肌）及TRAM皮瓣肌性成分共同覆盖[6, 33]。随着研究证实补片可优化带蒂皮瓣联合假体即刻置入时的囊袋控制效果[25, 34]，该理念被拓展至显微外科复合重建领域。因此，补片的应用使胸肌后平面复合式乳房重建术应运而生，其中假体下外侧支撑由脱细胞真皮基质或聚乳酸补片构成[24]。该方案可实现精准囊袋界定，为疗效优化奠定基础。此后，为降低手术创伤、简化流程，复合式胸肌前乳房重建术兴起，完全规避了胸大肌剥离操作[10, 26]。

不仅假体置入平面发生改变，术中操作顺序亦发生变化。早期临床研究报告采用先置入假体后转移皮瓣的流程，而目前采取先行皮瓣转移，待微血管吻合后完成再行假体置入的操作顺序。

14.5 手术技术

术前按照标准方式标记中线、乳房下皱襞、乳房上界及腹部皮瓣区域（图14.1）。采用成熟技术切取腹部皮瓣。切除乳房后，沿肌纤维方向分离第三肋软骨水平的胸大肌，随后切除第三肋软骨；若见较大肋间隙，则可选择保留肋骨。游离胸廓内血管后，将腹部皮瓣转移至胸壁，完成腹壁下深血管与胸廓内血管的显微吻合。随后将腹部皮瓣置入乳房切除后遗腔隙。此时用假体试模确定正式假体尺寸。值得注意的是，所选假体基底宽度通常较患者术前乳房宽度小 2~3cm，便于皮瓣定位并确保皮瓣完整覆盖假体前表面。确定假体尺寸后，将最终假体联合脱细胞真皮基质（ADM）置于无菌区域，以 ADM 包覆假体并用 2–0 聚乳酸羟基乙酸缝线固定（图 14.2）。需要注意的是，因假体尺寸差异可能无法实现完整包裹。假体-ADM 复合体经稀释碘伏溶液浸泡后置入乳房切除后遗腔隙。置入过程中须全程显露皮瓣血管蒂，避免对血管蒂的过度牵拉或扭曲。

确定假体理想位置后，使用 2-0 聚乳酸羟基乙酸缝线将 ADM 固定于胸壁以稳定假体。随后将腹部皮瓣覆盖于假体-ADM 复合体前表面，实现血管化组织的可靠覆盖（图 14.3），并以 2-0 缝线固定于胸壁。尽管假体体积普遍较小（150~210mL）[10, 24]，但其对重建乳房凸度的改善效果即刻显现（图 14.4）。图 14.5 展示了即刻复合重建术前与术后对照影像。

14.6 复合乳房重建术的优势

复合乳房重建术摒弃了乳房切除重建中非假体即自体组织的简单二元化模式，扩展了重建技术选项，使得乳房重建方案个体化程度更高。需要明确的是，该术式并非替代传统假体或自体组织重建，而是为特定患者群体提供更优化的重建解决方案。此类患者的特征为有意愿或需要行自体组织重建但供区组织量不足。评估患者

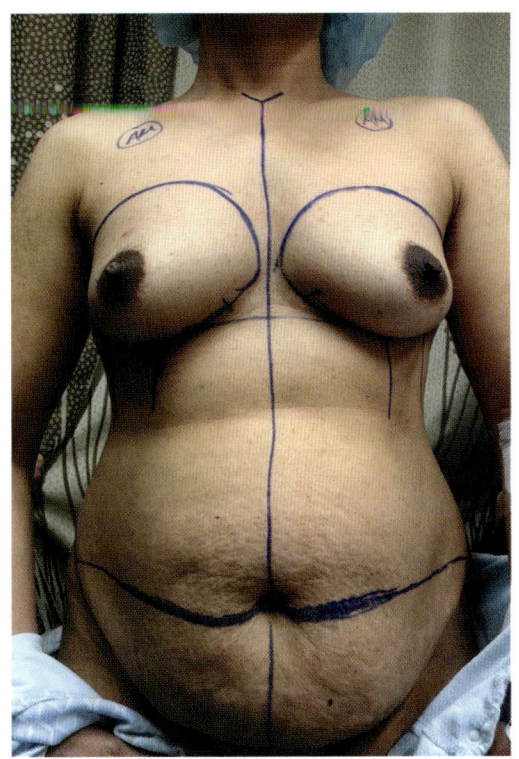

图 14.1 标准术前体表标记，包括中线、乳房下皱襞、乳房上界及腹部皮瓣轮廓。注意腹部皮瓣上缘经脐水平下方

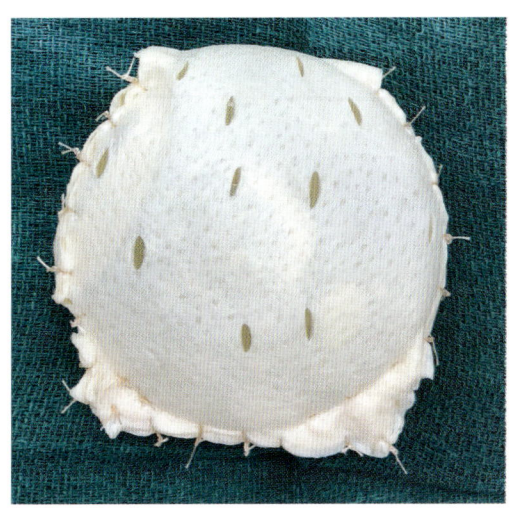

图 14.2 以脱细胞真皮基质包被的硅胶假体

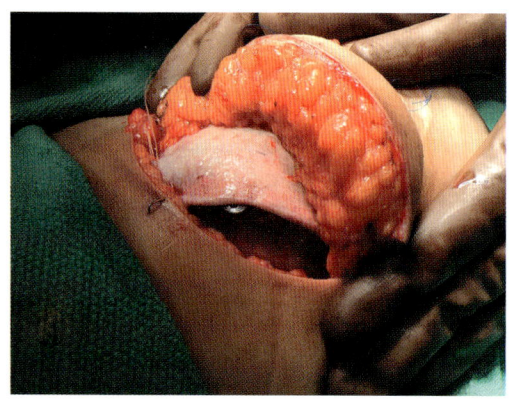

图14.3 胸肌前脱细胞真皮基质-假体复合物表面覆盖血供良好的软组织

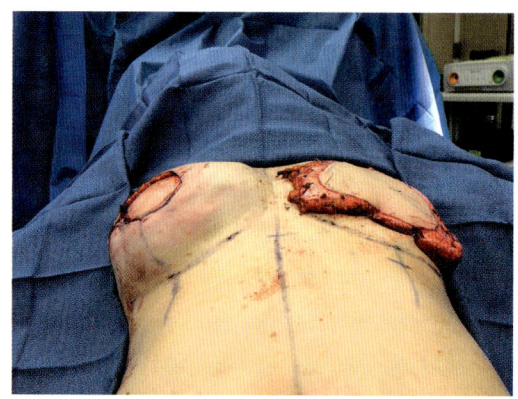

图14.4 术中可见假体对乳房凸度的成形作用

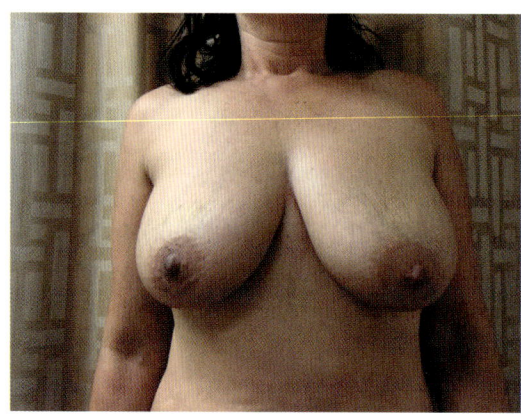

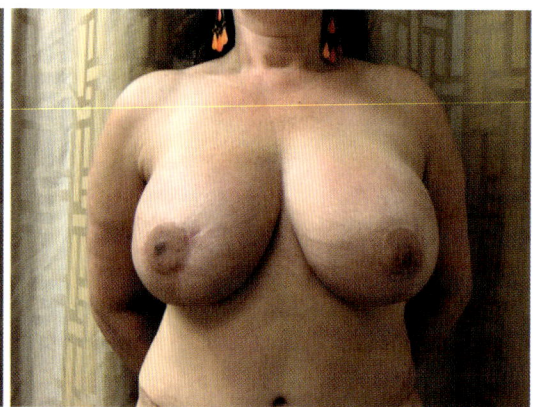

图14.5 49岁患者，行双乳保留乳头和乳晕的乳房切除术，联合使用175mL硅胶假体与游离腹部皮瓣行乳房重建术前与术后影像

是否适合行复合重建时，应重点评估腹部皮肤/软组织松弛程度，因其存在通常提示患者适于该重建模式。

复合重建术后血管化软组织的可靠覆盖能有效应对假体重建相关的诸多难题，尤其是假体显形及褶皱畸变。此外，自体组织占比的增加可降低远期假体相关并发症发生率。最后，与传统腹部皮瓣重建术相比，使用腹部皮瓣不仅能矫正脐下软组织松弛，并且术后腹部瘢痕位置显著更低[4]。

14.7 文献回顾

多项临床研究证实了显微外科复合乳房重建术的安全性。一项纳入19例患者（38例乳房重建）的研究表明，采用补片材料［尤其是脱细胞真皮基质（ADM）与聚乳酸羟基乙酸］进行即刻复合重建能有效控制假体位置，无假体移位、感染或皮瓣坏死报道。值得注意的是，该研究中的所有患者均采用胸肌后假体置入，并用补片加强下外侧支撑[24]。为减轻手术创伤并简化操作流程，一项针对 57 例患者（114 例乳房重建）的研究探讨了胸肌前复合重建的临床结局，验证了该术式的安全性[26]。然而，10% 以上的乳房切除术后皮瓣坏死率促使研究者提出改良方案——延迟 - 即刻重建法，即先通过常规胸肌前扩张器重建，再分阶段实施复合重建。一项针对 31 例患者（62 例乳房重建）的回顾性研究报道了该术式的临床结局[27]。值得关注的是，Ⅱ期重建患者无须二次更换假体矫正体积，印证了该术式在确定理想假体尺寸方面的优越性，同时未观察到术后皮瓣坏死病例[27]。近期研究进一步分析了复合重建的次级结局参数，如腹部瘢痕位置与供区美学评分。与传统皮瓣重建、复合重建与美容性腹壁成形术后的腹部外观相比，复合重建与腹壁成形术的腹部瘢痕位置明显低于传统腹部皮瓣重建，并且更低位的瘢痕位置与更高的腹部美学评分相关[4]。

值得注意的是，除传统背阔肌皮瓣或游离腹部皮瓣外，复合重建术亦可成功联合其他皮瓣实施。为减少切取背阔肌所致的供区并发症，胸背动脉穿支皮瓣（TDAP）与组织扩张器 / 永久假体的联合应用已获得成功[35]。此外，多项回顾性临床研究证实了脱细胞真皮基质在提供软组织支撑与调控假体位置方面的价值[25, 34]。

14.8 小结

复合乳房重建术因可弥补传统乳房重建术式不足，拓展了重建技术选项。尤其假体置入联合游离腹部组织移植术式展现了优异临床效果：源于腹部皮瓣的充足软组织可为假体提供稳定覆盖，有效降低假体触知感与皱褶风险；同时，假体能重建乳房的凸度且不损害皮瓣相关结局指标。此外，鉴于腹部供区不再是重建乳房体积的唯一来源，腹部皮瓣可设计于更低位，从而使瘢痕低位化并改善腹部美学外观。

与其他重建术式相同，患者选择是手术成功的关键。判断患者是否适用复合乳房重建术的核心指征为：腹部皮肤 / 软组织松弛且患者有修复意愿。推荐术中使用假体试模确定理想假体规格。尽管有不同术中操作流程的文献报道，目前我们倾向采取皮瓣转移并完成微血管吻合后在胸肌前置入假体的流程，因其有利于确定假体理想位置，并且对手术进程干扰最小。

参考文献

1. Alderman AK, Kuhn LE, Lowery JC, Wilkins EG. Does patient satisfaction with breast reconstruction change over time? Two-year results of the Michigan breast reconstruction outcomes study. J Am Coll Surg. 2007,204(1):7–12.

2. Hu ES, Pusic AL, Waljee JF, Kuhn L, Hawley ST, Wilkins E, et al. Patient-reported aesthetic satisfaction with breast reconstruction during the long-term survivorship period. Plast Reconstr Surg. 2009,124(1):1–8.

3. Nelson JA, Allen RJ Jr, Polanco T, Shamsunder M, Patel AR, McCarthy CM, et al. Long-term patient-reported outcomes following Postmastectomy breast reconstruction: an 8-year examination of 3268 patients. Ann Surg. 2019,270(3):473–83.

4. Li AY, Momeni A. Abdominal flap-based breast reconstruction versus abdominoplasty: the impact of surgical procedure on scar location. Plast Reconstr Surg Glob Open. 2020,8(9):e3112.
5. Albornoz CR, Bach PB, Mehrara BJ, Disa JJ, Pusic AL, McCarthy CM, et al. A paradigm shift in U.S. breast reconstruction: increasing implant rates. Plast Reconstr Surg. 2013,131(1):15–23.
6. Serletti JM, Moran SL. The combined use of the TRAM and expanders/implants in breast reconstruction. Ann Plast Surg. 1998,40(5):510–4.
7. Laporta R, Longo B, Sorotos M, Pagnoni M, Santanelli di Pompeo F. Breast reconstruction with delayed fat-graft-augmented DIEP flap in patients with insufficient donor-site volume. Aesthet Plast Surg. 2015,39(3):339–49.
8. Zhu L, Mohan AT, Vijayasekaran A, Hou C, Sur YJ, Morsy M, et al. Maximizing the volume of latissimus Dorsi flap in autologous breast reconstruction with simultaneous multisite fat grafting. Aesthet Surg J/Am Soc Aesthet Plast Surg. 2016,36(2):169–78.
9. Stalder MW, Lam J, Allen RJ, Sadeghi A. Using the retrograde internal mammary system for stacked perforator flap breast reconstruction: 71 breast reconstructions in 53 consecutive patients. Plast Reconstr Surg. 2016,137(2):265e–77e.
10. Momeni A, Kanchwala S. Hybrid Prepectoral breast reconstruction: a surgical approach that combines the benefits of autologous and implant-based reconstruction. Plast Reconstr Surg. 2018,142(5):1109–15.
11. Chu MW, Samra F, Kanchwala SK, Momeni A. Treatment options for bilateral autologous breast reconstruction in patients with inadequate donor-site volume. J Reconstr Microsurg. 2017,33(5):305–11.
12. Kanchwala SK, Glatt BS, Conant EF, Bucky LP. Autologous fat grafting to the reconstructed breast: the management of acquired contour deformities. Plast Reconstr Surg. 2009,124(2):409–18.
13. Khouri RK, Rigotti G, Khouri RK Jr, Cardoso E, Marchi A, Rotemberg SC, et al. Tissue-engineered breast reconstruction with Brava-assisted fat grafting: a 7-year, 488-patient, multicenter experience. Plast Reconstr Surg. 2015,135(3): 643–58.
14. Mayo JL, Allen RJ, Sadeghi A. Four-flap breast reconstruction: bilateral stacked DIEP and PAP flaps. Plast Reconstr Surg Glob Open. 2015,3(5): e383.
15. Slavin SA. Improving the latissimus dorsi myocutaneous flap with tissue expansion. Plast Reconstr Surg. 1994,93(4):811–24.
16. Biggs TM, Cronin ED. Technical aspects of the latissimus dorsi myocutaneous flap in breast reconstruction. Ann Plast Surg. 1981,6(5):381–8.
17. Figus A, Mazzocchi M, Dessy LA, Curinga G, Scuderi N. Treatment of muscular contraction deformities with botulinum toxin type a after latissimus dorsi flap and sub-pectoral implant breast reconstruction. J Plast Reconstr Aesthet Surg. 2009,62(7):869–75.
18. Button J, Scott J, Taghizadeh R, Weiler-Mithoff E, Hart AM. Shoulder function following autologous latissimus dorsi breast reconstruction. A prospective three year observational study comparing quilting and non-quilting donor site techniques. J Plast Reconstr Aesthet Surg. 2010,63(9):1505–12.
19. Roehl KR, Baumann DP, Chevray PM, Chang DW. Evaluation of outcomes in breast reconstructions combining lower abdominal free flaps and permanent implants. Plast Reconstr Surg. 2010,126(2):349–57.
20. Bach AD, Morgenstern IH, Horch RE. Secondary "hybrid reconstruction" concept with silicone implants after autologous breast reconstruction - is it safe and reasonable? Medical Sci Monit Int Med J Exp Clin Res. 2020,26:e921329.
21. Walters JA 3rd, Sato EA, Martinez CA, Hall JJ, Boutros SG. Delayed mammoplasty with silicone gel implants following DIEP flap breast reconstruction. Plast Reconstr Surg Glob Open. 2015,3(10):e540.

22. Pien IJ, Anolik R, Blau J, Hollenbeck ST. Delayed implant augmentation of breast free flaps. J Reconstr Microsurg. 2015,31(4):254–60.
23. Spear SL, Wolfe AJ. The coincidence of TRAM flaps and prostheses in the setting of breast reconstruction. Plast Reconstr Surg. 2002,110(2):478–86.
24. Momeni A, Kanchwala SK. Improved pocket control in immediate microsurgical breast reconstruction with simultaneous implant placement through the use of mesh. Microsurgery. 2018,38(5):450–7.
25. Borsen-Koch M, Gunnarsson GL, Udesen A, Arffmann S, Jacobs J, Salzberg A, et al. Direct delayed breast reconstruction with TAP flap, implant and acellular dermal matrix (TAPIA). J Plast Reconstr Aesthet Surg. 2015,68(6):815–21.
26. Kanchwala S, Momeni A. Hybrid breast reconstruction-the best of both worlds. Gland Surg. 2019,8(1):82–9.
27. Momeni A, Kanchwala S. Delayed-immediate hybrid breast reconstruction-increasing patient input and precision in breast reconstruction. Breast J. 2019,25(5):898–902.
28. Khansa I, Colakoglu S, Curtis MS, Yueh JH, Ogunleye A, Tobias AM, et al. Postmastectomy breast reconstruction after previous lumpectomy and radiation therapy: analysis of complications and satisfaction. Ann Plast Surg. 2011,66(5):444–51.
29. Chang DW, Barnea Y, Robb GL. Effects of an autologous flap combined with an implant for breast reconstruction: an evaluation of 1000 consecutive reconstructions of previously irradiated breasts. Plast Reconstr Surg. 2008,122(2):356–62.
30. Yun JH, Diaz R, Orman AG. Breast reconstruction and radiation therapy. Cancer Control. 2018,25(1):1073274818795489.
31. Zhao R, Tran BNN, Doval AF, Broadwater G, Buretta KJ, Orr JP, et al. A multicenter analysis examining patients undergoing conversion of implant-based breast reconstruction to abdominally based free tissue transfer. J Reconstr Microsurg. 2018,34(9):685–91.
32. Sinnott CJ, Persing SM, Pronovost M, Hodyl C, McConnell D, Ott YA. Impact of Postmastectomy radiation therapy in Prepectoral versus subpectoral implant-based breast reconstruction. Ann Surg Oncol. 2018,25(10):2899–908.
33. Miller MJ, Rock CS, Robb GL. Aesthetic breast reconstruction using a combination of free transverse rectus abdominis musculocutaneous flaps and breast implants. Ann Plast Surg. 1996,37(3):258–64.
34. Gunnarsson GL, Borsen-Koch M, Nielsen HT, Salzberg A, Thomsen JB. Bilateral breast reconstruction with extended thoracodorsal artery perforator propeller flaps and implants. Plast Reconstr Surg Glob Open. 2015,3(6):e435.
35. Hamdi M, Salgarello M, Barone-Adesi L, Van Landuyt K. Use of the thoracodorsal artery perforator (TDAP) flap with implant in breast reconstruction. Ann Plast Surg. 2008,61(2):143–6.

15 无补片胸肌前乳房重建术

编者：Eduardo González, Cicero Urban
译者：孙 政 孙德峰

15.1 引言

单期或分期扩张器/假体即刻置入乳房重建术的演变与并发症控制及美学效果优化息息相关。假体置入方式及辅助材料的应用作为关键因素，推动了整体术式理念的革新——即在保持低并发症发生率的前提下改善重建效果。

既往文献[1-3]报道曾尝试采用光面假体实施皮下重建，但受限于当时乳房切除术的激进性（皮瓣厚度控制不足及乳房切除范围局限），此类术式因效果欠佳且并发症高发而被弃用。Schlenker[4]报道的并发症包括皮肤坏死（13.5%）、假体外露（6.7%）、包膜挛缩（56%）、假体取出替换率（28%）等。此后，胸肌后重建术长期占据主流地位[5]。

因全胸肌后重建术式美学效果欠佳（尤其下极扩张困难），本团队自2004年起转向应用Serra-Renom[6]提出的双平面部分胸肌后术式。该术式虽可获满意效果，仍存在下极过度扩张风险，动态畸形与"窗幔效应"亦相对常见。

为规避上述并发症，合成或生物补片联合永久假体/扩张器的应用开始见诸报道[7-10]，核心目标在于延长胸大肌防止其回缩，控制乳房下皱襞形态及外侧缘稳定性，避免假体旋转并实现全包裹。需要明确的是，规范化的乳房切除术本应保持乳房下皱襞解剖完整性及皮肤覆盖形态，结合合适的假体即可规避上述问题。

虽然传统双平面技术（无论是否应用补片）已实现部分目标，但胸大肌剥离所致术后疼痛、动态畸形及放疗后包膜挛缩伴乳房轮廓异常等并发症仍频发。这些悬而未决的问题共同推动了胸肌前重建时代的重启。

胸肌前重建术是一种更快的手术方

E. González (✉)
Departamento de Mastología, Instituto de Oncología Ángel H Roffo, Universidad de Buenos Aires,
Buenos Aires, Argentina

C. Urban
Nossa Senhora das Graças Hospital and Centro de Doenças da Mama Curitiba (PR), Curitiba, Brazil

© The Author(s), under exclusive license to Springer Nature Switzerland AG 2023
R. Vidya, H. Becker (eds.), *Prepectoral Breast Reconstruction*,
https://doi.org/10.1007/978-3-031-15590-1_15

式，能够减轻疼痛和不适，同时实现快速康复。该术式保留了胸大肌，避免了动态畸形，通过精细剥离与血供制备良好的皮瓣，维持乳房自然形态与解剖边界。但其也存在一定争议，如可能引发波纹效应及假体可见度增加、脱出率升高，以及未使用补片包裹时更高的包膜挛缩发生率。

此时有必要就补片在该技术中的应用影响进行深入分析。补片主要分为两类，一类是由多种材料构成的合成补片，通常为慢吸收或不可吸收型[8-10]，主要功能是维持假体良好定位，其次旨在改善皮瓣营养状况与厚度，但后者通常难以实现；另一类为生物源性补片，取材于人（ADM）、猪、牛等，可促进组织血管化、营养代谢及皮瓣致密性，通过更佳的组织一致性减少波纹效应。值得注意的是，这类补片具有保护组织免受放疗影响及降低包膜挛缩率的重要功能。

目前有很多关于各类补片使用利弊及并发症的文献报道，其确切临床价值仍难明确，主要由于前瞻性研究证据稀缺。仅少数研究如 Ho 等[11] 的荟萃分析指出，与使用传统肌筋膜皮瓣的假体重建相比，ADM 辅助乳房重建术的血清肿、感染及重建失败的发生率更高，但降低包膜挛缩发生率的优势明显。

一项多中心前瞻性队列研究 iBRA（Potter 等[12]）对 1 357 例应用补片的乳房重建病例（1 133 例生物补片，243 例合成补片）进行分析，结果显示，合成补片组的感染率为 26%，假体脱落率为 10%。作者总结认为，此术式的并发症发生率均高于国家质量标准（National Quality Standards；再手术率、再入院率及假体脱落率 <5%，感染率 <10%）。

研究显示，胸肌前与胸肌后重建在并发症发生情况方面无明显区别。Chatterjee[13] 对 14 项研究（均使用生物或合成补片）进行荟萃分析，证实在合理筛选患者的情况下可支持上述结论；若叠加放疗因素，短期随访可见前胸肌前重建可获得更优的美容效果及更低的包膜挛缩率（约为原来的 1/4），可能与胸肌后重建中胸肌的纤维化相关[13, 14]。需要明确指出的是，这些研究均涵盖使用 ADM 的患者群体。

Ⅰ 期胸肌前直接假体置入乳房重建术目前被视为先进的重建技术，其安全性及可重复性已获验证，成为大多数乳房切除术后即时乳房重建的首选方案。本文的核心在于探讨在术中是否必须联合应用补片，抑或在所有临床情境中均可不依赖补片实现同等效果。

因此，本章旨在分析乳房切除术的手术技巧（无论术前存在有利或不利因素）对直接置入假体且未使用补片的乳房重建术的影响，并评估在放疗等后续治疗场景中该术式能否维持效果且不增加并发症。此外，我们将探究胸肌前技术中可能促使省略合成或生物补片应用的影响因素。

15.2 适应证与禁忌证

胸肌前乳房重建术的安全性基于严格的患者筛选，需要综合考虑术前合并症、乳房切除皮瓣存活度、放疗状态及肿瘤学标准。与其他手术相同，需要严格筛选合适的患者，并就技术选择、相关风险、获益及局限性进行充分沟通。

已报道多种基于假体的胸肌前乳房重建技术。该术式适用于拟行保留乳头及保留皮肤术式者，若皮瓣条件符合要求，可行Ⅱ期组织扩张器或Ⅰ期假体直接置入重建。胸肌前重建的适应证为：BMI<30、中小乳房体积、不吸烟、乳房轻度下垂，预防性乳房切除及乳腺中央区肿瘤患者[15, 16]。

胸肌前乳房重建的禁忌证包括：糖尿病控制不佳，肥胖（BMI>35）及吸烟者（现症或近期）。上述因素会导致患者微循环受损及软组织质量下降，显著增加皮瓣坏死、假体脱出或感染风险。另一需考量的因素是行乳房切除术时的放疗状态，建议既往接受过乳房放疗者避免采用该术式，因对其放射区域皮肤行组织扩张时存在切口裂开及感染的较高风险[17]。此类情况下，可选择两阶段胸肌后或胸肌前重建术，联合脱细胞真皮基质或脂肪移植以改善皮瓣血供。

从肿瘤学角度来说，术前需评估原发乳腺肿瘤位置。肿瘤侵犯皮肤或胸壁、炎性乳腺癌、Ⅳ期乳腺癌或伴侵袭性腋窝转移及大量腋窝淋巴结转移，亦应视为胸肌前乳房重建的禁忌证[17, 18]。此类患者通常存在较高的复发风险，可能延迟辅助治疗实施并增加复发监测难度。

根据本机构2021年的经验（发表于《Plastic and Reconstructive Surgery》），我们开展了"保留乳头乳房切除术中未应用脱细胞真皮基质或补片的胸肌前直接置入式即刻乳房重建"的多中心队列研究，纳入接受胸肌前直接置入式即刻乳房重建患者（治疗性或风险降低性），未使用任何类型补片（生物或合成），囊括所有腺体的乳房（无下垂或中度下垂）、不同脂肪层类型、身体质量指数、吸烟状态及既往放疗史患者，仅排除存在皮肤受累、乳房肥大或3~4级下垂、血运障碍（皮肤坏死或乳头-乳晕复合体高危者）患者。

15.3 手术技术

若乳房切除皮瓣符合要求，无论采用何种切口（乳晕周围、放射状、乳房下皱襞等），均可实施基于假体的胸肌前乳房重建。双侧乳房切除术中需确保切口对称。详细的术前规划（明确乳房边界及胸壁测量）是确保重建成功的关键步骤，尤其未使用补片时。此外，在非腺体组织存在区域（如上极，图15.1）保留脂肪组织至关重要。

目前，尚无前瞻性临床研究评估乳房切除皮瓣及乳晕-乳晕复合体（CAP）的最佳厚度。皮瓣厚度取决于患者体质及皮下组织量，需在维持足够血供与避免过厚（增加局部复发风险）之间取得平衡，尽可能避免残留乳腺组织（即使完全切除难以实现）[19]。为预防并发症，需综合考虑表15.1所列参数。

研究显示部分切口（如乳晕周围切口）并发症率较高，而其他切口更安全[20]。本团队采用两种乳房下切口变体：一种为常规褶皱处切口，无侧方或内侧延伸以保护更多穿支感觉神经（图 15.2）；另一种为外侧弧形切口，设计于乳房下皱襞上方 1~2cm 并延伸至腋前线，当前哨淋巴结阳性需行腋窝淋巴结清扫时可向上延至腋中线[21]（图 15.3）。

完成乳房切除术后，可采用临床体征（皮瓣色泽、温度、厚度及真皮层渗血情况）或吲哚菁绿血管造影等对皮瓣灌注进行评估，判断组织血供情况[22, 23]（图 15.4）。

若术中观察到皮瓣低灌注征象，应避免实施胸肌前重建，此时应选择胸肌后重建或应用扩张器的两阶段重建，确认皮瓣灌注适宜后方可继续进行重建[18]。

假体选择需基于多项临床评估参数，测量乳房基底与高度、下极保护度、下垂程度、皮肤弹性与冗余量等（图 15.5）。术中需复核相关测量值并用试模校准。所选假体包括 Mentor®313/323/333 型、Allergan / Natrelle®410 型（已禁用）、

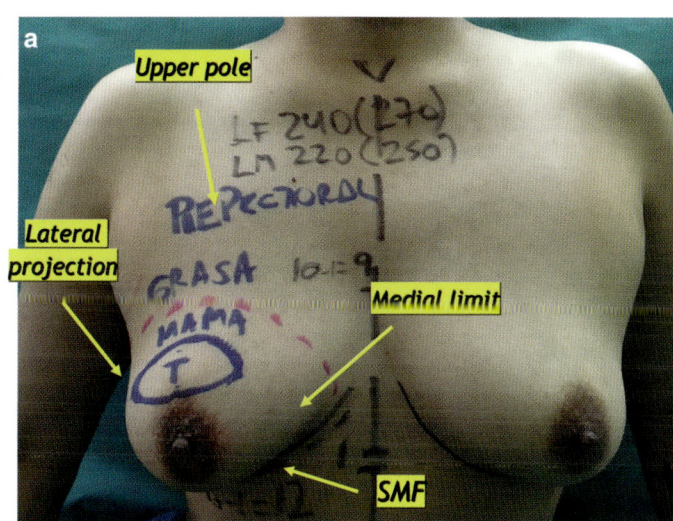
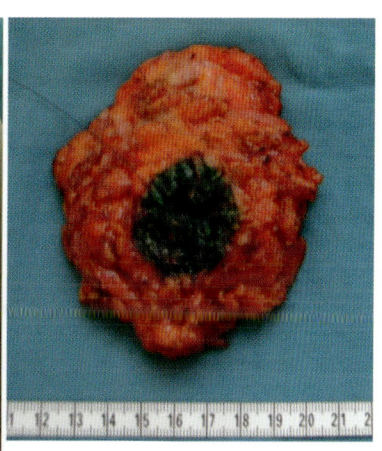
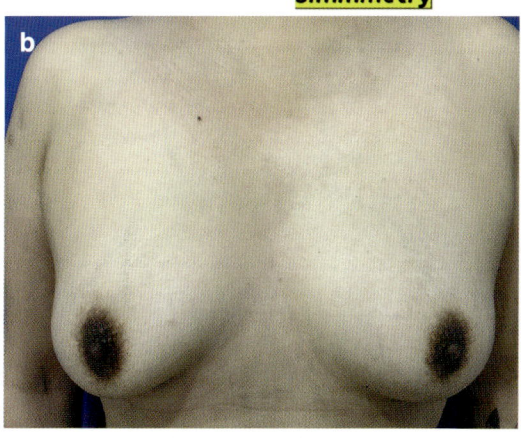
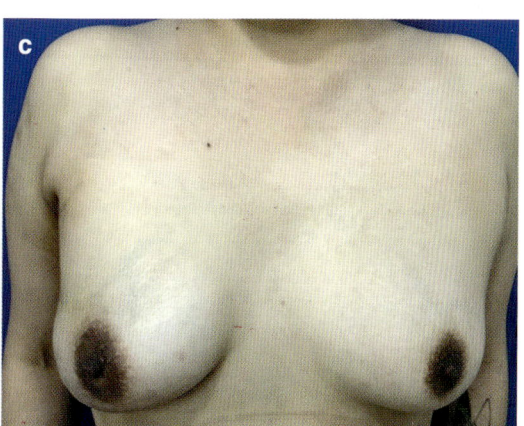

图 15.1 （a）高质量重建始于精准的乳房切除术：完整切除腺体组织同时保留乳房解剖边界，最大化脂肪组织存量。（b）右乳保留乳头乳房切除胸肌前重建术前。（c）术后效果

Motifu Ergonomix® 及 Potlytech® 等解剖型毛面假体，根据胸廓尺寸及期望乳房形态于胸肌前置入。

乳房切口采用可吸收缝线分两层闭合，脂肪层–皮下层与皮内缝合。对于单侧保留乳头乳房切除患者，若对侧乳房为中小体积且有 0~1 级下垂，术中同期行对称性调整；其他病例则于术后 6 个月（肿瘤治疗结束或放疗完成后 6 个月）行对称矫正手术。术后随访流程为：术后 4 周内每周复查，此后每 3 个月复查一次至术后 6 个月，1 年后每 4~6 个月随访。引流量低于 30mL/24h 时拔除引流装置。

表 15.1 如何预防并发症

胸肌前乳房重建 —— 如何预防并发症	
规划	解剖学
	术前影像学评估
	既往疾病（肥胖、吸烟、放疗史）
	策略选择（Ⅰ期手术、延迟手术、新辅助化疗等）
	技术选择
	切口设计
手术技术	皮瓣解剖
	乳房切除范围
	低温解剖方法
	存活能力评估方法（SPY 技术）
	腔隙选择
	假体选择（扩张器/假体）
	操作方式或术中技术调整
	引流

15.4 临床结果

我们于 2018 年 1 月至 2020 年 6 月在巴西 Curitiba，以及 2013 年 6 月至 2020 年 4 月在阿根廷 Buenos Aires 建立了多中心队列研究，纳入经乳房下皱襞切口（MFI）行保留乳头和乳晕乳房切除术（NSM）后立即行胸肌前假体直接置入重建的患者，未使用脱细胞真皮基质（ADM）或补片。该技术适用于所有尺寸及类型的乳房，包括预防性或治疗性手术。接受单侧或双侧 NSM 重建的患者也被纳入研究[24]。

共对 195 例连续病例采用上述术式完成了 280 例即刻乳房重建。患者平均年龄 45 岁，32.8% 处于绝经后。42 例（15.4%）为既往或现时吸烟者；92 例（32.9%）BMI 超过 25（超重或肥胖），7 例（5.4%）合并糖尿病。中位随访时间为 16.5 个月 ±17.43 个月。85 例（43.6%）采用该技术行双侧乳房切除即刻重建（IBR）；116 例（41.4%）为预防性乳房切除，164 例（58.6%）为治疗性乳房切除。68 例（24%）重建患者至少出现 1 种急性并发症，最常见的是假体取出（26 例乳房，9.2%），其他为持续性血清肿（19 例）、假体外露（23 例）、血肿（7 例），以及皮瓣或乳头–乳晕复合体（NAC）坏死（4 例）。轻度或中度表皮松解通常可自行消退。当发生皮肤或 NAC 坏死（依据感染或假体脱出风险判断）时，根据缺损类型采用不同修复技术干预（图 15.6）。假体取出中位时间为 64 天（12~180 天），主要原因包括皮瓣或 NAC 坏死及感染。与假体取出显著相关

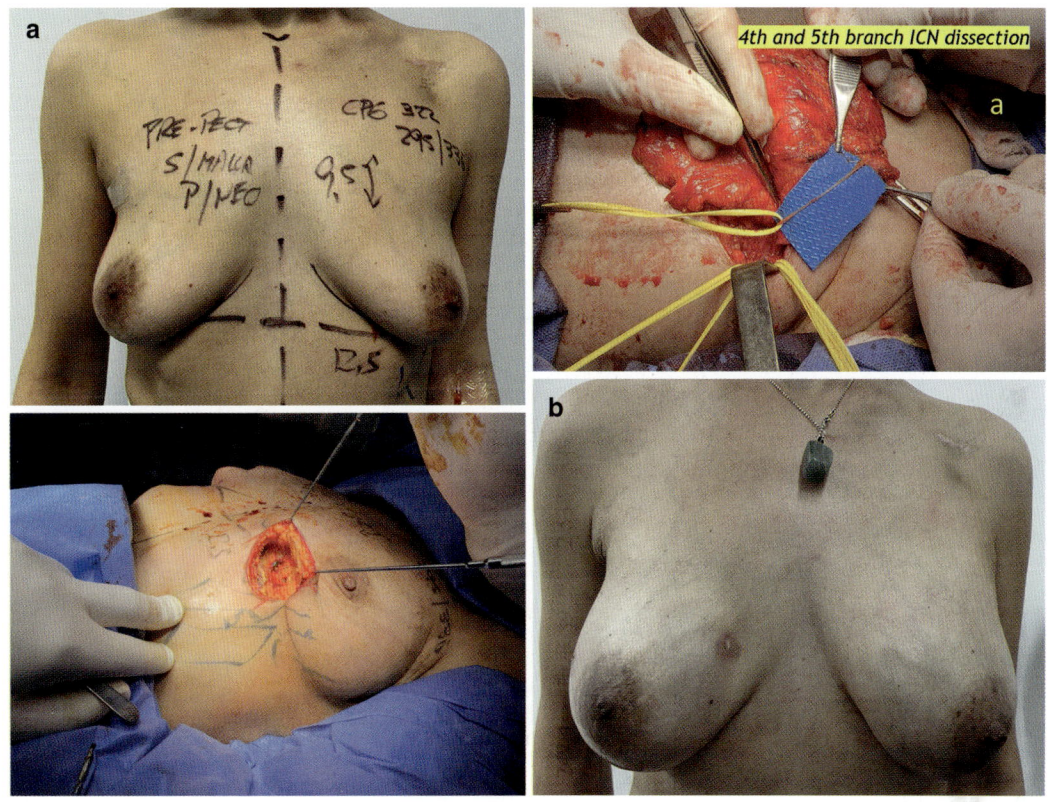

图 15.2 （a）双侧保留乳头乳房切除胸肌前重建术（新辅助治疗后 2+ 突变），采用经典乳房下皱襞切口（感觉神经保留）。（b）术后观

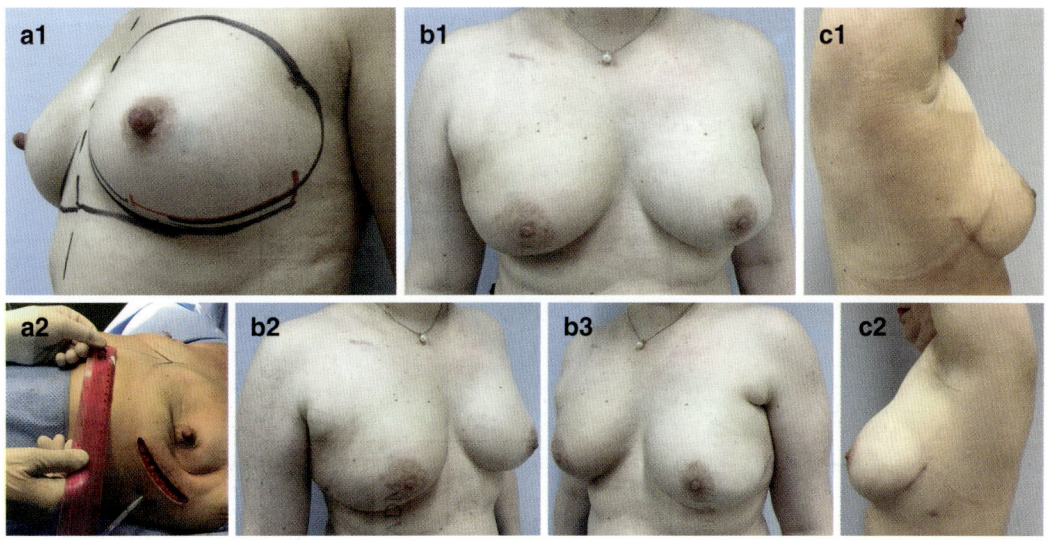

图 15.3 （a）乳房下外侧弧形切口（沿乳房下皱襞上方 1~2cm 至腋前线）。（b）终期效果，正位。（c）终期效果，侧位（瘢痕状态）

165

胸肌前乳房重建

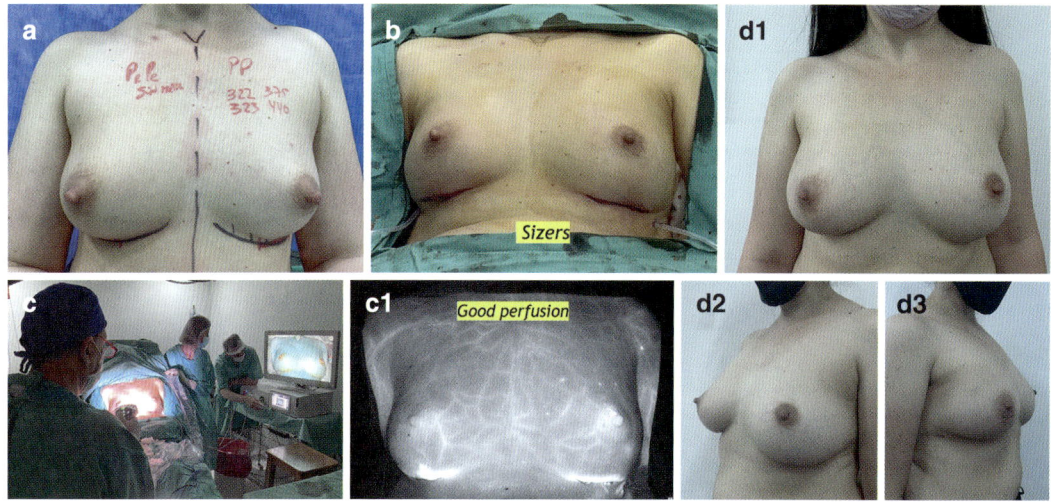

图 15.4 （a）双侧预防性保留乳头乳房切除胸肌前聚氨酯假体重建（右乳曾行保乳术+放疗）。（b）前间隙试模放置。（c）术中激光辅助吲哚菁绿荧光血管成像（LA-ICGA）。（d）术后 2 年无表皮松解或坏死

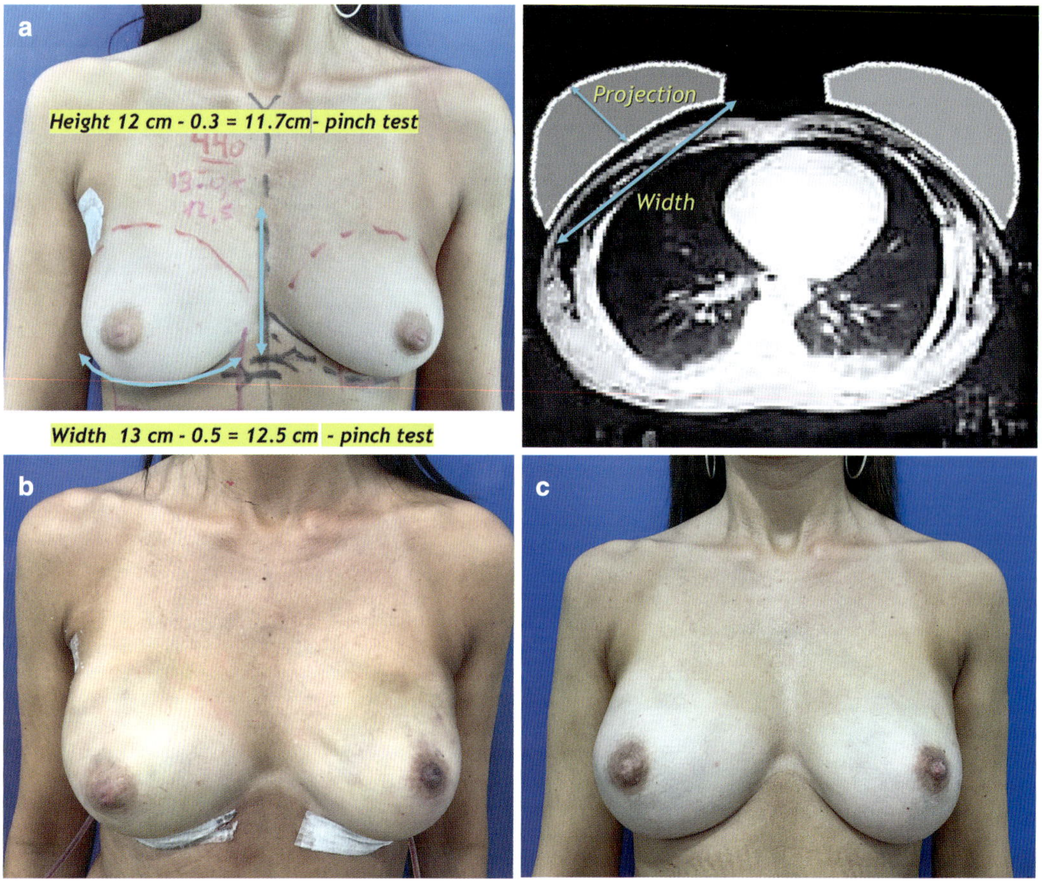

图 15.5 （a）假体选择策略。（b）双侧保留乳头乳房切除胸肌前重建术后 7 天。（c）术后 1 年效果

的风险因素为吸烟史（[OR]4.33；95%[CI]：1.81~10.37，P=0.0012），BMI超过25（OR 2.21；95%CI：0.98~4.99；P=0.077）及化疗（OR 2.23；95%CI：0.97~5.11；P=0.062）。其他因素如既往放疗、辅助放疗及糖尿病患者的假体脱出率也较高，但未达统计学显著性。腋窝淋巴结清扫、既往乳房手术史、乳房大小及下垂无相关性。

仅对随访超过6个月的病例（n=184）评估晚期并发症。15例乳房（8.1%）出现Ⅱ级波纹，7例（3.8%）出现需矫正的Ⅲ、Ⅳ级波纹（图15.7）。29例重建（15.7%）发生Baker Ⅱ~Ⅳ级包膜挛缩（图15.8），其中Baker Ⅱ级22例（11.9%）、Ⅲ级6例（3.3%）、Ⅳ级1例（0.5%）。126例乳房（45%）未出现包膜挛缩（图15.9）。44例乳房（15.7%）接受术后放疗，6例（13.6%）出现假体移位，11例（25%）无包膜挛缩（图15.10），Baker Ⅰ级7例（15.9%）、Ⅱ级8例（18.2%）、Ⅲ级3例（6.8%）（另有8例数据缺失）。观察到1例假体旋转。随访期内未发现动态畸形。美学评估（使用BCCT.core软件）[25]显示大部分患者（包括乳房较大者）效果

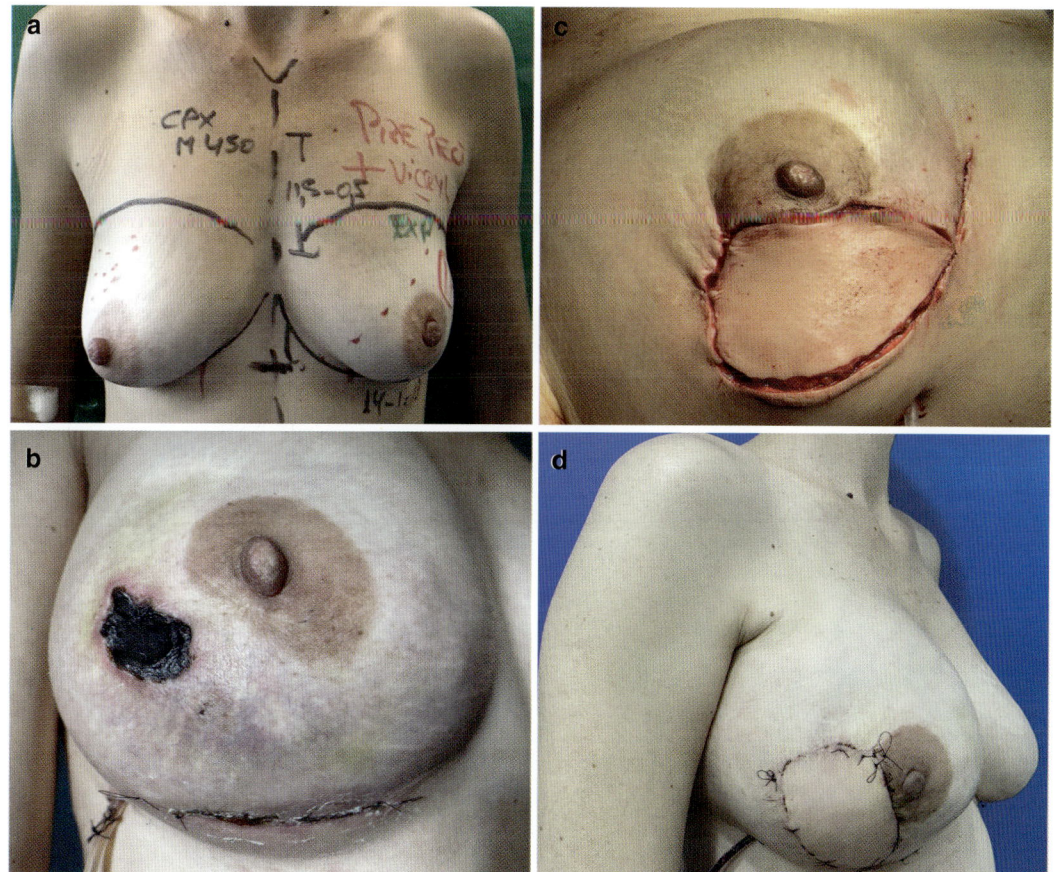

图15.6 （a）双侧保留乳头乳房切除无补片假体直接重建（DTI）。（b）右乳皮肤坏死。（c，d）背阔肌皮瓣移植保全假体

满意,乳房下皱襞切口隐蔽(图15.11)。

15.5 考量因素

NSM术后即刻重建存在多种技术选择,包括临时扩张器置入、假体直接置入或自体皮瓣重建。术式决策需综合考量术者经验、医疗机构可用材料及患者相关风险因素[如吸烟史、糖尿病、BMI、乳房特征(大小与下垂)及辅助抗癌治疗(放疗、化疗、内分泌治疗、淋巴结清扫)],上述因素可能增加美学效果不佳及并发症发生率增高的风险[26~30]。皮瓣灌注质量、血管完整性及乳房切除术操作水平,对胸

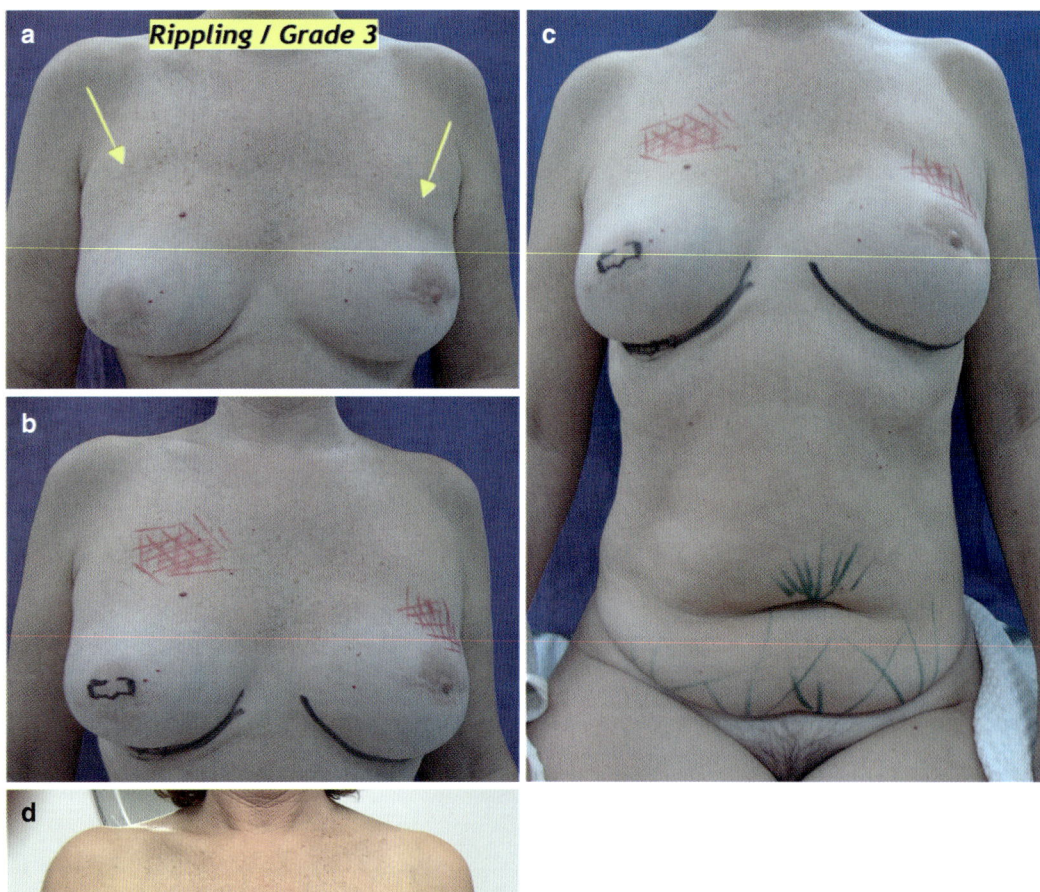

图15.7 (a)双侧保留乳头乳房切除无补片直接假体重建术后并发症(右侧假体褶皱伴乳头坏死)。(b,c)修复方案为脂肪移植+乳头重建。(d)终期效果

肌前重建成功至关重要[19~23]。

胸肌前术式的主要优势包括缩短手术时间，避免动态畸形，以及术后疼痛较轻（减少麻醉镇痛药需求并加速恢复），胸肌前术式的术后并发症发生率与部分肌覆盖技术相当。尽管多项研究证实了胸肌前假体乳房重建的优势，但多数研究主要关注两阶段组织扩张器法或需使用脱细胞真

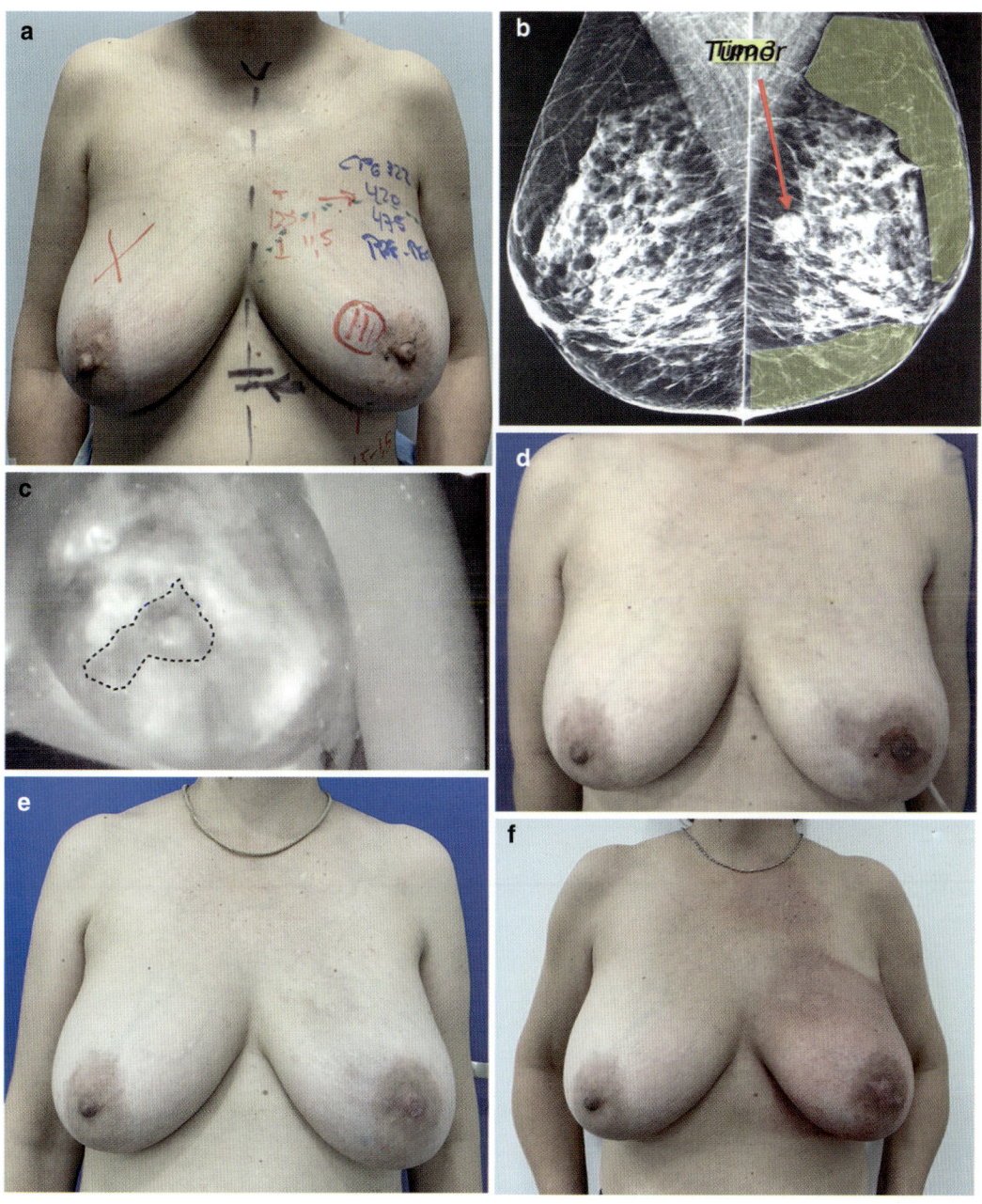

图15.8 （a）新辅助治疗后左侧保留乳头的乳房切除，无补片胸肌前重建。（b）3型脂肪结构乳腺X线表现。（c）术中血管成像示中度低灌注。（d）乳头-乳晕复合体部分坏死。（e）全层修复。（f）放疗结束

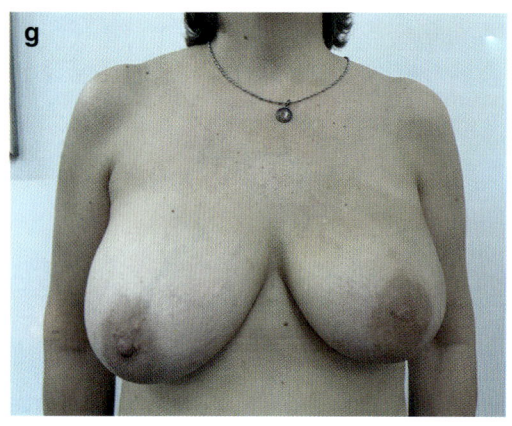

图 15.8（续） （g）放疗 1 年后轻度不对称与 Baker Ⅱ级包膜挛缩

皮基质（ADM）、补片支撑的假体直接置入术[30, 31]。Li 等对 16 项对比研究进行荟萃分析，发现胸肌前与胸肌后术式在总体并发症、假体脱出、血清肿、乳头或皮瓣坏死、血肿、再手术、伤口裂开及伤口-皮肤感染、波纹形成方面无统计学差异，并且胸肌前组 Breast Q 评分更高，术后疼痛更轻[32]。

胸肌前重建并非适用于所有患者。理想人群通常为中小乳房且无下垂或轻度下垂者，同时需排除其他风险因素（如肥胖、吸

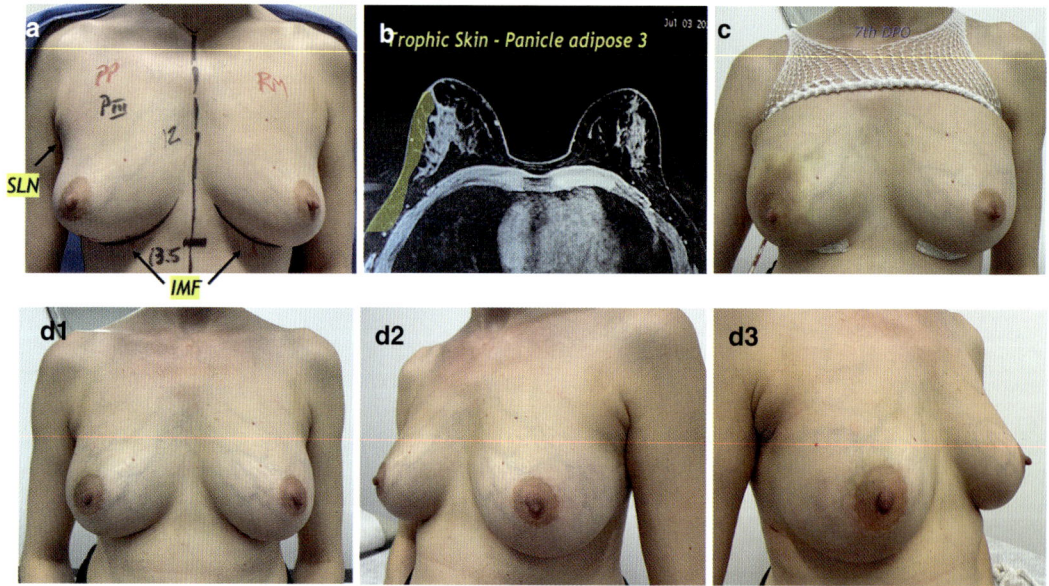

图 15.9 （a）右侧保留乳头乳房切除无补片胸肌前重建联合对侧隆乳。（b）MRI 显示 3 型脂肪结构。（c）术后 7 天。（d）术后 1 年无包膜挛缩

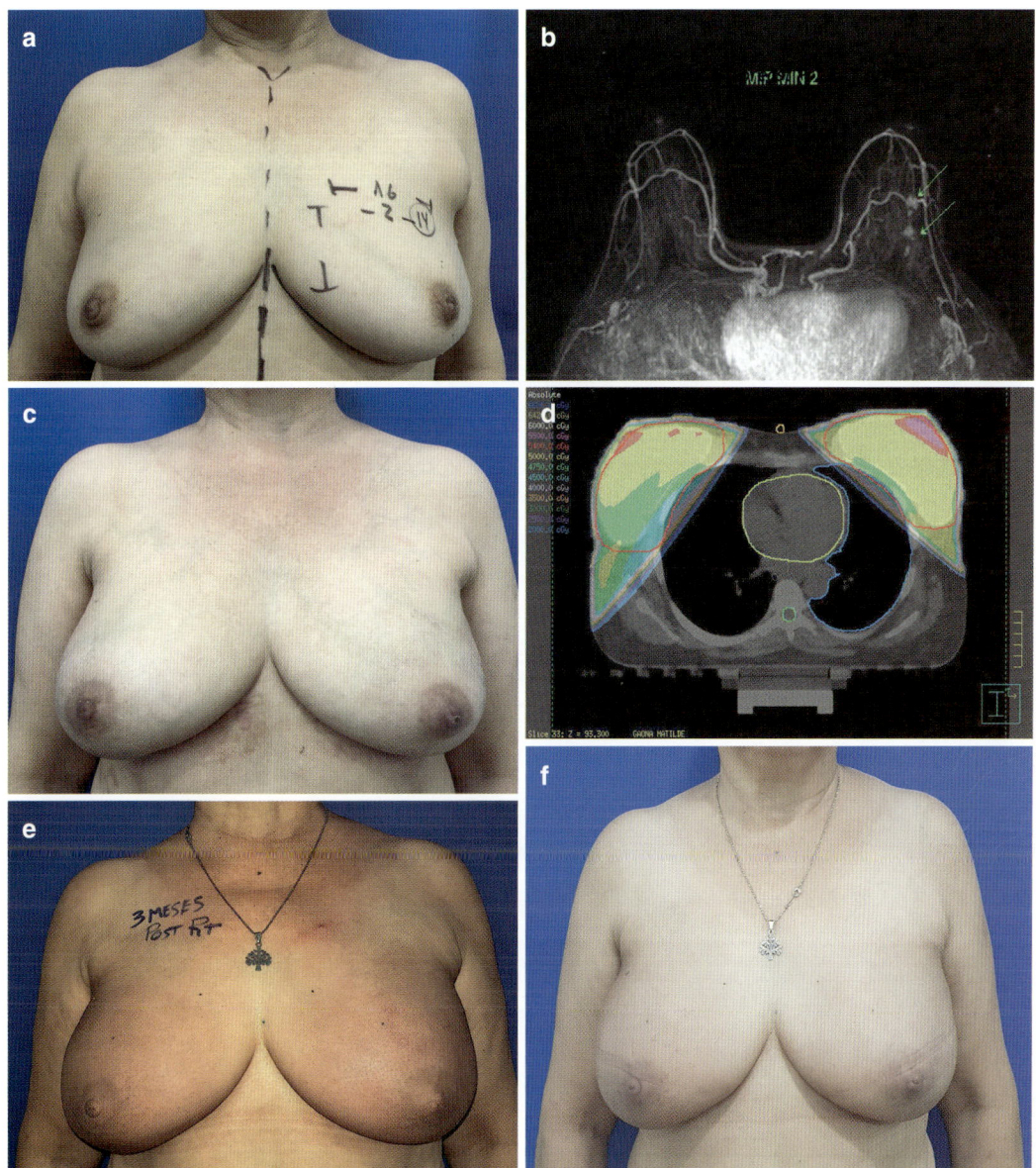

图15.10 （a）三阴性乳腺癌新辅助治疗后双侧保留乳头乳房切除联合无补片胸肌前重建。（b）MRI 示右乳完全缓解，左乳部分缓解。（c）术后21天。（d）双侧辅助放疗规划。（e）全层修复。（f）放疗结束。（e）放疗后即刻效果。（f）放疗后1年无包膜挛缩且对称性良好

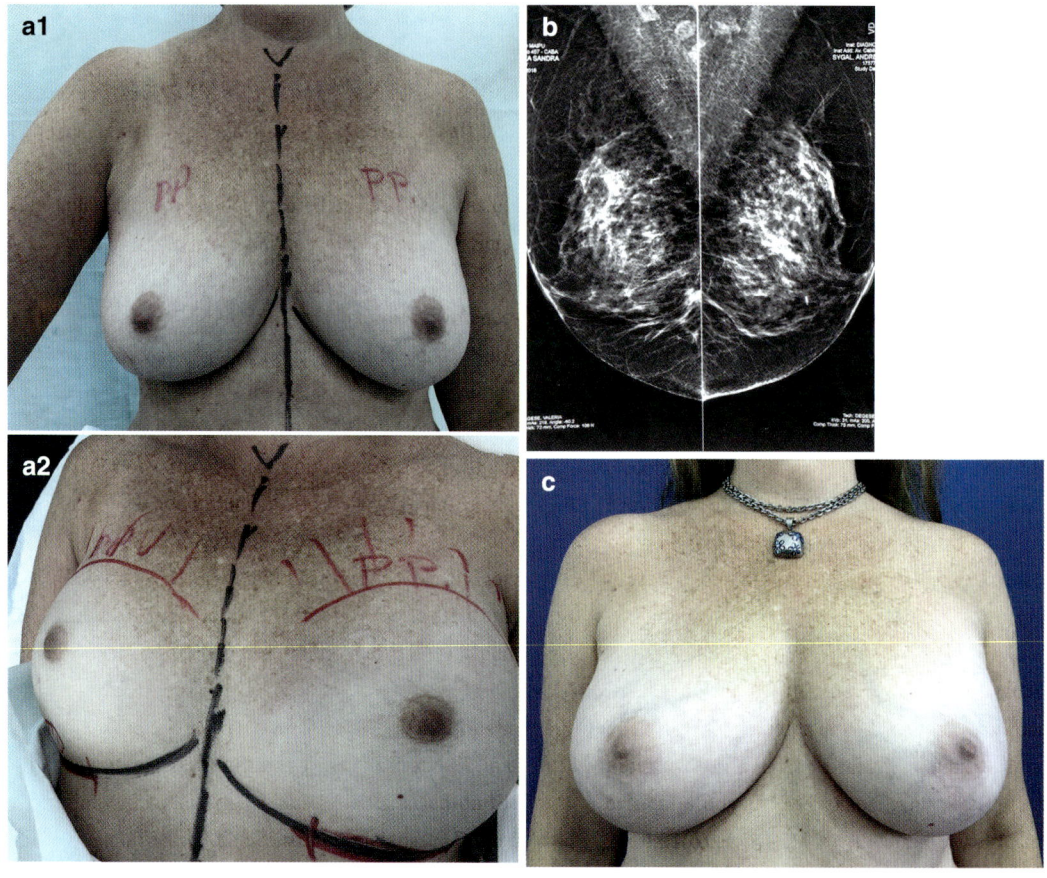

图 15.11 （a）BRCA1 突变携带者双侧保留乳头乳房切除无补片重建。（b）3 型脂肪结构乳腺 X 线表现。（c）终期美学效果优

烟、糖尿病及既往乳房放疗）[8-23, 26-34]。即便符合上述条件，许多术者仍倾向分阶段重建[26-29]。本研究未按此标准筛选患者。最常见早期并发症为假体取出，多与皮瓣坏死、感染及吸烟相关。本组假体取出率为 9.2%，与保留皮肤乳房切除胸肌后重建（SSM）及使用 ADM/补片的胸肌前重建研究结果接近[29-32, 34]，仅 1 例发生假体旋转。预期无肌肉覆盖时高发的显著波纹（Ⅲ-Ⅳ级）仅见于极少数病例（7/184 例乳房）。波纹/褶皱出现时需考虑皮瓣厚度、假体-乳房切除体积比例及假体黏聚度等因素，虽然普遍认为胸肌前重建中此类现象较常见，但缺乏明确数据支持。本研究显示其发生率亦较低。

包膜挛缩是假体重建术后常见并发症，常与放疗相关。Chu 等文献综述指出，术前/术后放疗均显著增加假体丢失风险[35]。肌肉纤维化可促进放疗后挛缩的发生。Sobti 等发现胸肌后组较胸肌前组包膜挛缩发生率更高（$n=28$，51.8%；$n=12$，30.0%；$P=0.02$）。对于放疗患者，胸肌后假体直接置入（DTI）发生包膜挛缩的风险约为胸肌前组的 4 倍（$P<0.01$）。本

研究中，15.7%（29例）患者出现Baker Ⅱ~Ⅳ级包膜挛缩，其中14例接受辅助放疗，未放疗组仅6.3%（15例乳房）发生包膜挛缩[13]。

补片及脱细胞真皮基质（ADM）可作为假体与乳房切除后皮瓣间的血管化再生组织层，有助于稳定重建乳房形态[29]。虽ADM被整形外科医师广泛使用，但Salibian等的研究表明，乳房切除皮瓣足够厚且严格保留天然乳房下皱襞时无须使用ADM，250例未使用ADM的胸肌前重建病例（随访10年）的结果显示，7.6%患者发生明显的包膜挛缩，0.8%出现假体移位，85.2%患者达到优良美学效果[31]。Heidemann等对NSM后行假体直接置入（DTI）ADM重建患者的并发症发生情况的系统综述与荟萃分析表明，ADM可能增加急性并发症风险[36]，报道的乳头-乳晕复合体（NAC）坏死率为4%，感染率为12%，血清肿的发生率为5%，血肿的发生率为1%，均与本组研究相当，需进一步论证ADM与急性并发症的关联性。ADM与补片成本昂贵（1 000~20 000美元），本组280例胸肌前DTI乳房重建未使用此类材料，但其并发症发生率及疗效与使用组相似。目前无ADM及补片支持的胸肌前DTI重建相关数据仍有限。

皮瓣坏死为主要并发症之一，发生率为3%~7%。Daar等的荟萃分析显示经乳房下皱襞切口（IMF）行NSM，术后NAC坏死发生率为6.82%[28]。本研究中仅4例（1.4%）发生NAC坏死，20例（7.1%）出现皮瓣坏死。乳房切除皮瓣因厚度、尺寸及灌注差异而变化，故皮瓣评估是胸肌前重建成功的关键决定因素。与灌注质量相比，乳房切除操作水平及皮瓣厚度并非首要考量，消瘦及年轻患者皮瓣通常较薄，超重/肥胖及年长患者皮瓣多较厚。正常乳房皮下组织厚度因人而异（2~3cm），当皮瓣较厚且灌注良好时，可选择于胸肌前置入永久假体或组织扩张器。

15.6　小结

2013~2020年，我们通过多中心队列研究纳入了治疗性或风险降低性胸肌前假体直接置入即刻乳房重建病例（无生物或合成补片辅助），包含各种类型的乳房（无下垂或中度下垂）、不同皮下脂肪层分布、不同BMI（吸烟与否）及有/无放疗史患者。

该技术相关并发症的发生率与文献报告的ADM、补片使用组或胸肌后重建组无显著差异，波纹及包膜挛缩的发生率亦未增加。数据表明，该技术具有应用前景及安全性，并且因无需ADM或补片的Ⅰ期手术更具经济效益优势，亦避免了动态畸形。本研究仅为短期及长期结果的初步数据，尚需大样本对比研究验证。

要点

- 手术并发症发生率与使用合成补片、ADM或胸肌后重建组相似。
- 波纹发生率不高于其他技术。
- 包膜挛缩发生率不高于其他技术。
- 放疗患者的包膜挛缩发生率与其他技术相当且不影响乳房形态，可较好地维持对称性。

- 无动态畸形。
- 该技术为无需ADM或补片的Ⅰ期手术，安全可行且节省成本。

参考文献

1. Freeman BS. Subcutaneous mastectomy for benign breast lesions with immediate or delayed prosthetic replacement. Plast Reconstr Surg. 1980,65(3):371–2.
2. Freeman BS. Technique of subcutaneous mastectomy with replacement; immediate and delayed. Br J Plast Surg. 1969,22(2):161–6.
3. Snyderman RK, Guthrie RH. Reconstruction of the female breast following radical mastectomy. Plast Reconstr Surg. 1971,47(6):565–7.
4. Schlenker JD, Bueno RA, Ricketson G, Lynch JB. Loss of silicone implants after subcutaneous mastectomy and reconstruction. Plast Reconstr Surg. 1978,62(6):853–61.
5. Gruber RP, Kahn RA, Lash H, Maser MR, Apfelberg DB, Laub DR. Breast reconstruction following mastectomy: a comparison of submuscular and subcutaneous techniques. Plast Reconstr Surg. 1981,67(3):312–7.
6. Serra-Renom JM, Fontdevila J, Monner J, Benito J. Mammary reconstruction using tissue expander and partial detachment of the pectoralis major muscle to expand the lower breast quadrants. Ann Plast Surg. 2004,53(4):317–21.
7. Breuing K, Warren S. Immediate bilateral breast reconstruction with implants and inferolateral AlloDerm slings. Ann Plast Surg. 2005,55(3):232–9.
8. Namnoum JD. Expander/implant reconstruction with AlloDerm: recent experience. Plast Reconstr Surg. 2009,124(2):387–94.
9. Colwell A. Direct-to-implant breast reconstruction. Gland Surg. 2012,1(3):139–41.
10. Dieterich M, Faridi A. Biological matrices and synthetic meshes used in implant-based breast reconstruction: a review of products available in germany. Geburtshilfe Frauenheilkd. 2013,73(11):1100–6.
11. Ho G, Nguyen TJ, Shahabi A, Hwang BH, Chan LS, Wong AK. A systematic review and meta-analysis of complications associated with acellular dermal matrix-assisted breast reconstruction. Ann Plast Surg. 2012,68(4):346–56.
12. Potter S, Conroy EJ, Cutress RI, Williamson PR, Whisker L, Thrush S, Skillman J, Barnes NLP, Mylvaganam S, Teasdale E, Jain A, Gardiner MD, Blazeby JM, Holcombe C, iBRA Steering Group; Breast Reconstruction Research Collaborative. Short-term safety outcomes of mastectomy and immediate implant-based breast reconstruction with and without mesh (iBRA): a multicentre, prospective cohort study. Lancet Oncol. 2019,20(2):254–66.
13. Sobti N, Weitzman RE, Nealon KP, Jimenez RB, Gfrerer L, Mattos D, Ehrlichman RJ, Gadd M, Specht M, Austen WG, Liao EC. Evaluation of capsular contracture following immediate prepectoral versus subpectoral direct-to-implant breast reconstruction. Sci Rep. 2020,10(1):1137.
14. Chatterjee A, Nahabedian MY, Gabriel A, Macarios D, Parekh M, Wang F, Griffin L, Sigalove S. Early assessment of post-surgical outcomes with pre-pectoral breast reconstruction: a literature review and meta-analysis. J Surg Oncol. 2018,117(6):1119–30.
15. Sigalove S, Maxwell GP, Sigalove NM, Storm-Dickerson TL, Pope N, Rice J, et al. Prepectoral implant-based breast reconstruction. Plast Reconstr Surg. 2017,139(2):287–94.
16. Sbitany H, Piper M, Lentz R. Prepectoral breast reconstruction: a safe alternative to submuscular prosthetic reconstruction following nipple-sparing mastectomy. Plast Reconstr Surg. 2017,140(3):432–43.
17. Sbitany H. Important considerations for performing prepectoral breast reconstruction. Plast Reconstr Surg. 2017,140(6S):7S–13S.
18. Nahabedian MY. Current approaches to prepectoral breast reconstruction. Plast Reconstr Surg.

19. Kaidar-Person O, Boersma LJ, Poortmans P, Sklair-Levy M, Offersen BV, Cardoso MJ, de Ruysscher D. Residual glandular breast tissue after mastectomy: a systematic review. Ann Surg Oncol. 2020,27(7):2288–96.
20. Carlson GW, Chu CK, Moyer HR, Duggal C, Losken A. Predictors of nipple ischemia after nipple sparing mastectomy. Breast J. 2014,20(1):69–73.
21. Blechman KM, Karp NS, Levovitz C, Guth AA, Axelrod DM, Shapiro RL, Choi M. The lateral inframammary fold incision for nipple-sparing mastectomy: outcomes from over 50 immediate implant-based breast reconstructions. Breast J. 2013,19(1):31–40.
22. Gurtner GC, Jones GE, Neligan PC, Newman MI, Phillips BT, Sacks JM, Zenn MR. Intraoperative laser angiography using the SPY system: review of the literature and recommendations for use. Ann Surg Innov Res. 2013,7(1):1.
23. Lauritzen E, Damsgaard TE. Use of Indocyanine Green Angiography decreases the risk of complications in autologous and implant-based breast reconstruction: A systematic review and meta-analysis. J Plast Reconstr Aesthet Surg. 2021,74(8):1703–17.
24. Urban CA, Gonzalez E, Fornazzari A, et al. Prepectoral direct-to-implant breast reconstruction without placement of acellular dermal matrix or mesh after nipple sparing mastectomy. Plast Reconstr Surg 2022,150(5):973–983. doi: https://doi.org/10.1097/PRS.0000000000009618
25. Hart A, Doyle K, Losken A, Carlson GW. Nipple malposition after bilateral nipple-sparing mastectomy with implant-based reconstruction: objective postoperative analysis utilizing BCCT. core computer software. Breast J. 2020 Jul; 26(7):1270–5.
26. Weber PW, Haug M, Kurzeder C, et al. Oncoplastic Breast Consortium consensus conference on nipple-sparing mastectomy. Breast Cancer Res Treat. 2018,172:523–37.
27. Storm-Dickerson T, Sigalove N. Prepectoral breast reconstruction: the breast surgeon's perspective. Plast Reconstr Surg. 2017,140:43S.
28. Daar DA, Abdou SA, Rosario L, et al. Is there a preferred incision location for nipple-sparing mastectomy? A systematic review and meta-analysis. Plast Reconstr Surg. 2019,143:906e.
29. Storm-Dickerson T, Sigalove NM. The breast surgeons' approach to mastectomy and prepectoral breast reconstruction. Gland Surg. 2019,8(1):27–35.
30. Manrique OJ, Huang TCT, Martinez-Jorge J, et al. Prepectoral two-stage implant-based breast reconstruction with and without acellular dermal matrix: do we see a difference? Plast Reconstr Surg. 2020,145:263e.
31. Salibian AH, Harness JK, Mowlds DS. Staged suprapectoral expander/implant reconstruction without acellular dermal matrix following nipple-sparing mastectomy. Plast Reconstr Surg. 2017,139:30–9.
32. Li L, Su Y, Xiu B, et al. Comparison of prepectoral and subpectoral breast reconstruction after mastectomies: a systematic review and meta-analysis. Eur J Surg Oncol. 2019,45:1542–50.
33. Vidya R, Iqbal FM, Becker H, Zhadan O. Rippling associated with pre-pectoral implant-based breast reconstruction: a new grading system. World J Plast Surg. 2019,8:311–5.
34. Louw RPT, Nahabedian MY. Prepectoral breast reconstruction. Plast Reconstr Surg. 2017,140: 51S.
35. Chu CK, Davis MJ, Winocour SJ, et al. Implant reconstruction in nipple sparing mastectomy. Semin Plast Surg. 2019,33:247–57.
36. Heidemann LN, Gunnarsson GL, Salzberg CA. Complications following nipple-sparing mastectomy and immediate acellular dermal matrix implant-based breast reconstruction—a systematic review and meta-analysis. Plast Reconstr Surg Glob Open. 2018,6:e1625.

16 胸肌前皮肤缩减术式

编者：Glenda Giorgia Caputo and Maurizio Governa

译者：李 彤

16.1 引言

皮肤缩减乳房重建术是一种较新的乳房切除/重建技术，涉及在胸肌前置入假体。Nava 等于 2006 年描述了本术式，假体被置于包含胸大肌及通过乳房下极去表皮化形成的皮肤-脂肪瓣的腔隙内[1]。2016 年，《整形与重建外科》报道[2]，此技术改良后无须分离胸大肌；将假体置于胸肌前间隙，下界为由依 Wise 法术前设计行乳房切除术时保留的皮肤-脂肪瓣构成的囊袋，上界为真皮基质；所述真皮基质缝合至胸肌筋膜，从而确保覆盖假体上极。

胸肌前重建的优势显而易见：由于无须分离肌肉，手术创伤更小，因而术后出血风险更低。此外，避免了肌下重建术中由胸大肌收缩引起的假体移位（肌下重建的典型并发症），患者的舒适度似乎得到了改善。事实上，胸肌前重建未出现常规肌下假体置入后的明显异物感[3]。

即便如此，本术式仍存在若干潜在并发症，首要的是乳房切除皮瓣可能发生缺血性损伤，导致患者面临假体外露及重建失败的风险。本章将阐述缩皮法乳房重建术的适应证、手术技术、常见并发症及其处理措施，并提出了若干降低并发症发生风险的建议。

16.2 适应证

要实现良好的乳房重建效果，必须从准确的患者选择和严谨的手术技术着手。该术式适用于因局灶性、多灶性或中心性乳腺癌（需排除炎性乳腺癌）需行乳房切除且伴有巨乳症及乳房下垂的患者（经捏持试验证实皮下脂肪厚度 >1cm 且乳房下极皮肤无肿瘤侵犯），也可作为巨乳症或重度乳房下垂患者（即存在乳房缩小术或乳房悬吊术指征的非肿瘤患者）行预防性

G. G. Caputo (✉)
Plastic and Reconstructive Surgery-ASUFC Udine,
Udine, Italy

M. Governa
Plastic and Reconstructive Surgery-AOUI Verona,
Verona, Italy

© The Author(s), under exclusive license to Springer Nature Switzerland AG 2023
R. Vidya, H. Becker (eds.), *Prepectoral Breast Reconstruction*,
https://doi.org/10.1007/978-3-031-15590-1_16

乳房切除术时的重建方法。此前开展的术前术后乳房 Q 量表评估显示，缩皮法乳房重建患者的评分与乳房缩小术患者处于同一水平；换言之，两类患者报告的术后健康状态改善程度具有可比性。

早期应用该技术进行乳房重建时，认为术后接受放疗属于绝对禁忌证。近年来，基于对放疗后假体周围包膜组织学特征的新认识（与应用脱细胞真皮基质覆盖的皮下内置物形成的包膜相比，肌肉后间隙的包膜更厚且更具抗性）[4]，以及脱细胞真皮基质辅助假体乳房重建可降低包膜挛缩发生率的证据[5, 6]，我们修正了这一观点。不过，对于因象限切除联合放疗（QUART）后复发或继发肿瘤而行乳房切除术的病例仍需谨慎：此类患者因既往接受过放疗，其乳房切除皮瓣存在活力问题[7]，故应视为倒 T 形切口胸肌前重建的禁忌证。

在评估缩皮法乳房重建术的潜在适用人群时，需要完整采集病史，包括吸烟史、糖尿病史、心脏病史、高龄及高体重指数等可能增加术后并发症风险的要素。

16.3 手术技术

16.3.1 术前设计

根据常规 Wise 模板法在术前精准画线（图 16.1）：首先，自胸骨切迹至脐部标记正中垂直线（a）。沿锁骨自此线向外测量 7~9cm（具体长度需根据患者胸廓形态调整）：胸廓狭小、肩窄者宜取

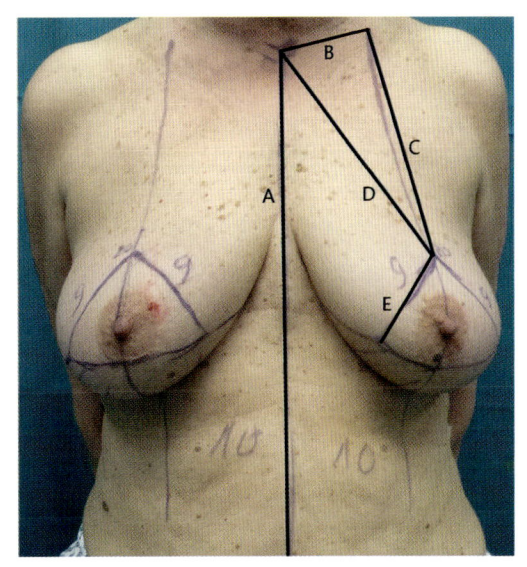

图 16.1 术前设计

7cm，胸肩宽大者则以 9cm 为佳（b）。自此点向乳头方向画线（c），并延伸至乳房下皱襞下方（画线时需用手上托乳房），继续向腹壁延伸。此点至胸骨切迹 – 脐正中线的距离应为 8~11cm（依胸廓宽度而定）。随后，标记乳头投影线与锁骨中线的交点：乳房下垂者自胸骨切向外 19~21cm，巨乳症者为 21~24cm（d）。上述测量值仅具参考意义，因胸骨切迹至乳头的距离应基于重建乳房预期缩小或抬升的幅度而定，确保与患者体型协调。换言之，重建乳房应"量体裁衣"，充分考虑患者的整体体态。故对体格健硕者实施乳房缩小时，应保留相对较大的乳房体积。此原则体现于胸骨切迹至乳头的距离设定。需要注意的是，过大假体（通常指体积 >500cm³ 者）不仅增加并发症风险，而且无法确保远期效果稳定，因假体在重力作用下其下垂程度会逐渐增加（详见下文假体选择部分相关内容）。

术前标记的最后阶段需将乳房向内、向外推移，以标定垂直瘢痕的内外侧臂。自新乳头位置向内外侧各画一条长 8~9cm 的线（E），此长度为垂直切口长度（6~7cm）与乳头－乳晕复合体半径（2cm）之和。术前 30 分钟常规静脉给予抗生素（头孢唑林 2g）。

16.3.2 切除步骤

浸润注射克林（Klein）溶液[8]，以实现无血术野并促进剥离平面水分离。具体范围需包括：①乳房区皮下层，即乳房切除术剥离平面（Cooper 韧带所在层面）；②下极区域全层表皮－真皮内层面，此处将形成假体周围囊袋皮瓣；③乳头－乳晕复合体所在部位真皮下层，该区域将作为全厚皮片移植供区（仅当乳晕后腺体标本术中冰冻病理检查示肿瘤细胞阴性时进行移植）。

此时进行真皮－脂肪瓣去表皮化操作。根据经验，保留乳房在原位状态下进行操作更为便捷。此外，用剪刀而非手术刀更利于单人操作（无须助手协助牵拉松弛的皮肤，此操作在使用冷刀去表皮时必不可少）。该步骤需遵循精细外科技术原则以减轻组织损伤，从而降低组织受损程度[9]。随后通过宽切口完成乳房切除、淋巴结清扫，腋窝切口采用皮下缝合，并与乳房切除区域分隔。至此术野完成准备，可进入重建阶段。

16.3.3 重建步骤

保留下极去表皮化区域的真皮瓣（图 16.2），用其与脱细胞真皮基质（ADM）补片联合构建真皮囊袋（图 16.3）；ADM/真皮瓣联合体用于覆盖解剖型假体上极，以可吸收缝线固定（图 16.4）。若 ADM 未预开孔，则应在助手牵拉其绷紧状态下用 11 号刀片穿刺打孔。此时可置入试模（如有条件）并以金属钉临时闭合切口，以评估创口闭合张力及双侧乳房对称性（双侧乳房切除术者需同期处理对侧，单侧乳房手术者需行对侧乳房缩小术）。体积评估应使患者取坐位（上半身前倾 45°~60°），如有荧光血管成像设备可注射吲哚菁绿评估皮瓣活性；血运欠佳的皮缘应予修剪，并可选择临时/永久性扩张器或更小、凸度更低的假体。若无荧光血管成像条件，则应通过临床检查判断皮瓣活力，以决定假体或扩张器选择[10]。要点在于全程坚持精细操作：从使用剪刀行乳房切除术、应用无创拉钩稳妥暴露术野，至避免过度牵拉（通常无须此举）。

最终的假体或扩张器置入后，可通过

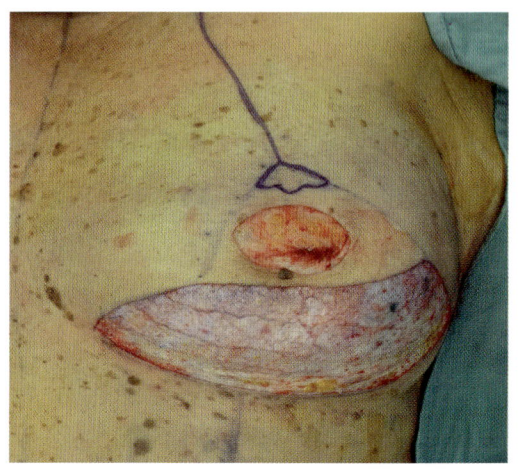

图 16.2　去表皮化下极保留

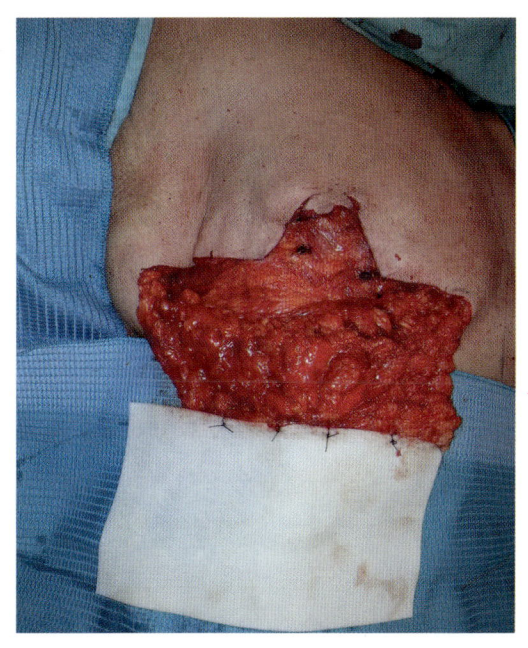

图 16.3 脱细胞真皮基质（ADM）与真皮瓣缝合

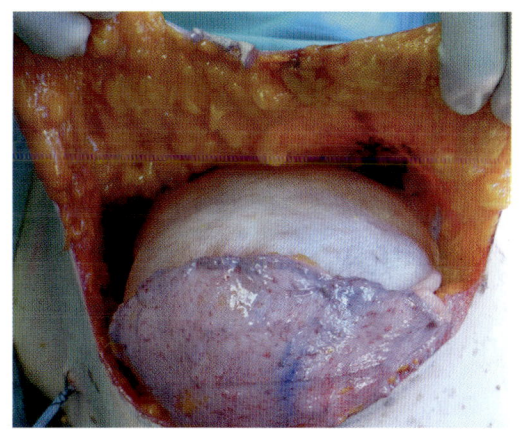

图 16.4 ADM–真皮复合瓣覆盖假体

外侧缝合真皮瓣与前锯肌筋膜闭合囊袋。为清晰界定乳房下皱襞，可沿皱襞切开真皮瓣基底（长度≤4cm）。随后将脱细胞真皮基质上缘以单根可吸收缝线固定于胸大肌前筋膜，囊袋内放置引流管，最后按倒 T 形缝合皮肤（图 16.5）。

乳头重建可于新乳房最凸点（对应于倒 T 形垂直臂尖端）用箭头形皮瓣等术式

来完成。若术中乳晕后腺体冰冻病理检查结果为阴性，则在标记新乳晕位置并行真皮内 Klein 液浸润后，将新乳头周围区域去表皮化以准备乳晕移植床（乳晕供区已于手术开始时切取并暂存于生理盐水中）。若无乳晕皮肤可供移植，可嘱患者愈后行纹饰着色处理。

假体选择需要考虑以下要点。根据经验，毛面解剖型假体可获得良好效果，但须谨记假体重建（尤其是皮下置入式）的成功率很大程度上取决于乳房切除皮瓣的血供状况。因此，并非所有病例均可即刻置入定容型假体。若皮瓣可靠性存疑，为避免切口裂开及延迟愈合风险，建议置入可调容型假体（后期进行生理盐水填充）[11]，或选择初始填充量最小的乳房扩张器（显然，后者需二次手术更换为永久假体）。通过维持假体/扩张器于低容状态，可降低缝合张力，提高切口愈合概率。同理，为降低倒 T 形切口中央区域张力，应优先选择中低凸度假体。假体的横径及垂直径需通过术前精确测量来确定，依据患者个

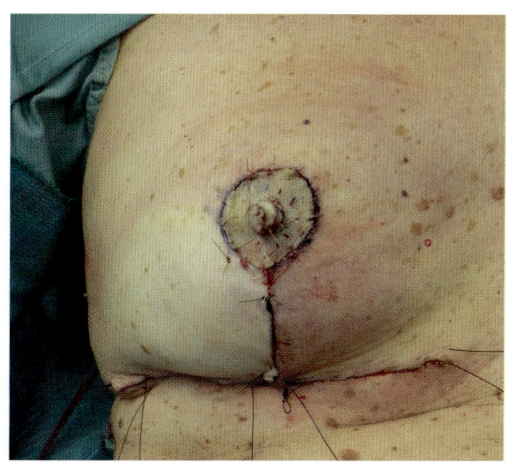

图 16.5 手术即刻重建乳房形态

体人体测量学特征调整，力求贴合自然乳房的基底形态。

16.4 术后管理

术后管理需密切关注愈合不良的细微征象，及时处理可避免进展为需要取出假体的严重并发症。本节基于本中心经验及关键行为学评估，列出术后监护重点事项。

1. 强烈建议术后 30 天内 24 小时持续穿戴专用术后塑形胸衣，但应避免对乳房上象限加压包扎；需确保胸衣弹性带不会过度压迫倒 T 形切口区域，必要时可适当松开乳房下缘弹力带。

2. 连续 2 日 24 小时引流量 <30mL 且切口边缘血运良好、愈合满意后，方可拔除引流管。

3. 重建乳头区域禁止使用加压敷料，但乳晕移植区需适度加压；建议将外科海绵裁剪成环形垫片以避开乳头施压，并于其上方覆盖非黏性敷料。

4. 皮肤愈合前限制患者上肢活动，以减轻切口张力及假体过度移位。

此类患者康复过程通常自然进展，恢复正常活动即可。事实上，由于未离断胸大肌，除参与短期健康教育小组会议（一般 5 次即可）外，多数病例无须特殊康复训练。有研究表明（未发表），胸肌前假体直接置入（DTI）患者较胸肌后 DTI 者所需康复强度较低：约 42% 的后者需个体化康复，前者仅约为 28%。

16.5 疗效与并发症

将假体置入真皮瓣 –ADM 复合囊袋（完全构建于皮下平面），可减轻传统胸大肌剥离所致的术后疼痛与不适感，重建乳房美学效果稳定，且假体无明显动态畸形（图 16.6，图 16.7）。此外，ADM 的应用可实现解剖型硅胶假体的个性化覆盖，从而降低传统术式的固有风险。所有患者术后上肢功能恢复迅速，及时出院并快速回归正常生活。需要指出的是，接受缩皮式乳房切除联合胸肌前假体重建的病例均为巨乳且体态丰腴者，假体上极轮廓虽被厚实的皮瓣遮蔽，必要时可于假体周围行二次脂肪填充术，同时矫正水平瘢痕处的"狗耳"畸形（图 16.8）。

尽管疗效显著，仍应重视潜在并发症。最常见者为倒 T 形切口交汇处延迟愈合，但术后早期即可识别局部真皮缺血灶（存在去表皮化乃至全层坏死风险）。发现明确缺血区时，应及时修剪坏死组织至创缘渗血，基于组织缺损范围及深度选择不同处理方案：

1. 创面较小且假体完全覆盖时，行皮肤直接缝合联合负压敷料（PICO®）[12]，酌情缩小假体体积。

2. 创面较小但假体外露时，以三联碘伏液[13]（50mL 碘伏、1g 头孢唑林及 80mg 庆大霉素溶于 500mL 生理盐水）充分冲洗，全层缝合关闭创口，缩小假体体积并覆盖负压敷料（PICO®）。

3. 创面较大而假体未外露（图 16.9）时，采用黑色聚氨酯海绵行负压吸引（75~100mmHg），持续 1~2 周后评估能否行直接缝合或植皮修复。

4. 在创面较大且假体仅在清创时由术者在无菌条件下暴露，可尝试保留假体/扩张器。创口以三联碘伏液彻底冲洗，缩小假体体积以降低张力，置引流管并多层缝合。若原采用单腔假体，需取出后更换为最小填充量扩张器或可调容假体。

5. 若创面较大且假体在清创前已外露（细菌污染风险高），需要取出假体，并根据个体情况制订重建方案。

另一种并发症是瘢痕组织变薄（图16.10），罕见且发生较晚——可能在瘢痕愈合数月后才出现。该现象与瘢痕分离相关，渐进性变薄可导致皮肤破损或形成小孔（与皮下突出点压力性坏死相关），常表现为轻微血清渗出。通常情况下，患者察觉胸衣突现黄色污渍时会联系就诊。多

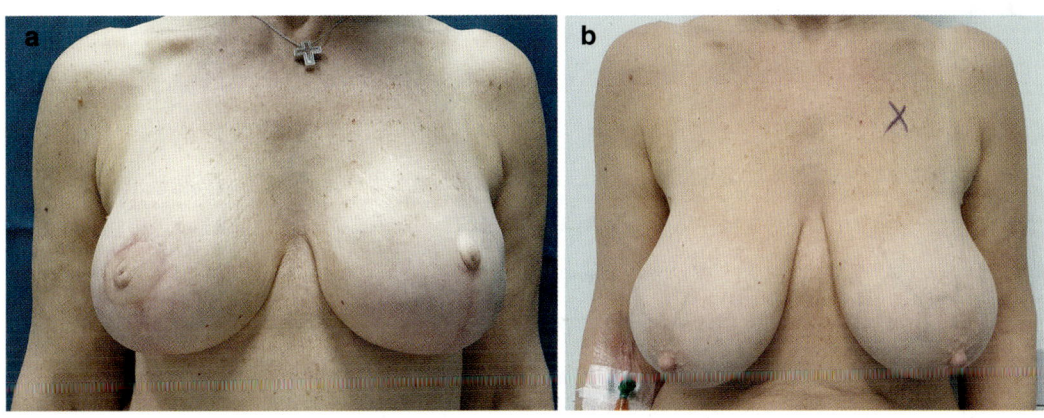

图 16.6 左侧缩皮式乳房切除胸肌前假体重建联合右侧乳房缩小术，术后 9 个月与术前正位观对比

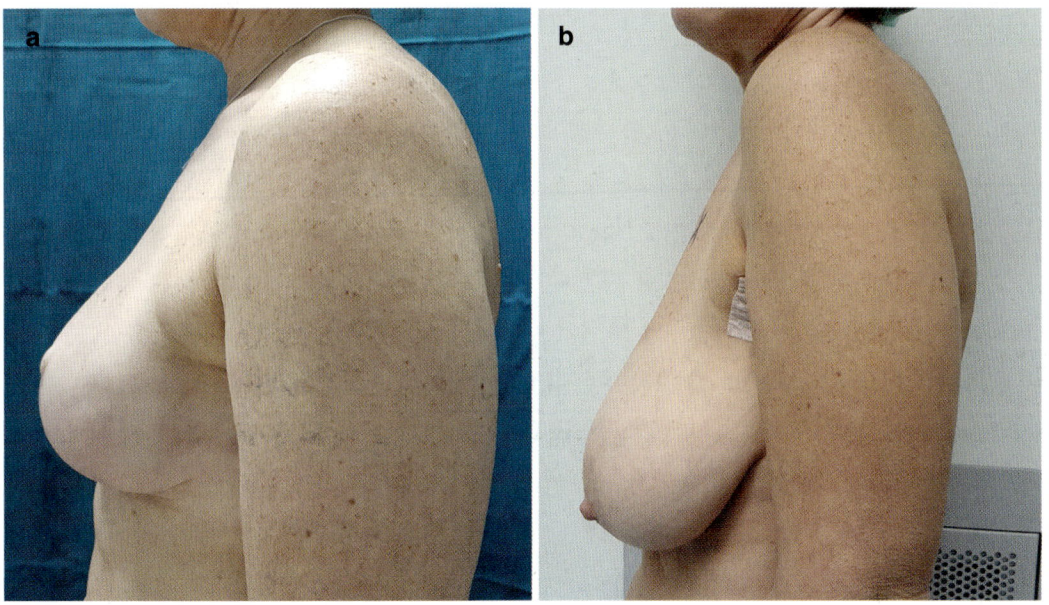

图 16.7 左侧缩皮式乳房切除胸肌前假体重建术，术后 9 个月与术前侧位观对比

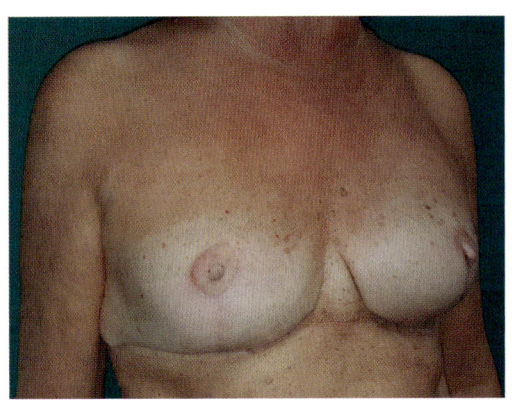 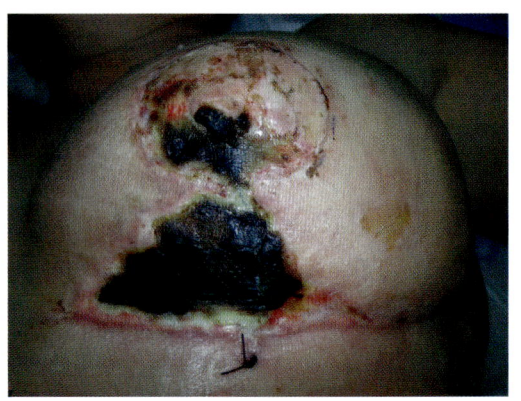

图 16.8　水平瘢痕外侧"狗耳"畸形　　　　图 16.9　乳房切除皮瓣全层坏死

数病例通过及时修剪皮缘（去除变薄皮肤）并行全层皮肤缝合即可解决问题。若瘢痕分离源于术后残留假体周围血清肿，建议放置细引流管，可与缝线同期拔除（约14天后）。

获得双侧乳房对称性是此类手术的主要目标之一，但单次手术常无法实现形态与体积的完美对称。因此，术后6个月待手术效果稳定时，需评估患者乳房体积分布的差异性。可能出现假体轮廓显露或外形不规则，原因包括乳房切除皮瓣厚度不均或继发脂肪坏死后皮下萎缩（图16.11）。此类情况可通过脂肪移植得到有效改善——通常单次填充即可解决问题。

某些情况下可能出现乳头萎缩。通常，若由血供不足所致，术后即可显现相关征象（图16.12）。该问题可通过Ⅱ期乳头再造解决，但患者多认为此类手术矫治非必需，转而倾向寻求专业文身师通过巧妙配色模拟三维乳头效果。

若重建技术操作欠规范或部分皮下缝线松脱，瘢痕可能高于乳房下皱襞。此问题见于瘢痕水平支与乳房下皱襞未准确对齐时（图16.13）。回顾重建手术步骤可发现准确定位乳房下皱襞的必要性：患者取坐位，沿皮瓣最外侧标记下皱襞，于皮瓣基底切开约4cm后，在此前锯肌间置入2-0 Vicryl 单线缝合。若此操作未能实现理想的轮廓，可沿整个乳房下皱襞行连续缝合。

16.6　现有文献回顾

近10年来，乳房切除即刻假体（DTI）重建技术已趋普及，主要归功于脱细胞真皮基质（ADM）技术及专为假体衬里设计的其他涂层材料的发展[14, 15]。这些创新技术变革了乳房重建手术范式，使得保留性乳房切除术病例的即刻 DTI 重建比例显著提升[16]。该术式在乳腺外科的适应证持续拓宽，并且良好患者接受度较高[17]。ADM 辅助 DTI 重建始于假体肌下置入技术：用基质材料覆盖假体下极，与胸大肌连续以完整构建置入腔隙[18]。近年来，又引入了肌肉保护技术——假体置于皮下层，完全或部分由 ADM 覆盖，此举可消

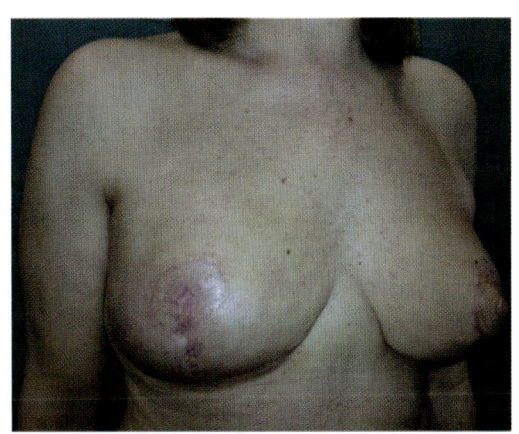

图 16.10 右侧乳房垂直瘢痕处皮下点状褥疮伴皮肤渗液

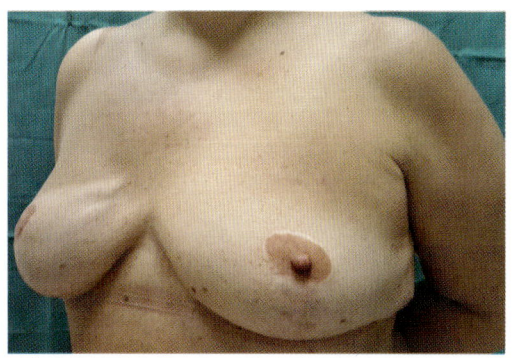

图 16.11 乳房右上象限因皮瓣厚度不均致形态不规则（褶皱显现）

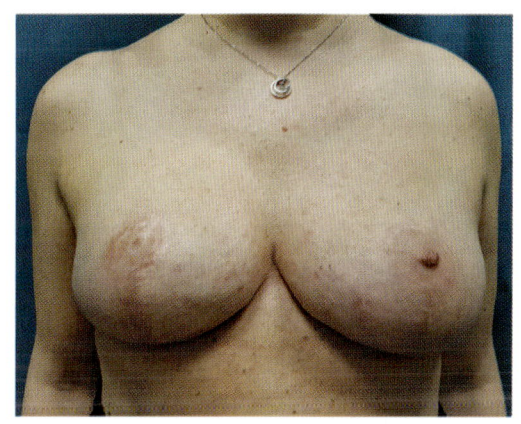

图 16.12 右侧乳头在重建术后萎缩

除动态畸形并获得更自然的外观[19, 20]。对于乳房肥大或下垂病例，传统的皮肤缩减切除术（假体肌下置入[21]）已被胸肌前术式取代[22, 23]。

技术要点

- 术前定位和画线须精准（倒 T 形垂直支长度不超过 9cm）。
- 用冷刀法切除乳房前（使用剪刀），术区应用 Klein 溶液充分浸润。
- 组织操作全程保持轻柔。
- 若 T 形切口转角处出现缺血征象，应修圆切缘；确保皮瓣基底对应区域为非去上皮化的三角形或半圆形。
- 选择假体容积不超过 500mL——假体过重将牵拉乳房切除皮瓣。
- 若皮瓣活性存疑，可置入可调节假体（Becker 假体）或扩张器，注水或注气充盈。若选择注气，推荐使用无菌 0.2μm 孔径滤器以降低细菌污染风险。
- 确认手术切口愈合良好后拔除引流管。
- 若创缘无愈合迹象，应立即修整创面并减少假体充盈度以降低张力——Ⅱ期愈合耗时漫长，且长期真皮层暴露或致假体外露。若为不可调节的单腔假体，应考虑更换为便于直接缝合的假体；若假体未暴露且真皮脂肪组织健康，修整后可实施 75~100mmHg 持续负压治疗（NPT）——此疗法可维持创面清洁并促使边缘靠拢（无负压时假体重量易致创缘分离）。
- 术后立即佩戴专用胸罩，首月需 24 小时全天使用。

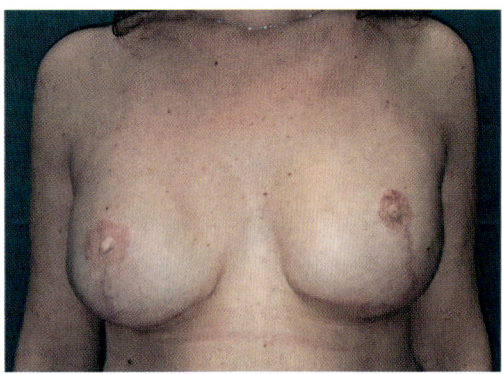

图 16.13　双侧缩皮式胸肌前假体重建术后水平瘢痕错位（位于乳房下皱襞上方）

参考文献

1. Nava MB, Cortinovis U, Ottolenghi J, et al. Skin-reducing mastectomy. Plast Reconstr Surg. 2006,118:603–10. discussion 611
2. Caputo GG, Marchetti A, Dalla Pozza E, et al. Skin-reduction breast reconstructions with Prepectoral implant. Plast Reconstr Surg. 2016,137（6）:1702–5.
3. Nahabedian MY. Current approaches to prepec¬toral breast reconstruction. Plast Reconstr Surg. 2018,142（4）:871–80.
4. Kim IK, Park SO, Chang H, Jin US. Inhibition mechanism of acellular dermal matrix on capsule formation in expander-implant breast reconstruction after Postmastectomy radiotherapy. Ann Surg Oncol. 2018,25（8）:2279–87.
5. Salzberg CA, Ashikari AY, Berry C, Hunsicker LM. Acellular dermal matrix-assisted direct-to-implant breast reconstruction and capsular contracture: a 13-year experience. Plast Reconstr Surg. 2016,138（2）:329–37.
6. Elswick SM, Harless CA, Bishop SN, et al. Prepectoral implant-based breast reconstruction with Postmastectomy radiation therapy. Plast Reconstr Surg. 2018,142（1）:1–12.
7. Shukla L, Morrison WA, Shayan R. Adipose-derived stem cells in radiotherapy injury: a new frontier. Front Surg. 2015,2:1. Published 2015 Jan 28
8. Klein JA. The tumescent technique. Anesthesia and modified liposuction technique. Dermatol Clin. 1990,8（3）:425–37.
9. Caputo GG, Franchini Z, Maritan M, et al. Daily serum collection after acellular dermal matrix-assisted breast reconstruction. Arch Plast Surg. 2015,42（3）:321–6.
10. Jeon FHK, Varghese J, Griffin M, Butler PE, Ghosh D, Mosahebi A. Systematic review of methodologies used to assess mastectomy flap viability. BJS Open. 2018,2（4）:175–84. Published 2018 May 28
11. Kedar D, Inbal A, Arad E, Gur E, Barnea Y. Immediate breast reconstruction in high-risk cases using an ana¬tomically shaped permanent expandable implant. J Plast Reconstr Aesthet Surg. 2019,72（3）:401–9.
12. Galiano RD, Hudson D, Shin J, et al. Incisional negative pressure wound therapy for prevention of wound healing complications following reduction mammaplasty［published correction appears in Plast Reconstr Surg Glob Open. 2018 Mar 23;6（2）:e1720］. Plast Reconstr Surg Glob Open 2018,6（1）:e1560. Published 2018 Jan.
13. Culbertson EJ, Felder-Scott C, Deva AK, Greenberg DE, Adams WP. Optimizing breast pocket irriga¬tion: the breast implant-associated anaplastic large cell lymphoma （BIA-ALCL） era. Aesthet Surg J. 2020,40（6）:619–25.
14. Salzberg CA. Direct-to-implant breast reconstruction. Clin Plast Surg. 2012,39（2）:119–26.
15. Dieterich M, Paepke S, Zwiefel K, et al. Implant-based breast reconstruction using a titanium-coated poly¬propylene mesh （TiLOOP bra）: a multicenter study of 231 cases. Plast Reconstr Surg. 2013,132（1）:8e–19e.
16. Vidya R, Masiá J, Cawthorn S, et al. Evaluation of the effectiveness of the prepectoral breast reconstruction with Braxon dermal matrix: first multicenter European report on 100 cases. Breast J. 2017,23（6）:670–6.

17. Vidya R, Green M. Minimal pain with prepectoral implant based breast reconstruction. Plast Reconstr Surg. 2019,143（1）:236e.
18. Breuing KH, Colwell AS. Inferolateral AlloDerm hammock for implant coverage in breast reconstruction. Ann Plast Surg. 2007,59:250255.
19. Antony AK, Poirier J, Madrigrano A, Kopkash KA, Robinson EC. Evolution of the surgical technique for "breast in a day" direct-to-implant breast reconstruction: transitioning from dual-plane to Prepectoral implant placement. Plast Reconstr Surg. 2019,143（6）:1547–56.
20. Mirhaidari SJ, Azouz V, Wagner DS. Prepectoral versus subpectoral direct to implant immediate breast reconstruction. Ann Plast Surg. 2020,84（3）:263–70.
21. della Rovere GQ, Nava M, Bonomi R, Catanuto G, Benson JR. Skin-reducing mastectomy with breast reconstruction and sub-pectoral implants. J Plast Reconstr Aesthet Surg. 2008,61:1303–8.
22. Thuman J, Freitas AM, Schaeffer C, Campbell CA. Prepectoral wise-pattern staged implant-based breast reconstruction for obese or ptotic patients. Ann Plast Surg. 2019,82（6S Suppl 5）:S404–9.
23. Maruccia M, Elia R, Gurrado A, et al. Skin-reducing mastectomy and pre-pectoral breast reconstruction in large Ptotic breasts. Aesthet Plast Surg. 2020,44（3）:664–72.

17 并发症：降低与管理

编者：Jaume Masià and Cristhian D. Pomata

译者：李 栋 李 超

17.1 引言

切除乳房后使用异体材料重建的技术始于20世纪60年代后[1]。自应用以来，该技术的缺陷主要与假体被置于极薄皮下的操作相关。因此，由于并发症发生率、重建失败率较高，胸肌前术式逐渐被摒弃[2-4]。

经过数十年的发展，为获得更优的假体乳房重建效果，首先需优化改良乳房切除技术以提升皮肤与皮下组织瓣的留存质量；其次应推动假体设计技术的显著进步，包括高性能外壳、高黏附性凝胶、微/纳米级表面纹理的应用；以及开发更多适应垂直与水平位移的假体轮廓形态。然而，21世纪初出现的脱细胞真皮基质（ADM）等生物材料[5]与脂肪移植术的整合应用，彻底革新了假体乳房重建技术，使得在保留皮肤或保留乳头和乳晕的乳房切除术后进行胸肌前重建成为可能[6, 7]。

尽管胸肌前术式的安全性及高成功率已得到广泛验证[6, 8]，其仍存在并发症风险[9, 10]。目前已明确胸肌前假体乳房重建（PPIBR）的多种不良事件的诱发因素，因此术者需采取风险防控策略以降低并发症发生风险，并在并发症发生时予以有效处理，避免重建失败。

17.2 并发症类型

胸肌前假体乳房重建（PPIBR）术后并发症类型与半个世纪前初期术式基本一

J. Masià
Department of Plastic Surgery, Santa Creu i Sant Pau Hospital - Universitat Autònoma de Barcelona, Barcelona, Spain

Unit of Advanced Breast Reconstruction and Lymphedema Treatment, Clínica Planas, Barcelona, Spain
e-mail: jmasia@santpau.cat

C. D. Pomata (✉)
Unit of Advanced Breast Reconstruction, Clínica Planas, Barcelona, Spain
e-mail: cpomata@clinicaplanas.com

© The Author(s), under exclusive license to Springer Nature Switzerland AG 2023
R. Vidya, H. Becker (eds.), *Prepectoral Breast Reconstruction*,
https://doi.org/10.1007/978-3-031-15590-1_17

致，仅各类别的发生率有所变化。总体上来说，PPIBR 术后不良事件可分为早期与晚期两类。早期并发症主要与手术操作相关，包括血清肿、血肿、乳头或皮肤的缺血或坏死、感染、切口裂开及假体外露。近年的研究还报道了与使用真皮修复材料相关的炎性反应——红乳综合征（red breast syndrome），亦归类为早期并发症。晚期并发症主要涉及假体与切除术区皮瓣的相互作用，表现为影响美学效果的不良效应，如包膜挛缩、波纹样畸形、假体错位、显影或触感异常等。报告的并发症发生率存在较大差异，可能与并存疾病、术式选择偏差、附加材料应用及放疗介入等因素相关[6-9]。表 17.1 列出了 Salibian 等 2017 年系统综述[11]、Wagner 等 2019 年研究[7]及 Masia 等 2020 年基于 ADM 的 PPIBR 多中心大样本数据[6]中报道的并发症发生情况。

17.3　并发症的危险因素

PPIBR 术后并发症的术前危险因素包括高龄、现时吸烟、糖尿病控制不佳、使用免疫抑制药物、病态肥胖症、巨乳症或乳房下垂等[6, 12~16]。既往乳房手术史及化疗史也被认为与并发症发生率高相关[6, 9]。这些危险因素主要与早期并发症相关。PPIBR 联合放疗是另一个争议焦点，既往乳腺放疗会增加缺血性并发症风险，而乳房切除术后放疗也被证实是晚期并发症的显著危险因素[6, 12, 17]。然而，导致

PPIBR 并发症发生率呈指数级上升的核心因素，是术者在实施乳房切除术及处理内置物/生物材料方面经验不足。

17.4　早期并发症

PPIBR 的早期并发症多于术后即刻发生，也可能在术后 2~3 个月内出现，通常分为无须手术干预的轻微并发症，以及需要再次入院或非计划重返手术室处理的严重并发症。此类事件若处理不当可能导致乳房重建失败，故采取必要预防措施至关重要。

17.4.1　血清肿

浆液性液体聚积是 PPIBR 术后最常见并发症之一，原因尚未完全明确，可能为淋巴液与炎性渗出液的混合液。影响因素包括：手术引发的组织炎症反应，异物（内置物及 ADM）置入产生的刺激，以及乳房切除术联合腋窝清扫形成的死腔（促进浆液蓄积）。此外，巨乳和/或肥胖患者常存在较大乳房切除皮瓣和/或外侧组织冗余，这两者均可增加死腔形成与浆液渗出风险。既往乳房美容手术史或使用免疫抑制药物亦与血清肿风险升高相关[18]。

17.4.1.1　预防措施

浆液蓄积通常被视为预期不良事件，为降低其发生率已形成多种预防策略。经典预防措施包括使用负压引流，避免肩关节主动运动等。另外，通过精细的手术操作（选用合适切剥设备）可减轻术后炎症

表 17.1 胸肌前假体置入乳房重建术（PPIBR）的并发症发生率

Semma	Salibian 等, 2016[8]			Wagner 等[7]				Masia 等[6]			
	总 PPIBR	PPIBR-ADM	PPIBR-网片	总 PPIBR	PPIBR-无	PPIBR-ADM	PPIBR-ADM/网片	PPIBR-ADM	PPIBR-ADM 非放疗	PPIBR-ADM 放疗
感染	2.9%	8.9%	0.0%	5.1%	6.9%	5.9%	4.1%	7.7%	7.0%	11.1%
轻微感染（抗生素）	2.3%	-	6.3%	2.6%	1.8%	3.8%	3.5%	4.8%	3.1%	5.1%
严重感染（手术）	1.2%	2.2%	0.0%	-	-	-	-	-	-	-
伤口愈合问题	2.3%	4.4%	1.6%	-	-	-	-	-	-	-
裂开	-	-	-	-	-	-	-	4.6%	4.5%	4.0%
红胸综合征	-	-	-	-	-	-	-	3.3%	3.5%	2.0%
坏死	-	-	-	-	-	-	-	3.2%	3.1%	4.0%
完全 NAC 坏死	1.1%	2.5%	0.0%	2.7%	-	-	-	-	-	-
部分 NAC 坏死	4.5%	5.0%	4.2%	-	4.2%	-	-	-	-	-
主要脂肪坏死	1.8%	0.0%	1.6%	5.4%	4.5%	-	-	-	-	-
血肿	2.3%	2.2%	3.1%	2.4%	3.0%	2.5%	2.7%	2.1%	2.2%	2.0%
内置物丢失	4.1%	6.7%	3.1%	3.3%	-	7.2%	5.9%	6.5%	5.6%	11.1%
波纹	4.7%	-	-	-	-	-	-	2.8%	3.1%	0.5%
包膜挛缩	1.2%	0.0%	0.0%	8.8%	12.4%	2.3%	2.4%	2.1%	1.7%	5.1%
内置物移位/旋转	0.0%	-	-	-	-	-	-	0.2%	0.2%	0.0%
内置物可见	4.3%	-	-	-	-	-	-	-	-	-
内置物可触及	8.5%	-	-	-	-	-	-	-	-	-

ADM：脱细胞真皮基质；NAC：乳头-乳晕复合体

反应，腋窝清扫术中正确识别淋巴管可减少术后淋巴液渗出。此外，消除死腔的技术（如使用组织封闭剂、荷包缝合或外部加压）亦可降低血清肿发生风险。

负压引流

预防浆液蓄积最常用闭式负压引流技术，引流管常置于乳房下皱襞与腋窝处并维持高压力梯度。拔管时机尚未达成共识，通常需持续至24~48h引流量不足20~25mL。长期留置引流管可能刺激炎性渗出进而加重浆液蓄积，并且易造成患者不适并增加感染风险，故建议术后7天内拔除引流管，并于拔管前预防性应用抗生素。

荷包缝合

通过固定乳房切除皮瓣以减少死腔并非新技术，可在不同部位（腋窝、外侧壁或贯穿乳房下皱襞至手术切口）实施以形成适形腔隙。多种荷包缝合技术已被证实可显著降低血清肿发生率，其中带刺缝线因其自锚定特性（无须多次打结）现已成为最佳选择。需注意荷包缝合可能造成皮肤暂时性凹陷，但通常可自行恢复[19]。

组织封闭剂

纤维蛋白封闭剂自20世纪40年代开始应用于外科手术[20]。鉴于乳腺及腋窝淋巴结切除术中会离断大量微小血管与淋巴管，理论上此类封闭剂可通过促进止血及组织贴合而减少术后浆血性渗出[21]。动物乳房切除模型研究表明，纤维蛋白封闭剂可减少血清肿形成[22, 23]，但其在人类乳腺癌手术中的应用仍存争议[24-26]。尽管纤维蛋白胶额外获益未达统计学显著性[27]，最新前瞻性随机临床试验证实氰基丙烯酸酯黏合剂可降低乳房切除术后血清肿发生率，同时缩短引流时间，减少浆液穿刺需求[28]。

手术切割设备

乳房切除术中使用的切割器械特性也会影响浆液生成量。电刀虽为最常用切割工具，但其组织损伤与急性炎症反应较重，血清肿发生率显著高于手术刀锐性分离[29, 30]。PEAK PlasmaBlade（等离子刀）为革新性电外科设备[31]，通过脉冲式射频在绝缘刀片边缘产生等离子介导放电，实现近似手术刀的无创性切割效果，并且刀片温度接近体温，能有效减少浆液渗出，进而缩短引流时间与住院时长[32, 33]。

腋窝清扫技术

腋窝淋巴结清扫术中识别淋巴管具有双重意义：既可防止淋巴液蓄积，又能通过即刻修复受损淋巴管降低肢体淋巴水肿风险。术中采用吲哚菁绿淋巴显影与专利蓝V染料显色识别淋巴管。即使未行腋窝淋巴结清扫，处理乳腺腋尾时仍需精细操作，辨别较粗大淋巴管后予以夹闭或双极电凝处理，以防止术后死腔内淋巴液积聚。

避免肩部主动活动

肩关节主动运动可能导致假体、乳房切除皮瓣与胸大肌间发生摩擦，加剧异物反应并延长炎症期，故建议术后至少1周内避免早期主动肩部活动，同时推迟功能训练[19]。

外部软压迫

使用软质加压绷带或手术胸罩可减少假体在乳房切除腔隙内的移动（刺激炎性

反应）。若行腋窝淋巴结清扫,加压包扎有助于缩小死腔[19, 34]。

17.4.1.2 处理措施

尽管采取预防措施,拔管后仍可能出现血清肿,表现为切口波动感或张力增加,可能导致切口裂开及假体外露。持续存在的血清肿还会影响 ADM/补片整合,并且在乳房切除术后新生血管不丰富的腔隙环境中易继发感染。对有临床意义的血清肿,现行处理方法是经皮穿刺抽吸联合预防性应用抗生素[18]。由于反复抽吸可能诱发感染,对难治性血清肿病例可选用多西环素、红霉素、乙醇或聚维酮碘等硬化剂行化学性硬化治疗[35, 36]。

17.4.2 血肿

任何乳房手术均存在术后出血风险,典型表现为乳房体积增大、皮肤瘀斑、引流量增加及剧烈疼痛。血肿常于术后 24 小时内发生,但亦可发生于术后 1 周或更晚时段。

某些药物（如抗血小板药、抗凝药及雄激素）可能增加出血风险。此外,高血压状态亦为危险因素。就术中操作而言,肿胀麻醉下切除乳房虽可减少术中失血,减轻围术期疼痛,但其术后血管收缩效应消退可能增加血肿风险。需要注意的是,乳房切除与重建分由两组术者实施的操作流程可能成为危险因素。

17.4.2.1 预防措施

血肿难以预测更凸显严格止血之的必

要[37]。术前静脉注射氨甲环酸可降低术后血肿风险[38]。

17.4.2.2 处理措施

若引流量持续增多或乳房体积急剧增大,应立即实施手术探查止血,清除血肿。该操作需要重返手术室（常采用全身麻醉）,多数情况下虽未见明确出血点,但遇活动性出血（如胸廓内动脉穿支等大血管损伤）应精准电凝或夹闭处理,随后以抗生素溶液彻底冲洗胸肌前腔隙清除残血,并重新置入引流管。

17.4.3 皮肤/乳头-乳晕复合体坏死

乳房切除皮瓣坏死是假体立即乳房重建术（PPIBR）潜在的灾难性并发症,尽管发生率不高,但仍构成重大挑战。由于皮肤与下方假体/ADM 之间缺乏血管化组织,该并发症易导致重建即刻失败。通常,多数皮瓣坏死发生于术后第 1 个月内。

诸多因素可导致乳房切除皮瓣坏死。过度去除皮下组织会改变灌注可导致皮瓣相对缺血。当使用过大的假体进行重建时,过大压力会加剧对皮瓣的损伤。吸烟及心血管、呼吸系统、外周血管疾病也会影响皮瓣组织的氧合与血管适应性。肥胖、糖尿病、高血压、放疗及类固醇给药与更高的皮肤坏死率相关。乳房体积过大是另一个重要因素,皮瓣过长更易发生远端缺血。同样,既往手术史可能增加并发症风险,因为瘢痕会影响乳头-乳晕复合体的血供。

17.4.3.1 预防

PPIBR 成功的最关键因素是高质量的乳房切除皮瓣，意味着皮瓣灌注充足。首要策略是尽可能纠正所有可能影响皮瓣灌注的基础疾病，吸烟者应至少术前戒烟 3 周。第二项关键预防措施是充分保留整个乳房的皮肤包裹层（皮肤及皮下组织），因乳房切除后皮瓣的血液供应完全依赖真皮下血管网。分离操作必须始终在浅筋膜前层与皮下组织之间的平面进行（即 Bisenberger 描述的平面），并维持至少 1cm 厚的皮下组织层。水分离技术有助于改善该分离平面的可视性。不建议使用电刀分离皮瓣，因其热损伤可能危及脆弱的皮下血管及表面皮肤包裹层。目前，峰值等离子刀是实施乳房切除的最佳软组织分离器械[31, 32, 39]。此外，使用拉钩时应谨慎控制对皮肤皮瓣的牵拉力及牵拉时长，避免血供中断，并确保两次牵拉之间有充足的时间让皮肤灌注恢复。

完成乳房切除后，必须系统评估乳房皮肤包裹层的可行性与质量，包括检查乳房切除皮瓣的灌注征象，如肤色、毛细血管充盈度、温度、肿胀度及真皮层出血情况。需要注意的是，厚实的乳房切除皮瓣未必代表灌注充分。因此，术中行吲哚菁绿联合激光血管造影对判断皮瓣活性具有重要指导价值。评估组织灌注时，可借助假体试模重构术后皮瓣将承受的张力。若术中应用含肾上腺素溶液辅助皮下剥离，可能影响灌注评估的可靠性。当皮肤灌注受损时，建议分阶段重建：首先在胸肌前置入组织扩张器，预留 2~3 周时间使皮瓣通过血管适应性建立充分灌注。切口处皮瓣张力（尤其是大量皮肤切除后）也需重点控制，因张力过高易诱发皮瓣边缘缺血。术后应避免使用过高压力敷料以维持皮瓣充分灌注。

17.4.3.2 治疗

根据坏死组织的严重程度及范围，皮肤坏死可采取手术或非手术治疗。术后若发现皮肤皮瓣或乳头缺血，可通过非手术技术改善组织灌注。硝酸甘油软膏可通过松弛皮下动静脉平滑肌壁增加皮肤局部血流量[40]。高压氧治疗亦可促进组织恢复[41]。

表浅坏死可使用相同非手术疗法，联合含银藻酸盐敷料等抗菌制剂降低细菌负荷[42]。此类表浅坏死通常通过坏死组织脱落及后续 II 期愈合完成修复。较大范围坏死可辅以创面管理装置（如负压敷料）加速愈合[43~45]。

累及乳房切除皮瓣全层的坏死需行手术清创并移除内置物。此时可根据术者经验采取个体化治疗策略处理组织缺损（图 17.1 及 17.2）。常规联合抗生素治疗。

17.4.4 感染

假体立即乳房重建术（PPIBR）中的感染属潜在灾难性并发症，常需通过再次手术移除假体。根据累及部位可分为表浅感染（仅累及皮肤及皮下浅层组织）与深部感染（累及软组织及接触假体/ADM 的结构）。该并发症多发生于术后 6 天至 6 周。

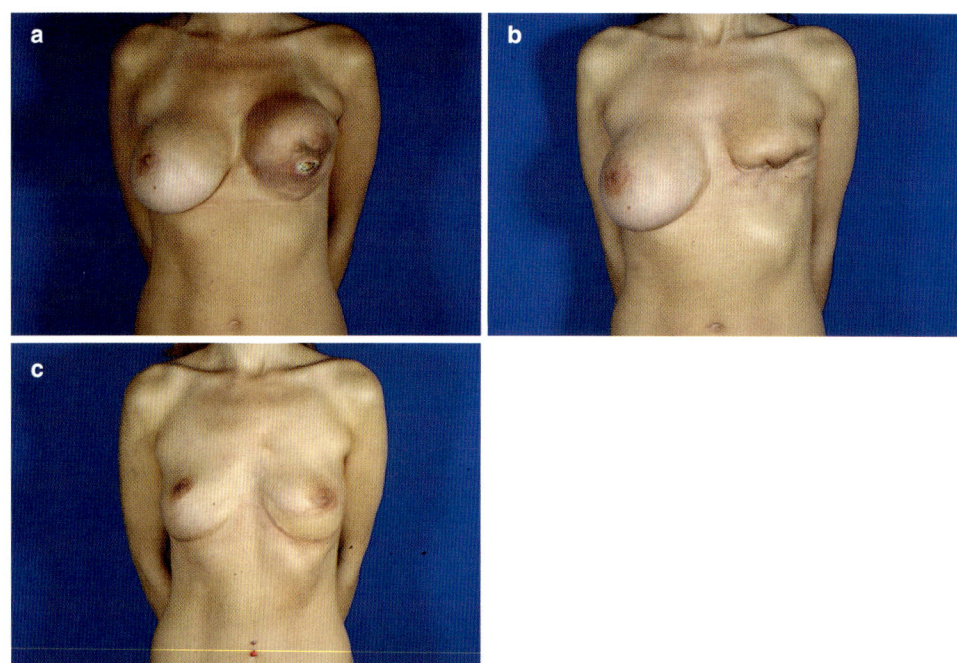

图 17.1 34 岁患者，既往于外院接受左乳保留乳头乳房切除即刻假体重建术。术后行放疗，疗程结束后因局部皮肤坏死及重度包膜挛缩就诊于我院（a）。Ⅰ期行假体取出术（b）。因乳房下极组织量不足难以塑造理想外形，Ⅱ期行腹壁下动脉穿支皮瓣（DIEAP）乳房重建术，同期实施对侧乳房缩小成形术（c）

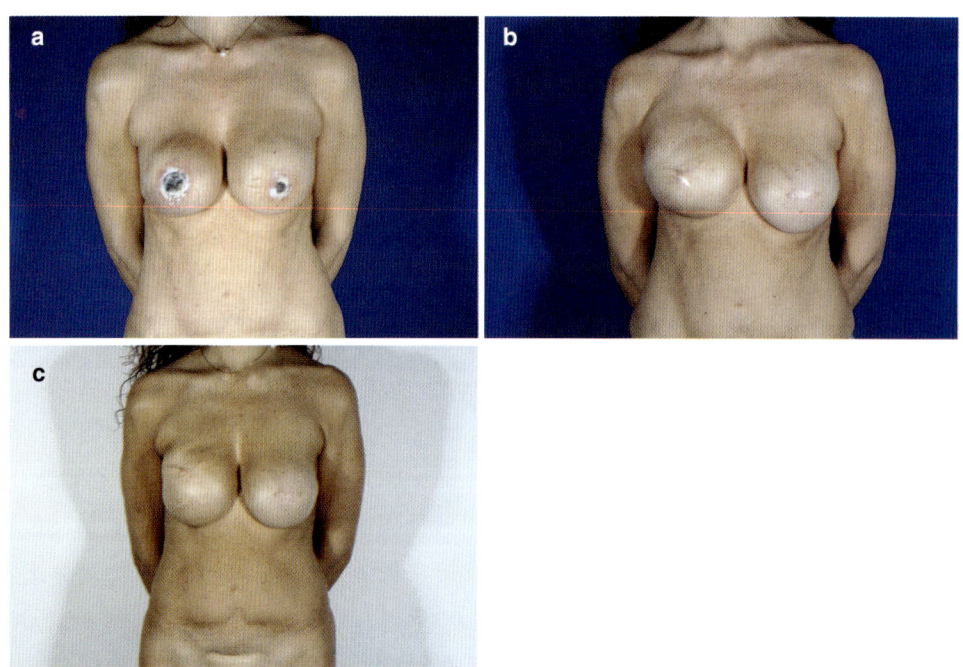

图 17.2 53 岁患者，既往于外院接受双侧保留乳头乳房切除即刻假体重建术，后因双侧乳晕坏死就诊于我院（a）。Ⅰ期行假体取出术，并行坏死组织清创及缺损关闭术（b）。Ⅱ期置入组织扩张器（c）；Ⅲ期置换为永久假体同时联合自体脂肪移植（d）

17.4.4.1 预防

术前预防策略除确认无局部或全身感染外，还包括通过规范术前淋浴（推荐使用抗菌剂）实现皮肤细菌去定植及预防性应用抗生素。术中预防措施包括：规范皮肤消毒；以贴膜敷料封闭乳头-乳晕复合体，避免术中乳头导管细菌污染术野；每60分钟更换无菌手套并在操作假体前换手套；用抗生素溶液冲洗胸肌前假体腔隙；通过乳房假体无菌包装纸质覆膜直接穿刺注射抗生素溶液，以避免取假体时静电污染；抗生素溶液充分浸润ADM；减少假体及ADM暴露时间以降低污染风险；尽可能采用最小接触技术；引流口远离手术切口（自胸肌前间隙向外穿出而非由外向内），避免皮肤菌群引入乳房切除腔隙；配备适宜的层流通风系统。术后护理应注重创面日常管理，综合防控血清肿、血肿及皮肤坏死[46,47]。

17.4.4.2 治疗

局限于轻度蜂窝织炎且无分泌物及全身感染征象的表浅手术部位感染，可通过静脉应用抗生素来治疗，直至肿胀、红斑消退，后继续口服抗生素7~10天并密切监测（无须移除假体）。若表浅皮肤坏死伴感染，局部可联合应用含银水胶体敷料及负压治疗。

出现深部皮下感染时，需以抗生素溶液大量冲洗，必要时行清创术并移除假体方可治愈。虽部分术者尝试通过开放冲洗假体腔避免移除内置物，但可能无效，并且假体滞留感染环境会增加患者系统性感染风险。假体移除后，须待抗生素治疗结束4~6个月以上，并且乳房组织充分愈合并软组织松解后，方可重新置入扩张器/假体。

17.4.5 切口裂开

切口裂开亦是PPIBR常见的早期并发症，定义为手术切口各层的部分或完全分离，通常由切口关闭不当或假体过大导致张力过大所致。血清肿及血肿亦可显著增加切口张力。乳房下部皮瓣菲薄（受重力作用压力更高）是另一类易致切口裂开的因素。皮肤损伤或溃疡、切口皮肤坏死及表浅感染，亦是切口裂开的重要诱因。患者合并症对切口愈合影响显著，吸烟、肥胖、糖尿病、高血压、贫血、营养不良或低白蛋白血症及放疗均是切口延迟愈合的风险因素。年龄>65岁与类固醇药物使用亦与切口愈合迟缓相关。

17.4.5.1 预防

预防手术切口裂开的首要策略是避免切口张力，为此须特别注意避免置入过大的假体，尤其对于乳房较小且乳房切除皮瓣紧张者。其次，切口缝合应遵循三层缝合原则：首先，将乳腺组织及Scarpa筋膜锚定于胸壁；其次，采用可吸收缝线行皮下组织层缝合，最后进行皮内缝合；最后，可应用氰基丙烯酸酯胶封闭切口表面，并使用胶带加强皮肤闭合。术后1周内限制肩关节主动活动亦有助于避免切口张力。此外，需针对血清肿、血肿、皮肤坏死和感染采取适当预防措施，以消除手术切口张力。

17.4.5.2 处理

轻微或浅表切口裂开须立即处理，治疗核心在于消除导致切口张力过大的因素。若因假体过大所致，应考虑更换较小假体。对于两阶段乳房重建患者，可通过部分排空扩张器来降低切口张力。当切口裂开合并血清肿、血肿或皮肤坏死时，成功处理这些并发症可促进切口愈合。

17.4.6 红色乳房综合征

红乳综合征（RBS）是一种与脱细胞真皮基质（ADM）应用于保留乳头乳房切除即刻重建（PPIBR）相关的炎症性反应，特征表现为 ADM 对应皮肤区域的红斑，临床表现类似蜂窝织炎或乳房切除皮瓣浅表感染。目前，关于其病因存在多种假说，但均未能阐明导致 RBS 发生和消退的生理学机制[48]。

17.4.6.1 预防及处理

为降低 RBS 发生率，有学者建议在将 ADM 置入乳房切除腔隙前，常规用无菌生理盐水冲洗后浸渍抗生素溶液[49]。处理要点在于鉴别 RBS 与感染。尽管二者病理机制不同，但可能同期发生且具有相似临床表现。RBS 患者通常无疼痛主诉，皮肤触诊无局部温度升高，可与蜂窝织炎术相鉴别。对所有 PPIBR 术后红斑均应行抗生素治疗。若 7 天后红斑无变化且未出现发热，则考虑为 RBS，可停用抗生素，因其红斑常于数周至数月内自行消退[48]。

皮质类固醇可缩短病程，亦有使用孟鲁司特成功治疗 RBS 的报道[49]。

17.4.7 假体外露

假体外露与重建失败密切相关，是上述早期并发症发展的结局。假体暴露可由切口裂开、严重皮肤坏死或手术部位感染引起，因此，预防并正确处理上述所有潜在并发症（血清肿、血肿、感染、皮肤坏死、切口裂开及红乳综合征）是保证保留乳头乳房切除即刻重建（PPIBR）获得成功的关键。

17.5 晚期并发症

晚期并发症多在术后数周（约 3 个月后）显现，通常由乳房切除操作不佳和早期并发症导致，主要影响重建乳房的美学效果，多数需手术矫正。以下分别阐述常见晚期并发症及其防治措施。

17.5.1 包膜挛缩

包膜挛缩是 PPIBR 最常见的晚期并发症之一，表现为重建乳房形态扭曲及位置上移[50]。临床征象包括乳房逐渐变硬或有束紧感，可伴有慢性疼痛。临床评估是判断包膜挛缩存在及分级的最简便的有效方法，目前普遍采用改良 Baker 分级标准（表 17.2）[51]。包膜挛缩病因尚未完全阐明，可能与假体周围腔隙或正在形成的包膜附近发生炎症反应有关，可导致胶原纤维及肌成纤维细胞异常沉积[52, 53]。血清肿、血肿、感染及放疗均为包膜挛缩的

表 17.2 假体乳房重建术后包膜挛缩分类[50]

IA 级	乳房重建术后外观完全自然，无法辨识曾行乳房重建
IB 级	重建乳房质地柔软，通过查体或视诊可察觉假体存在
II 级	重建乳房轻度硬化，假体可出现肉眼或触诊可辨识的形态异常
III 级	重建乳房中度硬化，假体易被察觉，但术后效果仍可被接受
IV 级	重度包膜挛缩，伴不可接受的美学缺陷和/或需手术干预的显著临床症状

潜在危险因素。另有研究报道，使用光面假体会增加包膜挛缩风险[54]。

17.5.1.1 预防

预防包膜挛缩的首要措施是采用可靠精细的乳房切除术式，保证皮下组织有充分的厚度。应采取综合措施来降低血清肿、血肿及感染风险。关于假体表面处理，多数研究认为聚氨酯泡沫覆盖假体较光面或毛面假体可显著降低包膜挛缩发生率[55]。此外，PPIBR 术中应用 ADM 已被证实与低包膜挛缩率相关[7]，具体机制尚未完全阐明，推测 ADM 可显著降低假体周围组织肌成纤维细胞浓度[56]。

17.5.1.2 处理

轻度包膜挛缩首选非手术疗法，包括假体机械移位、体外超声及药物干预（抗生素、维生素 E、类固醇、非甾体消炎药、化疗药及白三烯抑制剂），但均未取得满意疗效。伴慢性疼痛和/或乳房形态、位置显著改变的严重包膜挛缩（Baker III~IV 级）需要手术治疗，可放射状切开松解包膜（包膜切开术）或完全切除包膜组织（包膜切除术）；建议同时更换假体，尽可能全面覆盖 ADM，并严格执行早期并发症预防策略。

17.5.2 假体移位

假体乳房重建术的晚期并发症之一，是乳房假体随时间发生位移，从而丧失在乳房内的正常解剖位置。假体可向任意方向移位（上方、下方、外侧、内侧），甚至可出现假体翻转（光面假体）。病因包括乳房切除腔隙明显大于假体容积、缺血性或坏死性损伤导致的皮瓣回缩反应，或放疗对重建乳房组织产生的影响——后者常与包膜挛缩密切相关。

17.5.2.1 预防

预防策略主要基于以下三点：乳房切除腔隙与假体容积适配度的精细调整；将包裹假体的脱细胞真皮基质（ADM）确切固定于胸壁适当位置；术后采取预防措施避免乳房切除皮瓣坏死。术后常规穿戴弹性适度的压力胸罩以维持假体稳定性和既定解剖位置。术后 2~3 周应避免剧烈体力活动。

17.5.2.2 处理

假体移位需通过假体复位手术进行矫正，某些病例需行包膜松解术联合对侧包膜成形术，通过重建理想腔隙维度完成假体解剖位置重塑。具体操作包括：适度缩小并界定乳房切除腔隙范围，以及实施针对性的假体复位固定操作。

17.5.3 波纹效应

假体乳房重建术（PPIBR）术后波纹效应也是常见的晚期并发症，常引发患者严重不满。波纹效应指假体表面形态不规则，导致在乳腺表面出现可见的轮廓异常，在乳房的内上象限或外下象限区域尤为显著。早期仅存在触诊异常，手指轻抚乳腺表面可感知假体边缘；若病情进展，则会出现肉眼可见的褶皱或折叠。波纹效应的高危因素包括：低 BMI（<20）、乳腺皮肤及皮下脂肪菲薄者（捏持试验厚度<2cm）[57]。生理盐水假体及低黏聚性硅凝胶假体因更易发生形态学改变，波纹效应发生率最高；使用毛面假体同样存在更高风险，因其表面材质与乳腺组织及包膜的黏附作用可导致牵拉性波纹效应。乳房切除腔隙大于假体尺寸是另一高危因素[58]。

17.5.3.1 预防

预防波纹效应的首要措施是通过皮下正确平面进行分离操作，保持乳房切除皮瓣有足够的厚度。其次，推荐选择新型高黏聚性硅凝胶假体，现有研究表明，聚氨酯假体表面处理技术的波纹效应风险最低。第三，可采用脱细胞真皮基质（ADM）为假体提供支撑和覆盖，在假体与皮肤皮瓣之间构建更优化的接触界面，从而隐藏波纹效应。关键环节还包括根据乳房切除腔隙大小选择适配假体，避免冗余皮肤导致波纹现象。此外，建议闭合乳房下皱襞切口时同步行腔隙紧缩术[57, 58]。

17.5.3.2 处理

基于 Vidya 等提出的分级系统（表17.3）[57]，II~III 级波纹效应可通过自体脂肪移植有效矫正——既可恢复乳房切除皮瓣厚度，亦可掩盖表面形态异常（图17.3）。对 IV 级波纹效应，单纯行脂肪移植可能无法完全纠正，常需联合包膜松解术或部分包膜切除术。另一替代技术涉及在包膜后层与深层胸肌间构建新腔隙以重置假体，形成双层包膜覆盖结构[57, 58]。术后可应用透明薄膜敷料轻柔加压包扎，以实现皮肤皮瓣表面压力均匀。

表17.3 假体乳房重建术后波纹效应分级系统[56]

级别	描述
1 级	静息及运动状态下均无波纹效应可见
2 级	静息及运动状态下可触及轻度波纹，但不可视
3 级	静息及运动状态下可见中度波纹
4 级	重度——持续性波纹效应导致静息及运动状态下均存在明显畸形

17.5.4 假体边缘显形

假体内上或外侧边缘显形是 PPIBR 术后另一常见并发症，好发于皮下组织菲薄的消瘦患者。该问题最有效的解决方案为自体脂肪移植，通过重塑胸壁与再造乳房间的轮廓过渡实现形态自然化（图17.3）。

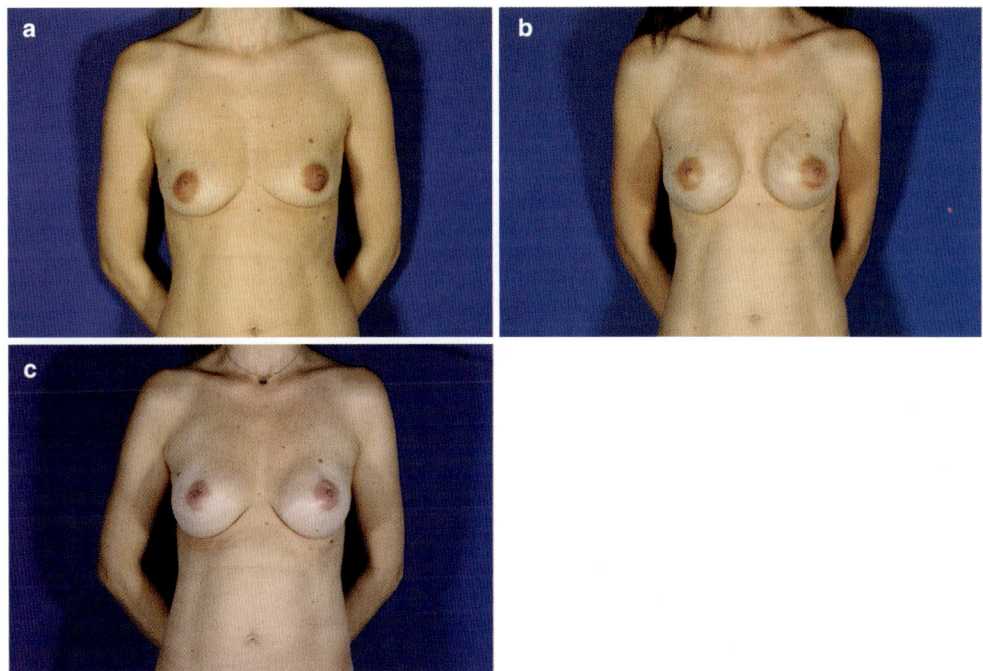

图 17.3　36 岁患者，既往接受双侧保留乳头乳房切除即刻假体重建术。术前影像（a）。术后 8 个月，患者出现乳房波纹效应显形及假体边缘轮廓异常（b），遂行双乳自体脂肪移植术（c）

17.6　小结

乳腺癌的综合治疗不仅要实现良好的肿瘤学疗效，还需兼顾美学重建效果。建立有效的早期并发症预防策略对避免重建失败，降低可能影响重建后期美学表现的并发症风险至关重要。成功的即刻假体乳房重建（PPIBR）需要严格把握患者适应证，实施科学合理的术前规划，遵循精细的手术操作技术规范，以及依据本章提出的规范进行术中精准决策，并在术后予以规范的护理措施。

参考文献：

1. Snyderman RK, Guthrie RH. Reconstruction of the female breast following radical mastectomy. Plast Reconstr Surg. 1971,47（6）:565–7.
2. Schlenker JD, Bueno RA, Ricketson G, Lynch JB. Loss of silicone implants after subcutaneous mastectomy and reconstruction. Plast Reconstr Surg. 1978,62（6）:853–61.
3. Gruber RP, Kahn RA, Lash H, Maser MR, Apfelberg DB, Laub DR. Breast reconstruction following mastectomy: a comparison of submuscular and subcutaneous techniques. Plast Reconstr Surg. 1981,67（3）:312–7.
4. Ward DC, Edwards MH. Early results of subcutaneous mastectomy with immediate silicone prosthetic implant for carcinoma of the breast. Br J Surg. 1983,70（11）:651–3.
5. Salzberg CA. Nonexpansive immediate breast reconstruction using human acellular tissue matrix graft（AlloDerm）. Ann Plast Surg. 2006,57（1）:1–5.
6. Masià J, iBAG Working Group. The largest

multicentre data collection on prepectoral breast reconstruction: the iBAG study. J Surg Oncol. 2020,122（5）:848–60.
7. Wagner RD, Braun TL, Zhu H, Winocour S. A systematic review of complications in prepectoral breast reconstruction. J Plast Reconstr Aesthet Surg. 2019,72（7）:1051–9.
8. Dave RV, Vucicevic A, Barrett E, Highton L, Johnson R, Kirwan CC, et al. Risk factors for complications and implant loss after prepectoral implant-based immediate breast reconstruction: medium-term outcomes in a prospective cohort. Br J Surg. 2021,108（5）:534–41.
9. Chatterjee A, Nahabedian MY, Gabriel A, Macarios D, Parekh M, Wang F, et al. Early assessment of postsurgical outcomes with pre-pectoral breast reconstruction: a literature review and meta-analysis. J Surg Oncol. 2018,117（6）:1119–30.
10. Salibian AA, Frey JD, Karp NS. Strategies and considerations in selecting between subpectoral and prepectoral breast reconstruction. Gland Surg. 2019,8（1）:11–8.
11. Salibian AA, Frey JD, Choi M, Karp NS. Subcutaneous Implant-based Breast Reconstruction with Acellular Dermal Matrix/Mesh: A Systematic Review. Plast Reconstr Surg Glob Open. 2016,4（11）:e1139.
12. Colwell AS, Tessler O, Lin AM, Liao E, Winograd J, Cetrulo CL, et al. Breast reconstruction following nipple-sparing mastectomy: predictors of complications, reconstruction outcomes, and 5-year trends. Plast Reconstr Surg. 2014,133（3）:496–506.
13. Munhoz AM, Aldrighi CM, Montag E, Arruda EG, Aldrighi JM, Gemperli R, et al. Clinical outcomes following nipple-areola-sparing mastectomy with immediate implant-based breast reconstruction: a 12-year experience with an analysis of patient and breastrelated factors for complications. Breast Cancer Res Treat. 2013,140（3）:545–55.
14. Hart A, Funderburk CD, Chu CK, Pinell-White X, Halgopian T, Manning-Geist B, et al. The impact of diabetes mellitus on wound healing in breast reconstruction. Ann Plast Surg. 2017,78（3）:260–3.
15. Vidya R, Berna G, Sbitany H, Nahabedian M, Becker H, Reitsamer R, et al. Prepectoral implant-based breast reconstruction: a joint consensus guide from UK, European and USA breast and plastic reconstructive surgeons. Ecancermedicalscience. 2019,13:927.
16. Rifkin WJ, Kantar RS, Cammarata MJ, Wilson SC, Diaz-Siso JR, Golas AR, et al. Impact of diabetes on 30-day complications in mastectomy and implant-based breast reconstruction. J Surg Res. 2019,235:148–59.
17. Spear SL, Hannan CM, Willey SC, Cocilovo C. Nipple-sparing mastectomy. Plast Reconstr Surg. 2009,123（6）:1665–73.
18. Jordan SW, Khavanin N, Kim JYS. Seroma in prosthetic breast reconstruction. Plast Reconstr Surg. 2016,137（4）:1104–16.
19. van Bemmel AJM, van de Velde CJH, Schmitz RF, Liefers GJ. Prevention of seroma formation after axillary dissection in breast cancer: a systematic review. Eur J Surg Oncol. 2011,37（10）:829–35.
20. Sierra DH. Fibrin sealant adhesive systems: a review of their chemistry, material properties and clinical applications. J Biomater Appl. 1993,7（4）:309–52.
21. Moore MM, Freeman MG. Fibrin sealant in breast surgery. J Long-Term Eff Med Implants. 1998,8（2）:133–42.
22. Lindsey WH, Masterson TM, Spotnitz WD, Wilhelm MC, Morgan RF. Seroma prevention using fibrin glue in a rat mastectomy model. Arch Surg. 1990,125（3）:305–7.
23. Eroğlu E, Oral S, Unal E, Kalayci M, Oksüz O, Tilmaz M. Reducing seroma formation with fibrin glue in an animal mastectomy model. Eur J Surg Oncol. 1996,22（2）:137–9.
24. Gioffrè Florio MA, Mezzasalma F, Manganaro T, Pakravanan H, Cogliandolo A.［The use of fibrin glue in the surgery of breast carcinoma］.

G Chir. 1993,14（4–5）:239–241.

25. Moore MM, Nguyen DH, Spotnitz WD. Fibrin sealant reduces serous drainage and allows for earlier drain removal after axillary dissection: a randomized prospective trial. Am Surg. 1997,63（1）:97–102.

26. Gilly FN, François Y, Sayag-Beaujard AC, Glehen O, Brachet A, Vignal J. Prevention of lymphorrhea by means of fibrin glue after axillary lymphadenectomy in breast cancer: prospective randomized trial. Eur Surg Res. 1998,30（6）:439–43.

27. Miri Bonjar MR, Maghsoudi H, Samnia R, Saleh P, Parsafar F. Efficacy of fibrin glue on seroma formation after breast surgery. Int J Breast Cancer. 2012,2012:643132.

28. Vasileiadou K, Kosmidis C, Anthimidis G, Miliaras S, Kostopoulos I, Fahantidis E. Cyanoacrylate adhesive reduces seroma production after modified radical mastectomy or Quadrantectomy with lymph node dissection-a prospective randomized clinical trial. Clin Breast Cancer. 2017,17（8）:595–600.

29. Srivastava V, Basu S, Shukla VK. Seroma formation after breast cancer surgery: what we have learned in the last two decades. J Breast Cancer. 2012,15（4）:373–80.

30. Keogh GW, Doughty JC, McArdle CSM, Cooke TG. Seroma formation related to electrocautery in breast surgery: a prospective randomized trial. Breast. 1998,7（1）:39–41.

31. Loh SA, Carlson GA, Chang EI, Huang E, Palanker D, Gurtner GC. Comparative healing of surgical incisions created by the PEAK PlasmaBlade, conventional electrosurgery, and a scalpel. Plast Reconstr Surg. 2009,124（6）:1849–59.

32. Dogan L, Gulcelik MA, Yuksel M, Uyar O, Erdogan O, Reis E. The effect of plasmakinetic cautery on wound healing and complications in mastectomy. J Breast Cancer. 2013,16（2）:198–201.

33. Sowa Y, Inafuku N, Kodama T, Morita D, Numajiri T. Preventive effect on seroma of use of PEAK PlasmaBlade after latissimus Dorsi breast reconstruction. Plast Reconstr Surg Glob Open. 2018,6（12）:e2035.

34. O'Hea BJ, Ho MN, Petrek JA. External compression dressing versus standard dressing after axillary lymphadenectomy. Am J Surg. 1999,177（6）:450–3.

35. Sood A, Kotamarti VS, Therattil PJ, Lee ES. Sclerotherapy for the management of seromas: a systematic review. Eplasty. 2017,17:e25.

36. Throckmorton AD, Askegard-Giesmann J, Hoskin TL, Bjarnason H, Donohue JH, Boughey JC, et al. Sclerotherapy for the treatment of postmastectomy seroma. Am J Surg. 2008,196（4）:541–4.

37. Seth A, Hirsch E, Kim J, Dumanian G, Mustoe T, Galiano R, et al. Hematoma after mastectomy with immediate reconstruction an analysis of risk factors in 883 patients. Ann Plast Surg. 2012,71:20–3.

38. Banuelos J, Weissler JM, Harless CA, Jacobson SR, Van Tran N, Nguyen M-DT, et al. Intravenous tranexamic acid in implant-based breast reconstruction safely reduces hematoma without thromboembolic events. Plast Reconstr Surg Glob Open. 2019,7（8 Suppl）:87.

39. Ruidiaz ME, Messmer D, Atmodjo DY, Vose JG, Huang EJ, Kummel AC, et al. Comparative healing of human cutaneous surgical incisions created by the PEAK PlasmaBlade, conventional electrosurgery, and a standard scalpel. Plast Reconstr Surg. 2011,128（1）:104–11.

40. Gdalevitch P, Van Laeken N, Bahng S, Ho A, Bovill E, Lennox P, et al. Effects of nitroglycerin ointment on mastectomy flap necrosis in immediate breast reconstruction: a randomized controlled trial. Plast Reconstr Surg. 2015,135（6）:1530–9.

41. Fredman R, Wise I, Friedman T, Heller L, Karni T. Skin-sparing mastectomy flap ischemia salvage using urgent hyperbaric chamber oxygen therapy: a case report. Undersea Hyperb Med.

2014,41（2）:145–7.
42. Robertson SA, Jeevaratnam JA, Agrawal A, Cutress RI. Mastectomy skin flap necrosis: challenges and solutions. Breast Cancer Targets Ther. 2017,9:141–52.
43. Matusiak D, Wichtowski M, Pieszko K, Kobylarek D, Murawa D. Is negative-pressure wound therapy beneficial in modern-day breast surgery? Contemp Oncol. 2019,23（2）:69–73.
44. Kim JH, Kim YS, Kim YW, Kim YJ, Chun YS, Park HK, et al. A single-use negative-pressure wound therapy device can reduce mastectomy skin flap necrosis in direct-to-implant breast reconstruction. Arch Aesthet Plast Surg. 2020,26（1）:12–9.
45. Irwin GW, Boundouki G, Fakim B, Johnson R, Highton L, Myers D, et al. Negative pressure wound therapy reduces wound breakdown and implant loss in Prepectoral breast reconstruction. Plast Reconstr Surg Glob Open. 2020,8（2）:e2667.
46. Holland M, Lentz R, Sbitany H. Utility of postoperative prophylactic antibiotics in Prepectoral breast reconstruction: a single-surgeon experience. Ann Plast Surg. 2021,86（1）:24–8.
47. Papa G, Frasca A, Renzi N, Stocco C, Pizzolato G, Ramella V, et al. Protocol for prevention and monitoring of surgical site infections in implant-based breast reconstruction: preliminary results. Med Kaunas Lith. 2021,57（2）:151.
48. Nahabedian MY. Prosthetic breast reconstruction and red breast syndrome: demystification and a review of the literature. Plast Reconstr Surg Glob Open. 2019,7（5）:e2108.
49. Wu PS, Winocour S, Jacobson SR. Red breast syndrome: a review of available literature. Aesthet Plast Surg. 2015,39（2）:227–30.
50. Nealon KP, Weitzman RE, Sobti N, Gadd M, Specht M, Jimenez RB, et al. Prepectoral direct-to-implant breast reconstruction: safety outcome endpoints and delineation of risk factors. Plast Reconstr Surg. 2020,145（5）:898e–908e.
51. Spear SL, Baker JL. Classification of capsular contracture after prosthetic breast reconstruction. Plast Reconstr Surg. 1995,96（5）:1119–23. discussion 1124
52. Siggelkow W, Faridi A, Spiritus K, Klinge U, Rath W, Klosterhalfen B. Histological analysis of silicone breast implant capsules and correlation with capsular contracture. Biomaterials. 2003,24（6）:1101–9.
53. Poeppl N, Schreml S, Lichtenegger F, Lenich A, Eisenmann-Klein M, Prantl L. Does the surface structure of implants have an impact on the formation of a capsular contracture? Aesthet Plast Surg. 2007,31（2）:133–9.
54. Stevens WG, Nahabedian MY, Calobrace MB, Harrington JL, Capizzi PJ, Cohen R, et al. Risk factor analysis for capsular contracture: a 5-year Sientra study analysis using round, smooth, and textured implants for breast augmentation. Plast Reconstr Surg. 2013,132（5）:1115–23.
55. Handel N, Silverstein MJ, Jensen JA, Collins A, Zierk K. Comparative experience with smooth and polyurethane breast implants using the Kaplan-Meier method of survival analysis. Plast Reconstr Surg. 1991,88（3）:475–81.
56. Tevlin R, Borrelli MR, Irizarry D, Nguyen D, Wan DC, Momeni A. Acellular dermal matrix reduces Myofibroblast presence in the breast capsule. Plast Reconstr Surg Glob Open. 2019,7（5）:e2213.
57. Vidya R, Iqbal FM, Becker H, Zhadan O. Rippling associated with pre-pectoral implant based breast reconstruction: a new grading system. World J Plast Surg. 2019,8（3）:311–5.
58. Pantelides NM, Srinivasan JR. Rippling following breast augmentation or reconstruction: Aetiology, emerging treatment options and a novel classification of severity. Aesthet Plast Surg. 2018,42（4）:980–5.

18　Ⅰ期胸肌前乳房重建术后临床、组织学及超声随访观察

编者：Maruccia Michele, Giudice Giuseppe, Gurrado Angela, Cazzato Gerardo, Elia Rossella

译者：宋书彬　宋　翔

18.1　引言

假体乳房重建是最常见的乳房切除即刻重建方式。乳腺癌治疗、乳房切除技术和重建方案的改进，进一步扩大了假体乳房重建的适应证[1]。

将假体置于胸肌前作为胸肌后术式的简化替代方案正得到逐步推广，旨在应对胸肌后假体放置术相关缺陷，包括：①肌力减退；②术后疼痛；③恢复期延长；④胸大肌（PPM）收缩时引发的乳房动态畸形。

反之，无须离断胸大肌（PPM）的胸肌前假体置入术需要实现内置物覆盖，以及基于组织支撑的内置物固定，使用脱细胞真皮基质（ADMs）、补片或自体真皮脂肪瓣来完成。随着脱细胞真皮基质及各类补片的临床普及，其与胸肌前假体放置技术的联合应用显著改善了美学效果[2]。

此外，当前对有家族性癌症高风险的年轻患者施行预防性乳房切除即刻乳房重建的案例日益增多[3]。此类患者通常期望规避胸肌离断相关并发症，胸肌前假体置入技术可保障其快速回归正常生活。

Ⅰ期胸肌前假体置入重建术以充分的皮肤灌注量维系组织活性为前提。患者是否适宜行胸肌前重建术主要依据皮肤灌注水平而非皮瓣厚度，对组织灌注系统的客观评估对确保手术成功具有决定性意义[4-6]。相对禁忌证包括合并未控制的糖尿病、病理性肥胖、近期或当前吸烟史等基础疾病患者，以及有术前放疗史者[7, 8]。

同所有乳房切除假体重建术式一样，肿瘤学考量不可或缺。胸肌前假体重建对

M. Michele (✉) · G. Giuseppe · E. Rossella
Division of Plastic and Reconstructive Surgery, Department of Emergency and Organ Transplantation, University of Bari Aldo Moro, Bari, Italy

G. Angela
Unit of Endocrine, Digestive, and Emergency Surgery, Department of Biomedical Sciences and Human Oncology, University Medical School "Aldo Moro" of Bari, Bari, Italy

C. Gerardo
Section of Pathology, University of Bari 'Aldo Moro', Bari, Italy

© The Author(s), under exclusive license to Springer Nature Switzerland AG 2023
R. Vidya, H. Becker (eds.), *Prepectoral Breast Reconstruction*,
https://doi.org/10.1007/978-3-031-15590-1_18

晚期癌症或任何肿瘤复发高风险的患者通常视为禁忌[9]。

18.2 主文部分

采用Ⅰ期胸肌前假体乳房重建（PPBR）患者的临床、影像学及组织学随访，对评估这项较新技术的安全性特征具有重要价值。研究旨在明确该术式的并发症发生率、功能预后及美学效果，并与传统胸肌后术式进行比较。

18.3 临床随访

接受PPBR的患者普遍诉诸不适感较轻，无须术后扩张，组织皮瓣水肿轻微，且对上肢功能基本无影响。此外，动态畸形现象可得到彻底改善（图18.1）。

美容效果及患者报告的结局数据同样呈现积极趋势，但仍需进一步的长期研究。多项病例系列研究显示，在通过评估量表获得的术后整体满意度、乳房局部满意度、心理社会适应度及性健康水平等方面，患者术后评分显著高于术前，上述领域的改善具有统计学意义[10, 11]。

重建外科医师既往更倾向胸肌后术式而非胸肌前术式，主要出于对包膜挛缩（CC）的顾虑。近期研究报告表明，临床应用新型补片后包膜挛缩发生率与胸肌后重建相近，可能得益于补片材料介导的炎症反应抑制效应[12, 13]。脱细胞真皮基质（ADM）可发挥假体与皮下组织间筛状屏障功能，协同降低炎症反应与包膜挛缩的发生率[14, 15]。

关于手术并发症的其他研究，最初有报道在小样本系列病例中采用即刻内置物和两阶段扩张器重建术，通过使用多种脱细胞真皮基质（ADMs）及补片进行胸肌后乳房重建，并发症发生率较低[2, 11, 16-19]。这些结果已在一项更大规模的多中心研究中获得验证[13]。

最近，由Barcelona医院发起的一项多中心回顾性研究汇集了30个中心使用Braxon脱细胞真皮基质实施胸肌后乳房重建的经验[20]。该研究在一年内总共回顾性收集了1 450例手术案例，旨在获取采用完整Braxon脱细胞真皮基质包裹行胸肌后乳房重建的大规模循证数据，以明确临床结局的实证性结论，进而优化患者筛选标准。患者平均随访时间为22.7个月（3~75.7个月）。

作者报告，糖尿病、吸烟及免疫抑制状态对并发症发生有影响，内置物重量亦是相关因素。包膜挛缩与术后放疗相关，但总体发生率较低（2.1%）。并发症导致假体取出率为6.5%。此外，针对并发症风险因素的多变量分析表明，使用免疫抑制药物（RR=4.56；P=0.017）、既往接受过乳房美容手术（RR=2.54；P=0.030）以及在胸肌后乳房重建（PPBR）中行腋窝淋巴结清扫患者（RR=1.67；P=0.039）的血清肿形成风险显著增加。肿瘤类型亦可能增加血清肿发生率（P=0.029）。感染更易发生于糖尿病患者（RR=4.026；P=0.003）和既往/现吸烟者（P=0.016），既往吸烟者RR=2.15，现吸烟者RR=2.08。腋窝

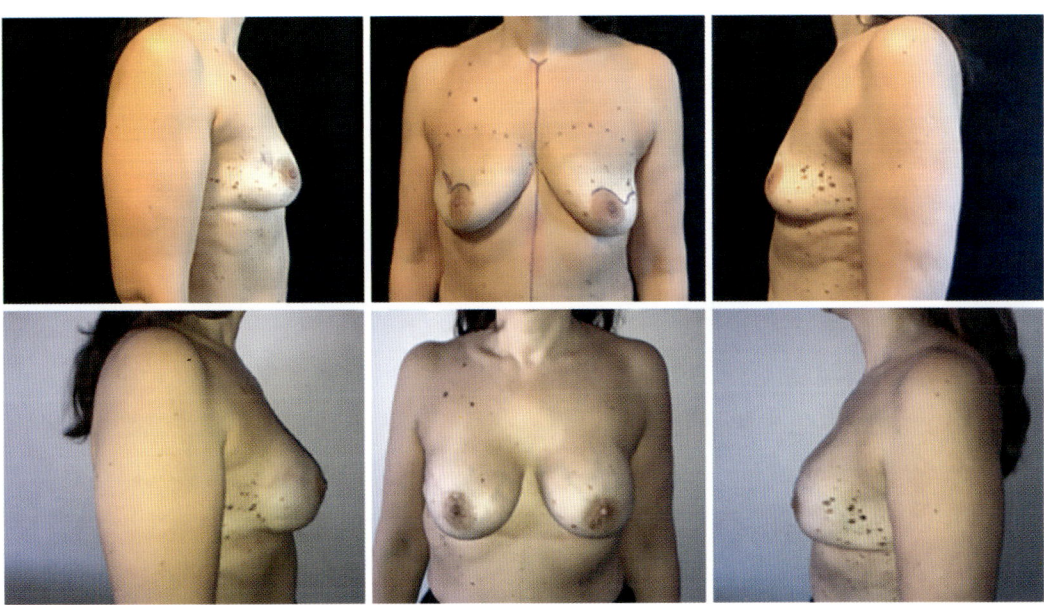

图 18.1　45 岁女性，右乳浸润性小叶癌合并左乳多发性微钙化灶，行双侧保留乳头—乳晕的乳房切除胸肌前重建术。术前视图（上图）与术后 1 年随访视图（下图）。选用的圆形硅胶乳房假体，容量为 300 mL，覆盖材料为 Braxon® 脱细胞真皮基质（ADM）

淋巴结清扫亦影响感染发生（RR=2.17；$P=0.009$）。单变量及多变量分析均显示，内置物体积增加与感染风险升高相关，感染组乳房平均体积为 409.3g，非感染组为 346.2g（$P=0.001$）。简而言之，数据分析提示该术式并发症发生率低且疗效持久，同时明确了导致术后并发症的风险因素。

从已发表的关于胸肌前假体重建术的病例系列研究中可轻易获取临床结局数据，相比之下，目前关于胸肌前与胸肌后假体重建术的对比研究有限。与胸肌后术式相比，胸肌前乳房重建术具有术后疼痛较轻、上肢功能恢复更快、BREAST-Q 美学评分更优以及经济成本更低等优势[21]。

亦有研究探讨了乳房切除术后放疗（PMRT）对胸肌前乳房重建的影响。PMRT 是乳房重建术后并发症的明确危险因素，尤易引发包膜挛缩和重建失败[22]。PMRT 与假体乳房重建术后二次修复手术率升高、美容效果降低及患者满意度下降密切相关[23]。

Sigalove 等及 Elswick 等分别基于 93 例和 52 例乳房的短期、回顾性数据分析发现，接受 PMRT 的胸肌前重建患者并未出现有统计学意义的不良结局风险增加[9, 24]。

此外，Sinnot 团队的研究结果表明，与接受胸肌前重建者相比，接受胸肌后乳房重建和 PMRT 的患者的包膜挛缩发生率显著升高[25]。

18.4　组织学随访

对因假体外露/感染行翻修术时获取

的假体周围组织进行组织学检查，结果显示脱细胞真皮基质与患者组织存在整合迹象。

取患者内置物的脱细胞真皮基质活检标本行光学显微镜观察。简要流程：样本经10%福尔马林溶液固定、脱水、透明化处理后包埋于石蜡，制备5μm厚的石蜡切片行苏木精-伊红染色。

组织学观察可见纤维硬化组织形成（图18.2中心及右上方），伴轻度慢性炎症浸润（以淋巴细胞和单核细胞为主）并存在出血浸润现象（图18.2右下方）及新生血管形成，为典型异物反应表现。

在高倍镜（10×）下可见上皮样肉芽肿性巨细胞性慢性炎性浸润包绕并整合脱细胞真皮基质，使其与宿主组织融合。尤其可观察到多个巨细胞围绕材料，呈"车轮状"排列（图18.3中心），部分巨细胞处于"吞噬"无定形基质的过程。此现象从组织学角度诠释了"异源"材料在人体组织内完成生理性分布的原动力。巨细胞周围可见"组织样肉芽"反应，表现为新生血管形成、红细胞外渗，伴有淋巴细胞、单核细胞及局灶性浆细胞浸润（图18.3）。

整合过程可分为两个不同阶段（图18.4）。视野右侧可见纤维硬化组织，源于异源真皮基质与细胞外基质的整合，并可见嗜酸性蛋白样物质残留。视野左侧可见具有肌成纤维细胞形态的细胞，这些细胞迁移至整合部位后有序排列以优化整合过程，从而增强移植物稳定性及弹性，最终获得更优的形态功能学效果。

上述发现与文献[16]报道一致，证实与合成补片（在皮下乳房重建中曾被视作更经济的生物基质替代物）相比，脱细胞真皮基质具有显著优势，但许多外科医生仍对非可吸收材料的置入存在顾虑[26]。严格来言，生物网状材料无论来源如何，均为通过特殊处理去除抗原细胞的支架结构，可通过促进宿主血管再生及细胞增殖以获得良好手术效果。

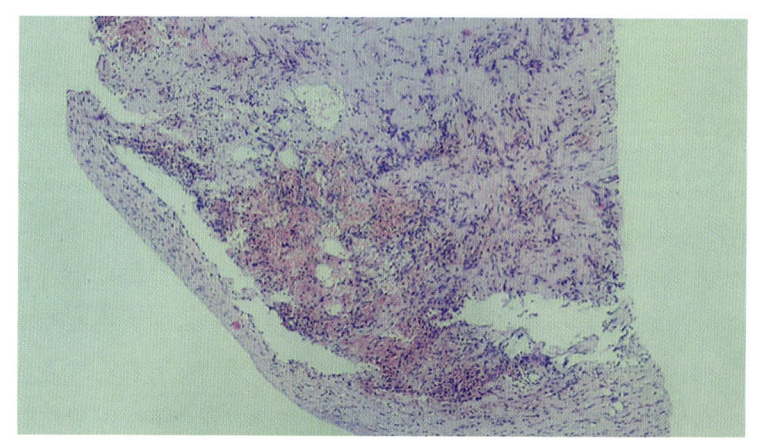

图18.2　假体周围组织活检（苏木精-伊红染色，4×）

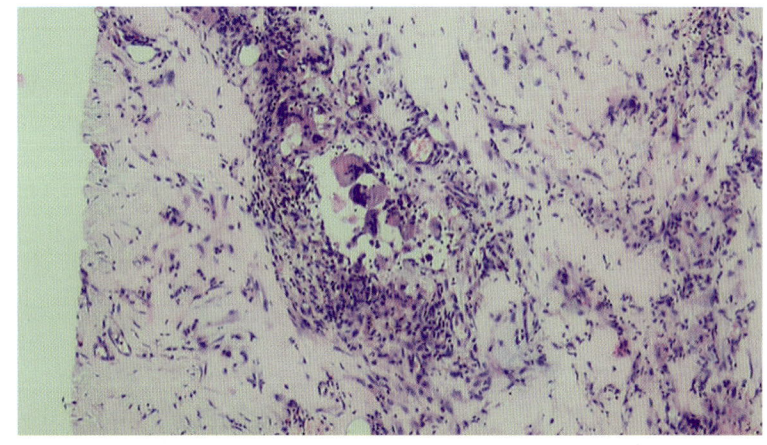

图 18.3 假体周围组织活检（苏木精-伊红染色，10×）

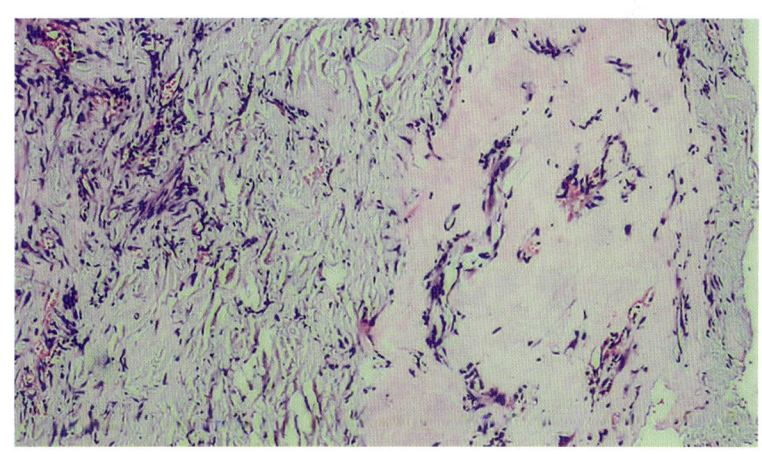

图 18.4 假体周围组织活检（苏木精-伊红染色，10×）

采用脱细胞真皮基质的组织学变化研究[14,27]进一步证实，由于缺乏抗原表位，脱细胞真皮基质能形成屏障以阻隔宿主对异物（扩张器/假体）的免疫应答，从而降低包膜形成与挛缩风险[28]。Komorowska-Timek 等[27]通过研究脱细胞真皮基质在放疗前后对包膜形成的影响，发现该基质可减轻放射相关炎症反应及假性上皮形成，从而延缓包膜形成及挛缩进程。组织学及临床观察显示，使用脱细胞真皮基质者的包膜挛缩发生率显著降低[29]。

18.5 超声随访

对接受假体乳房重建术（PPBR）患者的超声评估旨在观察脱细胞真皮基质与宿主组织整合的征象，包括生物膜的可见性及厚度、假体形态、假体边缘以及内外侧膜皱襞的存在。

此外，超声可监测随访期间局部手术并发症的发生，如假体周围积液、软组织异质性、脂肪坏死、血肿、血清肿、感染、淋巴囊肿，并有助于发现可疑疾病复发征象及辅助手术操作。

Parvini 等[30]首次采用超声造影

（CEUS）描述假体乳房重建术后脱细胞真皮基质（ADM）的血管生成情况，超声造影剂可增强血液流动信号，能够更敏感且更可重复地考察这些特性。对16例患者在术后随访1~18个月，证实了ADM乳房重建术后血管生成及组织形成的体内评估可行性。

假体乳房重建术后的早期超声评估常显示生物膜沿假体凸面延展，而在假体内外侧缘处生物膜松弛并形成部分褶皱与屈曲（图18.5，图18.6）。该特征在术后早期评估中较为明晰，可能与假体周围液体的存在有关（有时呈颗粒状），但随着时间推移，生物膜褶皱会逐渐融合（图18.7）。

18.6　现有文献简要综述

2014年，Bern等首次报道一种保留胸肌的乳房重建术式。该技术将乳房假

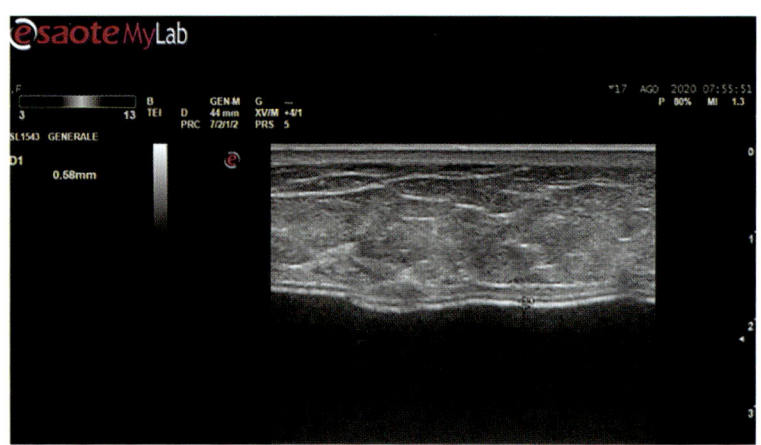

图18.5　术后早期评估（术后7天）显示生物膜呈现为假体周围低回声层

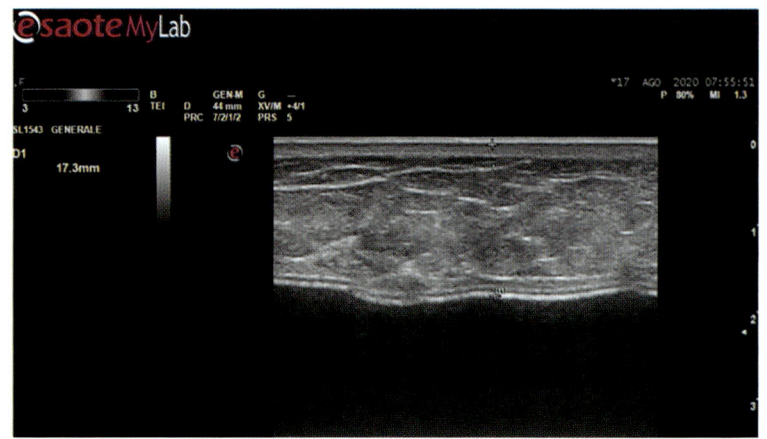

图18.6　术后早期评估（术后7天）可见皮下脂肪组织轻度不均匀增厚

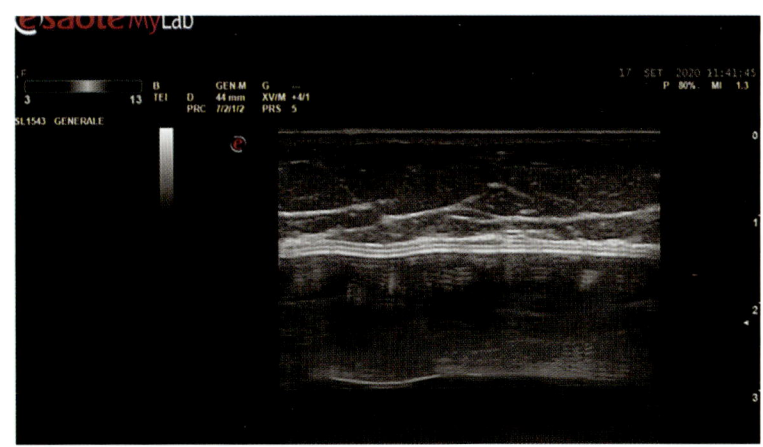

图 18.7　术后 18 个月评估显示假体周围低回声层消失，证实脱细胞真皮基质（ADM）已与宿主组织整合

体置于皮下，以 0.6mm 厚的预制猪源脱细胞真皮基质（ADM）（Braxon®；德国 Neustadt-Glewe 的 MBP Biologics 公司生产，意大利 Marcon 的 Decomed 公司持有许可证）[31] 完全包裹假体。这项创新技术旨在避免胸肌剥离引起的术后并发症（如肌痛、肩臂乏力），并通过更符合生理的假体定位来提升美学效果。

目前，该材料是欧洲乳腺中心胸肌前乳房重建术（PPBR）应用最广泛的材料，也是唯一配备特殊专利设计的 ADM，可实现标准化覆盖操作，减少变量干扰，使得不同机构间数据可比性增强[13]（图 18.8，图 18.9）。

英国已有 2 项国家审计描述了乳房重建的结局[32]。首次审计涵盖了 2008 年 1 月至 2009 年 3 月实施的乳房重建手术；假体重建队列包含 3 000 余例患者，总体并发症发生率为 14.7%，再次手术率为 4.6%，假体取出率为 9%，所有假体均置于胸肌后。近期开展的假体乳房重建评估（iBRA）研究[20] 纳入 2014 年 2 月至 2016 年 6 月接受假体重建的 2 108 例患者，其中 42 例（2.0%）采用胸肌前重建。总体再入院率和再次手术率约为 18%，3 个月假体取出率为 9%。胸肌前亚组的结果经独立分析显示与总体结局相当。

此外，通过 Wise 切口实施的皮肤缩减乳房切除（SRM）联合脱细胞真皮基质-假体重建的新术式，近期被推荐应用于大而下垂乳房患者的胸肌前重建。对大体积乳房实施 Wise 模式皮肤缩减切除联合即刻重建，除需缩减皮肤组织的巨乳症患者可能存在其他危险因素（如较高 BMI）[33] 外，本身也存在乳房切除皮瓣坏死及"T"形交界处裂开的固有风险。

Caputo 等[34] 提出分别利用真皮皮瓣及脱细胞真皮基质（ADM）构建完整的胸肌前囊袋，以覆盖乳房下极和上极区域。Thuman 等[35] 的研究表明，对于高 BMI 患者，采用 Wise 模式皮肤缩减术联合胸肌前两阶段乳房重建是可行的。

有文献[36] 报道了针对乳房肥大下垂患者实施 Wise 模式皮肤缩减乳房切除术

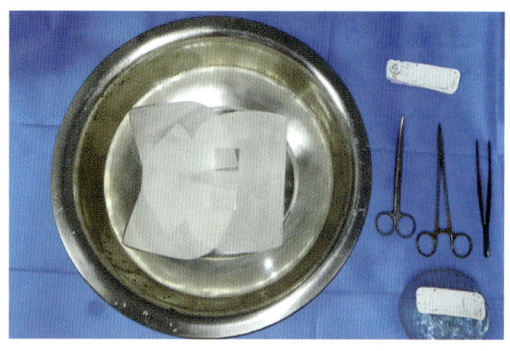

图18.8 Braxon® 置入套件。为使 ADM 融入组织且不引发过度炎症反应，产品最终阶段需进行升华处理。该处理使产品呈干燥态，使用前需快速复水 5~10 分钟。基础手术器械配合 2-0 薇乔缝线，先行构建硅胶试模腔隙，最终置入硅胶假体

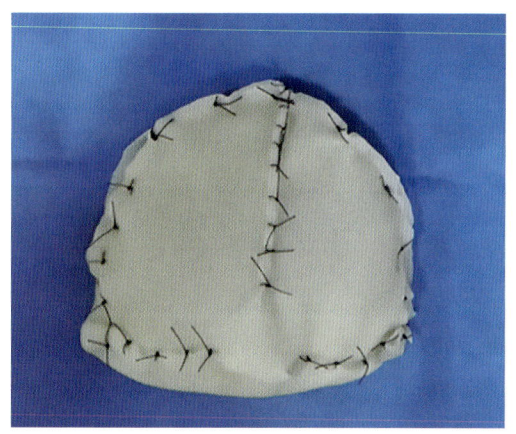

图18.9 Braxon®ADM 假体标准化包裹技术。需以单针缝线将 Braxon® 固定于胸大肌及上方皮瓣，确保基质与血管化组织紧密接触以获得初期稳定性

（SRM）联合胸肌前假体置入及 Braxon® 材料全覆盖的单期手术。该研究未观察到重大假体相关并发症，无须紧急重返手术室或非计划再入院。仅有 2 例伤口裂开经保守处理成功，无须取出假体。Wise 模式皮肤缩减切除联合胸肌前重建可适用于肥大下垂乳房，由此拓展了胸肌前假体重建的患者选择范围。获取下真皮悬吊带可发挥保护作用，且不显著延长手术时间。乳房切除皮瓣的血供状态仍是优化手术流程的关键。

研究证实，ADM 辅助单期胸肌前重建同样是双侧预防性乳房切除重建的理想手术方案。乳腺癌高危女性对治疗效果要求较高，在追求肿瘤学安全性的同时期待良好美学效果及无功能损伤。小、中体积乳房及肥大下垂乳房患者接受前述[36]保留乳头乳房切除术或 Wise 模式皮肤缩减乳房切除术后，均接受 Braxon® 覆盖假体重建术。总计 46 例重建术未见重大并发症及假体取出。术后 BREAST-Q 问卷调查显示患者对疗效满意，表明该重建术式能有效满足患者的临床需求和期望[37]。

18.7 新一代 ADM：三维基质

多数可用于胸肌前重建的生物基质呈扁平形态，须裁剪以适配乳房假体轮廓。其中，Braxon® 是唯一通过预设计实现与假体快速匹配且仅需微调的基质。自 2021 年起，Braxon® 基质的新版本 Braxon®Fast 上市，在保留 Braxon® 原有特性的同时升级为三维构型。依托 Volumatrix® 技术，Braxon®Fast 成为唯一采用穹顶形胶原蛋白片的生物基质，其前部曲度与假体凸面完美契合。通过连接穹顶的扁平胶原蛋白片形成封闭系统，实现假体全覆盖（图 18.10）。此创新三维构型在水合后仍保持稳定（图 18.11，图 18.12），同时也简化了假体包裹步骤：

将假体置入基质并严密包裹后，仅需以单线缝合两片皮瓣（Braxon®需缝合4片；图18.13），必要时可修剪多余基质（图18.14）。Braxon®Fast包裹假体的置入流程与Braxon®包裹假体相同：采用降落伞式缝线定位并固定于远离切口的胸大肌远端（图18.15），基质与皮下组织的缝合确保机械稳定性以及基质与血供良好存活组织的紧密接触。

Braxon®Fast的预弯形态还可提升美学效果：消除基质表面褶皱后，更易实现自然的重建效果（图18.16）。

18.8 新一代ADM：具有促脂肪生成作用的基质

生物材料领域的研究聚焦于开发能与人体组织相互作用并激活特定生物进程的生物活性基质。乳房重建的目标是再生手术损伤的皮下乳腺组织，从而通过治疗手段降低术后并发症（尤其是包膜挛缩）风险。在此背景下，胶原基质不仅需具备整合能力并形成柔软弹性包膜，还应支持乳腺组织中细胞活动以恢复其结构与成分。Braxon®与Braxon®Fast是专为乳腺组织优

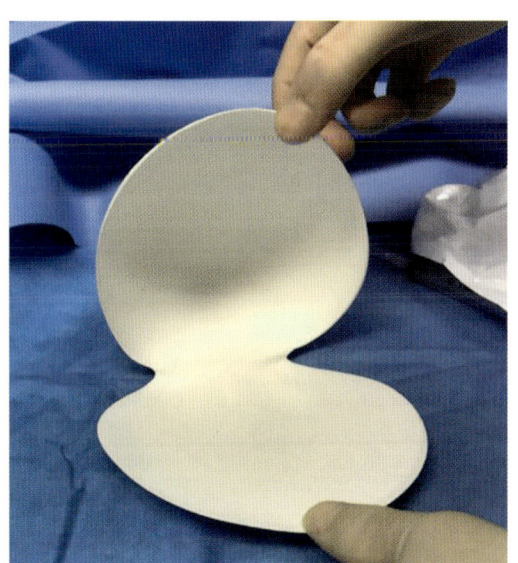

图18.10　Braxon®Fast ADM 干燥形态，呈现穹顶及平坦基底设计

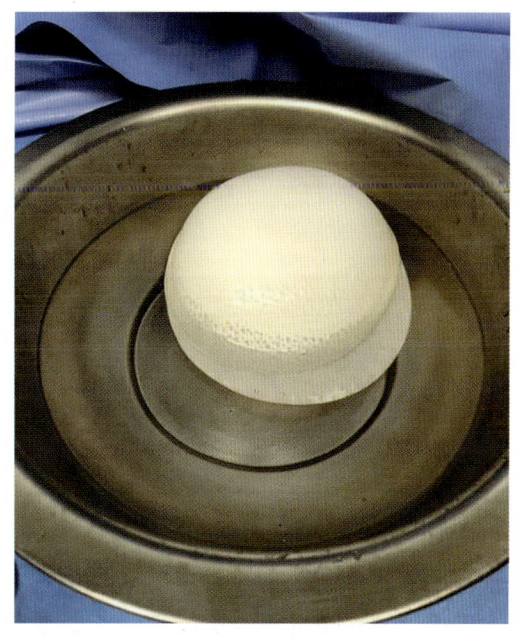

图18.11　Braxon®Fast 于生理盐液中复水

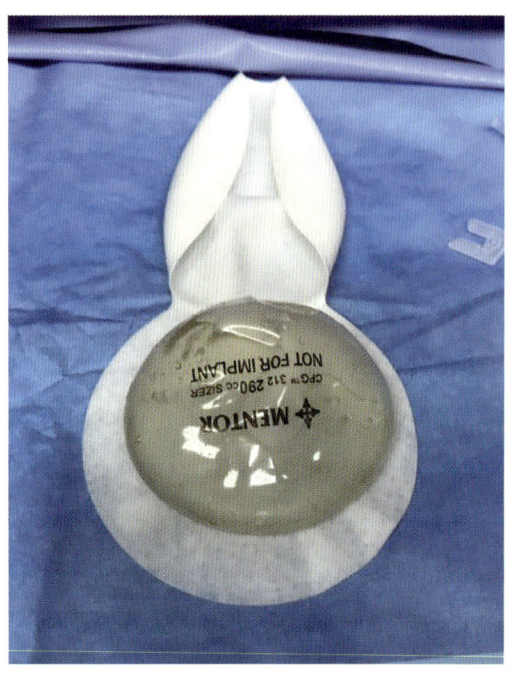

图18.12 ADM 表面试模放置。即使复水状态下，Braxon®Fast 仍保持穹顶三维形态

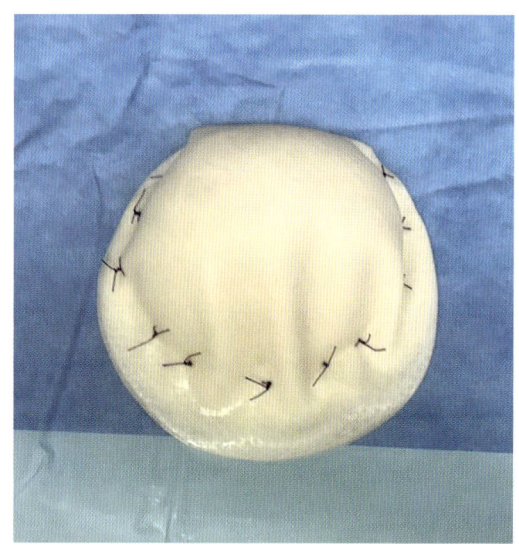

图18.14 修剪多余基质，于边缘保留足够组织用于胸大肌固定

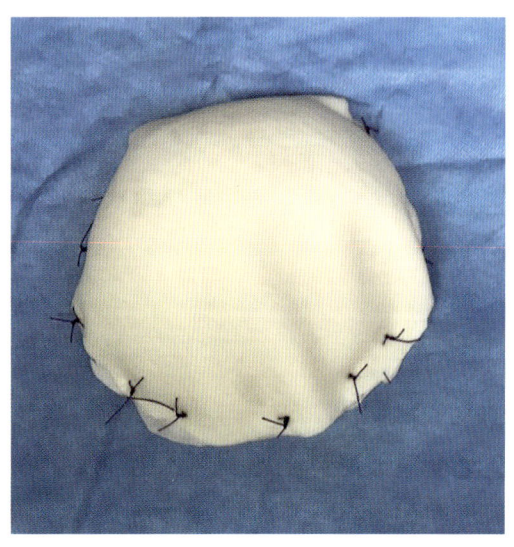

图18.13 Braxon®Fast ADM 假体标准化包裹技术。采用间断缝合连接两片膜瓣，并在假体周围形成紧贴覆盖。缝线须置于膜瓣重叠处，以避免基质张力过度及穿刺假体

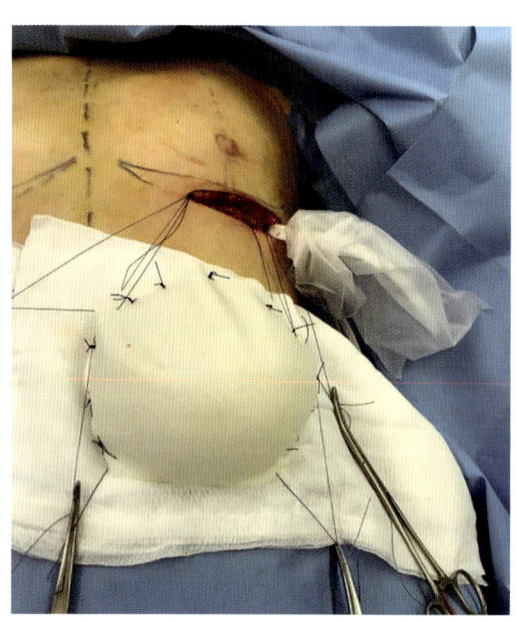

图18.15 采用伞降缝线技术置入 ADM 包裹假体

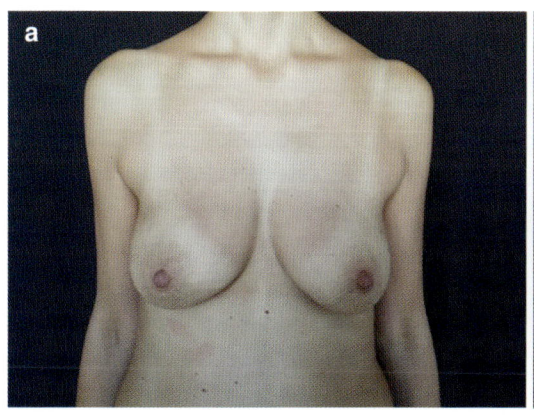
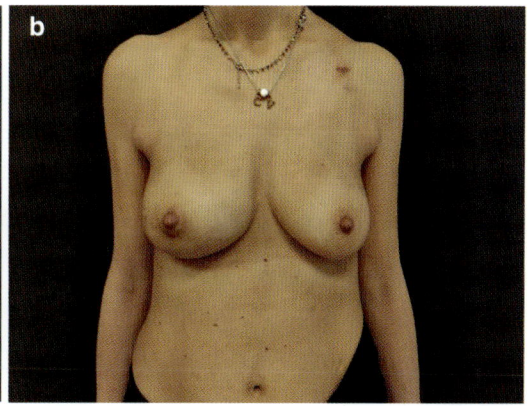

图 18.16 Braxon®Fast 假体置入患者术前（a）与术后（b）影像学资料。术后 2 年随访显示外观自然，无美学缺陷

化、特异性发挥此类再生功能的基质，特有的促脂肪生成特性（Adipomatrix® 技术）旨在恢复乳房脂肪组分。

不同基质（Braxon®、另一种市售 ADM 及心包膜）的体外及体内比较实验证实了材料的成脂潜能，观察到三种基质在孔隙率、显微结构及液体吸收能力方面存在差异。与人脂源性干细胞（ADSCs）共培养时，仅接触 Braxon® 膜的细胞在 7 天后出现脂质积聚，随着第 14 天细胞增殖进一步增加，提示成功实现成脂分化。置入小鼠 30 天后，Braxon® 是唯一被常驻细胞均匀定植且内部形成良好组织结构与血管化成熟脂肪细胞沉积的基质。其他两种膜在体外显示较弱（市售 ADM）或无（心包膜）成脂刺激能力，置入体内后亦未观察到脂肪组织生成[38]。由此可见，Braxon® 表现独特的成脂基质特性。尽管该生物刺激作用尚未有临床证据发表，但大量研究报道使用 Braxon® 的包膜挛缩发生率较低[15, 16, 20, 31, 32, 36, 37]。

该研究表明，材料来源（真皮或心包膜）及生产工艺差异会导致不同的生物学结果，此特性在临床选择时应予充分考虑。

18.9 小结与提示

- 脱细胞真皮基质（ADM）在假体重建中的应用，使胸肌前假体置入及假体完全覆盖成为可能，并获得优异的手术与美学效果。
- Braxon® 是目前唯一可体外实现假体全覆盖的预成型模板式 ADM。
- 胸肌前重建的组织学随访显示 ADM 整合的细胞学征象，如上皮样 – 肉芽肿性巨细胞慢性炎性浸润。
- 超声随访证实 ADM 整合，假体周围低回声基质层随时间逐渐消失。
- Braxon®Fast 因其三维预弯设计及成脂刺激特性，成为目前唯一且最先进的乳房重建专用优化 ADM。

参考文献

1. Rebowe RE, Allred LJ, Nahabedian MY. The evolution from subcutaneous to prepectoral prosthetic breast reconstruction. Plast Reconstr Surg Glob Open. 2018,6（6）:e1797.

2. Reitsamer R, Peintinger F, Klaassen-Federspiel F, Sir A. Prepectoral direct-to-implant breast reconstruction with complete ADM or synthetic mesh coverage—36-Months follow-up in 200 reconstructed breasts. Breast. 2019,48:32–7.

3. Cemal Y, Albornoz CR, Disa JJ, McCarthy CM, Mehrara BJ, Pusic AL, et al. A paradigm shift in U.S. breast reconstruction: part 2. The influence of changing mastectomy patterns on reconstructive rate and method. Plast Reconstr Surg. 2013,131（3）:320e–6e.

4. Jones G, Antony AK. Single stage, direct to implant pre-pectoral breast reconstruction. Gland Surg. 2019,8（1）:53–60.

5. Moyer HR, Losken A. Predicting mastectomy skin flap necrosis with indocyanine green angiography: the gray area defined. Plast Reconstr Surg. 2012,129（5）:1043–8.

6. Komorowska-Timek E, Gurtner GC. Intraoperative perfusion mapping with laser-assisted indocyanine green imaging can predict and prevent complications in immediate breast reconstruction. Plast Reconstr Surg. 2010,125（4）:1065–73.

7. Vidya R, Iqbal FM. A guide to prepectoral breast reconstruction: a new dimension to implant-based breast reconstruction. Clin Breast Cancer. 2017,17（4）:266–71.

8. Salibian AA, Frey JD, Karp NS. Strategies and considerations in selecting between subpectoral and prepectoral breast reconstruction. Gland Surg. 2019,8（1）:11–8.

9. Sigalove S, Maxwell GP, Sigalove NM, Storm-Dickerson TL, Pope N, Rice J, et al. Prepectoral implant-based breast reconstruction: rationale, indications, and preliminary results. Plast Reconstr Surg. 2017,139（2）:287–94.

10. Walia GS, Aston J, Bello R, Mackert GA, Pedreira RA, Cho BH, et al. Prepectoral versus subpectoral tissue expander placement: a clinical and quality of life outcomes study. Plast Reconstr Surg Glob Open. 2018,6（4）:e1731.

11. Casella D, Di Taranto G, Marcasciano M, Lo Torto F, Barellini L, Sordi S, et al. Subcutaneous expanders and synthetic mesh for breast reconstruction: long-term and patient-reported BREAST-Q outcomes of a single-center prospective study. J Plast Reconstr Aesthet Surg. 2019,72（5）:805–12.

12. Reitsamer R, Peintinger F. Prepectoral implant placement and complete coverage with porcine acellular dermal matrix: a new technique for direct-to-implant breast reconstruction after nipple-sparing mastectomy. J Plast Reconstr Aesthet Surg. 2015,68（2）:162–7.

13. Vidya R, Masià J, Cawthorn S, Berna G, Bozza F, Gardetto A, et al. Evaluation of the effectiveness of the prepectoral breast reconstruction with Braxon dermal matrix: first multicenter European report on 100 cases. Breast J. 2017,23（6）:670–6.

14. Hester TR, Ghazi BH, Moyer HR, Nahai FR, Wilton M, Stokes L. Use of dermal matrix to prevent capsular contracture in aesthetic breast surgery. Plast Reconstr Surg. 2012,130（5 Suppl 2）:126S–36S.

15. Polotto S, Bergamini ML, Pedrazzi G, Arcuri MF, Gussago F, Cattelani L. One-step prepectoral breast reconstruction with porcine dermal matrix-covered implant: a protective technique improving the outcome in post-mastectomy radiation therapy setting. Gland Surg. 2020,9（2）:219–28.

16. Onesti MG, Maruccia M, Di Taranto G, Albano A, Soda G, Ballesio L, et al. Clinical, histological, and ultrasound follow-up of breast reconstruction with one-stage muscle-sparing "wrap" technique: a single-center experience. J Plast Reconstr Aesthet Surg. 2017,70（11）:1527–36.

17. Maruccia M, Mazzocchi M, Dessy LA, Onesti MG. One-stage breast reconstruction techniques

18. Maruccia M, Di Taranto G, Onesti MG. One-stage muscle-sparing breast reconstruction in elderly patients: a new tool for retaining excellent quality of life. Breast J. 2018,24（2）:180–3.
19. Giudice G, Maruccia M, Nacchiero E, Elia R, Annoscia P, Vestita M. Dual plane breast implant reconstruction in large sized breasts: how to maximise the result following first stage total submuscular expansion. JPRAS Open. 2018,15:74–80.
20. Masià J, iBAG Working Group. The largest multicentre data collection on prepectoral breast reconstruction: the iBAG study. J Surg Oncol. 2020,122（5）:848–60.
21. Cattelani L, Polotto S, Arcuri MF, Pedrazzi G, Linguadoca C, Bonati E. One-step prepectoral breast reconstruction with dermal matrix-covered implant compared to submuscular implantation: functional and cost evaluation. Clin Breast Cancer. 2018,18（4）:e703–11.
22. Ricci JA, Epstein S, Momoh AO, Lin SJ, Singhal D, Lee BT. A meta-analysis of implant-based breast reconstruction and timing of adjuvant radiation therapy. J Surg Res. 2017,218:108–16.
23. Magill LJ, Robertson FP, Jell G, Mosahebi A, Keshtgar M. Determining the outcomes of post-mastectomy radiation therapy delivered to the definitive implant in patients undergoing oneand two-stage implant-based breast reconstruction: a systematic review and meta-analysis. J Plast Reconstr Aesthet Surg. 2017,70（10）:1329–35.
24. Elswick SM, Harless CA, Bishop SN, Schleck CD, Mandrekar J, Reusche RD, et al. Prepectoral implant-based breast reconstruction with post-mastectomy radiation therapy. Plast Reconstr Surg. 2018,142（1）:1–12.
25. Sinnott CJ, Persing SM, Pronovost M, Hodyl C, McConnell D, Ott Young A. Impact of postmastectomy radiation therapy in prepectoral versus subpectoral implant-based breast reconstruction. Ann Surg Oncol. 2018,25（10）:2899–908.
26. Logan Ellis H, Asaolu O, Nebo V, Kasem A. Biological and synthetic mesh use in breast reconstructive surgery: a literature review. World J Surg Oncol. 2016,14:121.
27. Komorowska-Timek E, Oberg KC, Timek TA, Gridley DS, Miles DAG. The effect of AlloDerm envelopes on periprosthetic capsule formation with and without radiation. Plast Reconstr Surg. 2009,123（3）:807–16.
28. Basu CB, Leong M, Hicks MJ. Acellular cadaveric dermis decreases the inflammatory response in capsule formation in reconstructive breast surgery. Plast Reconstr Surg. 2010,126（6）:1842–7.
29. Koltz PF, Frey JD, Langstein HN. The use of human acellular dermal matrix in the first stage of implant-based breast reconstruction simplifies the exchange procedure. Plast Reconstr Surg. 2013,132（4）:691e–2e.
30. Parvizi D, Haas F, Peintinger F, Hubmer M, Rappl T, Koch H, et al. First experience using contrast-enhanced ultrasound to evaluate vascularisation of acellular dermal matrices after implant-based breast reconstruction. Breast J. 2014,20（5）:461–7.
31. Berna G, Cawthorn SJ, Papaccio G, Balestrieri N. Evaluation of a novel breast reconstruction technique using the Braxon® acellular dermal matrix: a new muscle-sparing breast reconstruction. ANZ J Surg. 2017,87（6）:493–8.
32. Chandarana M, Harries S. Multicentre study of prepectoral breast reconstruction using acellular dermal matrix. BJS Open. 2019,4（1）:71–7.
33. Inbal A, Gur E, Lemelman BT, Barsuk D, Menes T, Leshem D, et al. Optimizing patient selection for direct-to-implant immediate breast reconstruction using wise-pattern skin-reducing mastectomy in large and ptotic breasts. Aesthetic Plast Surg. 2017,41（5）:1058–67.
34. Caputo GG, Marchetti A, Dalla Pozza E, Vigato E, Domenici L, Cigna E, et al. Skin-reduction breast reconstructions with prepectoral implant. Plast Reconstr Surg. 2016,137（6）:1702–5.

35. Thuman J, Freitas AM, Schaeffer C, Campbell CA. Prepectoral wise-pattern staged implant-based breast reconstruction for obese or ptotic patients. Ann Plast Surg. 2019,82（6S Suppl 5）:S404–9.
36. Maruccia M, Elia R, Gurrado A, Moschetta M, Nacchiero E, Bolletta A, et al. Skin-reducing mastectomy and pre-pectoral breast reconstruction in large ptotic breasts. Aesthetic Plast Surg. 2020,44（3）:664–72.
37. Maruccia M, Elia R, Tedeschi P, Gurrado A, Moschetta M, Testini M, Giudice G. Prepectoral breast reconstruction: an ideal approach to bilateral risk-reducing mastectomy. Gland Surg. 2021,10（10）:2997–3006. https://doi.org/10.21037/gs-21-339. PMID: 34804886; PMCID: PMC8575706.
38. Quintero Sierra LA, Busato A, Zingaretti N, et al. Tissue-material integration and biostimulation study of collagen acellular matrices. Tissue Eng Regen Med. 2022,19:477–90. https://doi.org/10.1007/s13770-021-00420-6.

19　胸肌前假体与放疗

编者：Rashmi Benda, Orit Kaidar-Person, Philip M. Poortmans
译者：张　良

19.1　引言

乳腺癌是全球女性最常见的恶性肿瘤，确诊时通常尚未转移，但约30%的早期乳腺癌患者最终会在发生转移[1]。乳腺癌治疗采用多学科联合治疗方案，包括手术、全身治疗和放疗（radiation therapy，RT），需根据个体情况来确定最佳治疗顺序[2]。根据Milan试验、NSABP、丹麦乳腺癌协作组（Danish breast Cancer Group）和EORTC等临床试验结果，对早期乳腺癌患者主要采用保乳手术（breast-conserving surgery，BCS）联合全乳放疗（即保乳治疗，breast-conserving therapy，BCT）的治疗模式，这些试验证实BCT的疗效与全乳切除术相当或具有非劣效性[3~7]。1990年，在美国国立卫生研究院（National Institutes of Health，NIH）召开的早期乳腺癌治疗共识发展会议上，专家小组指出：BCT应优先于全乳切除术，因其在保留乳房的同时可达到与全乳切除术同样的生存率[8]。后续研究进一步表明，对于早期乳腺癌患者，BCT不仅不亚于全乳切除术，其10年总生存率和相对生存率甚至优于全乳切除术。该结果被认为与BCT包含术后放疗有关，即通过放疗消除亚临床病灶[9]。然而在NIH声明发布10年后，相关文献显示早期乳腺癌患者的治疗呈现新趋势——超过三分之一的保乳适应证患者选择全乳切除术作为初始手术方案[10~13]。

此外，对非遗传性乳腺癌患者的单侧

R. Benda (✉)
Shore Regional Cancer Center, Requard Radiation Oncology, Easton, MD, USA
e-mail: Rashmi.Benda@umm.edu

O. Kaidar-Person
Breast Cancer Radiation Therapy Unit, Sheba Medical Center, Ramat Gan, Israel

Dept. Radiation Oncology (Maastro), GROW-School for Oncology and Reproduction, Maastricht University Medical Centre+,
Maastricht, The Netherlands

P. M. Poortmans
Department of Radiation Oncology, Iridium Netwerk, Wilrijk, Antwerp, Belgium

Faculty of Medicine and Health Sciences, University of Antwerp, Wilrijk, Antwerp, Belgium
e-mail: Philip.poortman@gza.be

© The Author(s), under exclusive license to Springer Nature Switzerland AG 2023
R. Vidya, H. Becker (eds.), *Prepectoral Breast Reconstruction*,
https://doi.org/10.1007/978-3-031-15590-1_19

病变行双侧乳房切除术的比例从 1998 年的 5.4% 上升至 2011 年的 29.7%，同期该群体行乳房重建术的比例也从 36.9% 增至 57.2%[14]。这一趋势与美国整形外科网站报告的寻求乳房增大术的健康人群（非乳腺癌患者）数量变化相似——2000 年至 2017 年的绝对增长率达 41%。这些现象不仅反映了公众对乳房美容手术的普遍需求，也提示保乳治疗适应人群手术方式选择可能受复发焦虑、放疗恐惧及乳房整形"文化"等因素的明显影响。尽管多项最新研究支持保乳治疗相较全乳切除术可改善患者总体生存[9, 15]且保乳仍是推荐治疗选择，但 1998 年至 2011 年美国的全乳切除术实施率仍从 36.9% 攀升至 57.2%，而欧洲地区的该比例呈下降趋势[16]。应对这一趋势的关键在于向患者、外科医师及其他医疗从业者有效传递临床研究最新证据，以扭转全乳切除术的滥用趋势，实现生存获益最大化，并缓解其对复发风险和放疗的过度担忧[14, 17]。

乳房切除术后放疗（postmastectomy irradiation，PMRT）主要应用于 ≥ 3 枚淋巴结转移患者。随着腋窝降级手术理念的普及，当前 1~3 枚淋巴结阳性患者接受 PMRT 的比例呈上升趋势[18, 19]。近期的回顾性研究指出，接受即刻重建的早期（淋巴结阴性）乳腺癌患者若未行 PMRT，其局部复发率将升高，研究认为该现象可能与残留乳腺组织及皮肤内潜在亚临床病灶相关[20]。鉴于即刻乳房重建患者中 PMRT 需求人群持续扩大，欧洲放射肿瘤学会（European Society for Radiotherapy and Oncology，ESTRO）发布了即刻假体置入乳房重建后 PMRT 的靶区勾画指南，旨在降低 PMRT 相关并发症发生率[21]。为确保乳腺癌手术与重建技术发展不影响肿瘤控制效果，开展多学科协作至关重要——放射医师须充分理解乳房切除与重建手术的技术难点，而乳腺整形外科医师亦须深刻认识放疗的作用及其应用于乳房重建患者的挑战。

19.2　乳房切除术后放疗的作用

1997 年，《新英格兰医学杂志》（NEJM）发表了 2 项探讨乳房切除术后放疗（post-mastectomy radiation therapy，PMRT）应用于 T3/4 期病灶和/或 ≥ 4 枚淋巴结阳性患者[22, 23]的研究。结果显示，对 1~3 枚淋巴结阳性患者实施胸壁及区域淋巴结根治性放疗可改善无病生存期（Disease-free Survival，DFS）与总生存期（overall survival，OS）。

20 年后，欧洲癌症研究与治疗组织（European Organisation for Research and Treatment of Cancer，EORTC）22 922-10 925 试验、加拿大主导的 MA.20 试验及丹麦全国性队列 DBCGIMN 研究进一步证实了内乳淋巴结预防性放疗的临床意义。入组标准包括经组织学确诊的单侧乳腺癌（Ⅰ~Ⅲ期）：原发灶位于中央区或内侧象限（无论腋窝淋巴结状态和局部手术范围），或原发灶位于外侧象限但伴腋窝淋巴结转移[24, 25]。这些研究结果将 PMRT 的适应证扩展至高危淋巴结阴性患者。

虽然放疗可延长患者的无病生存期（DFS）与总生存期（OS），但治疗计划中若未严格控制剂量，则可能诱发心脏相关并发症及死亡风险。对 20 世纪 90 年代前接受放疗患者进行 10 年随访发现，其全因死亡率明显升高。首项基于治疗年的心脏毒性荟萃分析显示，左侧乳腺癌放疗后心脏相关死亡率显著增加，随访每增加 5 年该风险会递增[26, 27]。Darby 等[28]研究发现，心脏平均放疗剂量每增加 1Gy，心脏相关死亡风险将以线性方式自治疗后 5 年开始持续升高（风险率达 7.4%/Gy），并且这一效应至少持续 20 年。尽管上述得出心脏毒性较高结论的研究采用的是二维（2D）放疗技术（该技术心脏受照剂量显著高于现代技术），但此类研究促使临床医生对心脏保护重视程度的提升，并通过优化放疗策略大幅降低心脏剂量，从而有效减少放疗远期并发症。

一项针对 HERA III 期随机临床试验前瞻性数据的回顾性分析显示，对于接受乳房切除术及曲妥珠单抗辅助治疗的 HER-2 阳性乳腺癌患者（n=1 633），若存在 1~3 枚淋巴结转移，PMRT 可降低局部区域复发风险。虽然其获益程度低于历史研究，但目前证据仍支持该人群接受 PMRT[29]。随着全身治疗进展（如抗 HER-2 药物的应用），未来或可筛选出无须 PMRT 的亚组患者。

NSABP-B51 试验将新辅助治疗后达到病理完全缓解的患者随机分组，分别接受胸壁、区域淋巴结 PMRT 或观察。尽管部分现行 PMRT 适应证患者未来可能无须放疗，但 PMRT 的临床应用仍将持续存在[30]。

19.3 放疗靶区与技术

保乳术后放疗（PMRT）对乳房重建提出了新挑战，其照射靶区需覆盖胸壁（包括乳房切除术后残留的皮下组织）、腋窝淋巴结 I～IV 水平未切除部分、胸肌间淋巴结及内乳淋巴结（internal mammary nodes，IMN）。大面积胸壁及区域淋巴结照射会增加放疗计划的复杂性。内乳淋巴结链是乳腺癌重要淋巴引流路径之一。基于扩大根治术的系列解剖学研究表明，约 75% 的乳腺淋巴引流至腋窝，25% 至内乳淋巴结。淋巴闪烁显像研究显示，28%~44% 乳腺癌患者存在内乳淋巴结引流，其中内/中央型肿瘤患者发生率高达 65%。1998 年，Zucali 等报道内/中央型乳腺癌患者远处转移率增加 30%，死亡率增加 20%，提示未治疗的 IMN 微转移灶可能导致远处转移[31]。将内乳淋巴结纳入照射范围，显著增加了放射的技术挑战（见图 19.1）。

而 ACOSOG Z0011 试验[32]与 AMAROS 试验[33]基本消除了标准腋窝淋巴结清扫术式，同时将低位腋窝淋巴结纳入照射范围，涵盖这些淋巴结也使得切线野后部覆盖范围增大。尽管有观点认为 ACOSOG Z0011 试验不允许区域淋巴结放疗，因此无须将这些区域纳入照射靶区，但仅行锁骨上淋巴结照射而忽略低位腋窝淋巴结的做法缺乏合理性。此外，虽然

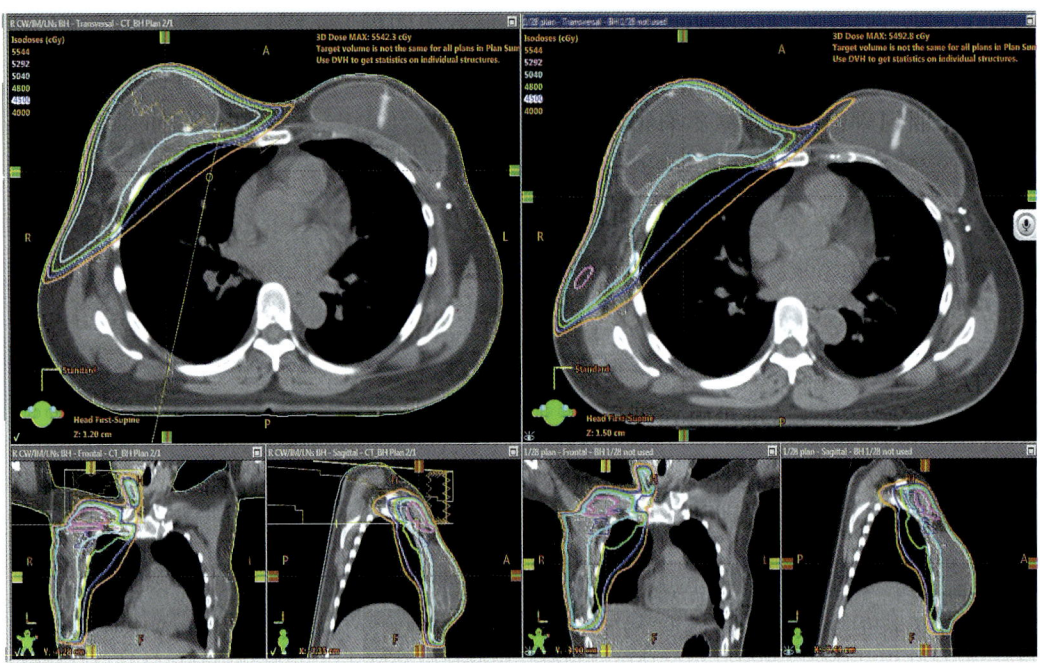

图 19.1 缩小对侧扩张器容积可优化放疗剂量分布：提升靶区覆盖同时消除热点。右图示处方剂量 5 040 cGy（热点区 105% 达 5 292 cGy）时，4 000 cGy 剂量线穿透对侧乳房。射束角度优化同时减少肌肉受照，或可缓解患者术后紧绷感

ACOSOG Z0011 试验不允许增加锁骨上照射野，但至少部分低位腋窝淋巴结仍接受局部至全程剂量。遗憾的是，因 ACOSOG Z0011 试验未前瞻性要求勾画这些淋巴结并采集剂量-体积直方图数据，无法佐证免除这些淋巴结放疗的依据。然而 Monica Murrow 团队发表的论文显示，即使不行术前腋窝影像学检查或常规淋巴结放疗，多数符合 Z0011 入选标准的患者仍可避免腋窝淋巴结清扫，同时获得良好区域控制效果[34]。除了（加拿大）British Columbia 省和丹麦试验外，EORTC 与 MA20 的近期数据进一步验证了广泛区域淋巴结放疗的合理性。

胸壁补量放疗存在一定争议。与保乳患者的乳腺补量不同，目前尚无评估胸壁补量疗效的随机对照试验。目前，胸壁补量放疗主要在美国应用，常规额外给予 5 次分割 10Gy 的补量照射，通常靶区覆盖乳房切除术瘢痕周围 2~3cm 范围的胸壁皮肤与皮下组织——该区域被认为是复发风险的最高区域。接受补量照射组假体暴露发生率为 7.6%，未补量组为 1.76%（$P=0.0025$）；包膜挛缩发生率分别为 13.4% 与 8.4%，呈现临界显著性差异（$P=0.059$）[35]。总体假体失败率，补量组为 35%，未补量组为 19%（$P<0.0001$）。该回顾性研究显示，即使对包括年轻、切缘阳性或存在淋巴脉管侵犯（LVI）等高危人群，胸壁补量放疗亦未能预防局部失

败。其他研究显示具有高风险特征患者的局部复发绝对比例有所下降，但未达统计学显著性[36]。目前缺乏该主题的前瞻性数据，因而临床实践存在差异，多数放疗科医师选择对切缘阳性患者行补量照射。

19.4 分割放疗方案

针对接受乳房切除术（无论是否行重建术）的乳腺癌患者，不同国家在总剂量与分割方案上存在差异。即刻乳房重建中最常应用的放疗方案仍为传统分割模式（总剂量50~50.4Gy/25~28次）[37]。与之相反，越来越多的国家采用中等程度大分割方案（如3周内分15次给予总剂量40Gy）对胸壁及区域淋巴结进行放疗，这一方案同样适用于乳房重建术后患者。该选择基于英国START A/B试验的长期数据，后者提示，与传统分割模式中等大分割方案相比，其在保乳术后放疗及无重建的保乳术后放疗（PMRT）中具有更低的毒性反应。尽管目前缺乏专门评估即刻乳房重建背景下大分割放疗的临床试验数据，但基于保乳治疗中大分割方案的长期数据以及英国、荷兰等国家的长期应用经验，没有理由认为其疗效会逊于传统分割方案[37,38,40,41]。Chen等[39]近期开展的研究回顾性分析了75例接受II期假体重建并行术后放疗的患者，所有患者于乳房切除的同时置入扩张器并使用去细胞真皮基质加强乳房下极区域，术后2周开始扩张，放疗前部分回抽扩张器，放疗结束后3个月更换为永久假体。放疗方案采用50.4Gy/28次或40.05Gy/15次两种模式，皮肤高复发风险患者追加填充物。靶区范围涵盖胸壁及区域淋巴结（包括腋窝、内乳及锁骨上淋巴结）。中位随访时间32.5个月，总体并发症发生率为22.7%，大分割放疗组并发症发生率（14.3%）显著低于传统分割组（38.5%，$P=0.017$），并且急性放射性皮炎严重程度与并发症发生率呈正相关［皮炎组 G0 3/28（10.7%），G1 5/33（15.2%），G2 7/10（70%），G3 2/4（50%），$P<0.001$］。

一项多中心前瞻性II期大分割PMRT试验的5年随访数据构成了正在进行的随机RT CHARM试验基础。该研究入组患者接受胸壁（或重建乳房）及区域淋巴引流区每日3.33Gy的大分割放疗（11次），可选择追加乳房切除瘢痕补量照射（4次）。主要终点为未发生3级及以上晚期非重建相关放射性毒性，次要终点包括局部及区域复发率、美容效果及重建并发症。毒性反应采用"不良事件通用术语标准"（CTCAE，v4.0）进行评价。43例患者计划行乳房重建，其中40例（93%）于放疗前接受重建（88%为临时扩张器，7%为即刻假体，5%为既往隆胸假体），3例(7%)为放疗后重建。43例患者中，35%出现与放疗相关的3或4级重建并发症。RT-CHARM是一项随机III期临床试验，针对假体重建PMRT患者，比较乳房切除联合重建术后42.56Gy/16次与50Gy/25次分割方案，不允许补量照射。若研究结果与其他乳腺癌试验类似，该方案或将成为新的标准分割模式。

19.5 乳房重建类型与放疗

乳房切除术后可采用不同术式进行重建。历史上，20 世纪 60 年代起可采用硅胶假体行重建[42]。早期重建通过将假体直接置于乳房切除术后皮下囊袋中来实现。尽管操作简单，但该技术会导致假体移位、褶皱、假体外露及挛缩等并发症，推测与假体表面组织覆盖不足有关。

2006 年，脱细胞真皮基质（acellular dermal matrix，ADM）的引入可将胸大肌下缘固定于乳房下皱襞，从而加强假体的下外侧支撑并减少下外侧移位。ADM 的应用促使整形外科医师重新考虑将假体置于胸肌前的优势，一项系统综述[43]比较了单纯胸肌前假体重建与联合 ADM 或补片的胸肌前重建的并发症发生情况，检索 PubMed 数据库自建库至 2017 年 3 月的文献，筛选接受胸肌前假体重建（是否联用 ADM/补片）的乳房切除术后患者研究，提取研究特征、并发症发生率及结局进行分析。使用 Newcastle-Ottawa 量表评估研究质量，并采用随机效应模型分析并发症特征，550 项研究中有 27 项符合纳入标准。1 881 例乳房中，联用 ADM 组的并发症发生率为 23.4%，而未联用其他内置材料组为 27.5%；联用与未联用 ADM 组的包膜挛缩率分别为 2.3% 和 12.4%。胸肌前重建中，联用 ADM 虽与更低的包膜挛缩率及总体并发症率相关，但假体丢失、感染及乳房切除皮瓣坏死发生率更高。不同研究结果存在差异且证据质量普遍较低。因结局评估方法存在异质性，需进一步开展对比研究并规范结局报告标准。

回顾性研究表明，与胸肌后置入相比，胸肌前重建在客观美学效果和患者预后方面均具优势[44-46]。有学者建议对计划接受术后放疗的患者优先采用胸肌前假体重建[45, 47]。早期研究显示，与胸肌后组织扩张器相比，胸肌前组织扩张器在放疗后发生上方位移的风险更低。然而，近期一项对比胸肌前与胸肌后置入组织扩张器的研究显示，两种重建方式（假体取出率分别为 15.4% 和 19.3%）的总体并发症发生率无统计学差异[48]。针对放疗后乳房重建患者的更多研究将有助于明确最佳治疗方案。乳房切除皮瓣的血供是决定胸肌前重建成功的关键要素：保留乳头-乳晕的乳房切除术后乳头区域始终存在低灌注现象，若皮肤血供同时受损，则需分阶段重建——于胸肌前平面置入组织扩张器，2~3 周待皮瓣血运改善后再行后续重建。

一项研究[49]评估了 33 例患者 52 例采用胸肌前重建的乳房，其中 65% 的乳房接受了放疗（2/3 采用永久假体进行放疗）。在平均 25 个月的随访期内，放疗组乳房出现 1 例血清肿及 1 例伤口裂开伴后续扩张器取出事件，两组均未发生包膜挛缩。

在一项回顾性研究中，Sinnot[50]报道胸肌后乳房重建术后包膜挛缩发生率为 52.2%，而胸肌前乳房重建在放疗后包膜挛缩率仅为 16.1%。此外，胸肌后组 12 例包膜挛缩病例中有 10 例分级达 3/4 级，而胸肌前组仅见 2 例良性病例。有研究表明，脱细胞真皮基质（ADM）扩大了内置物表面覆盖范围，具有保护作用。术后放疗期间，双平面组的扩张器移位率亦高于胸肌前组，推测与放疗诱发的肌纤维化及胸肌挛缩导致扩张器上移有关。批评者质疑胸肌前假体置入重建研究的随访时间较短。值得注意的是，胸肌前重建需为内置物制作囊袋，即便使用 ADM 仍易残留较厚皮瓣，可能导致更多残余乳腺组织及真皮淋巴管中潜在亚临床肿瘤细胞存留[51]。

Becker 等[52,53]的研究为胸肌前 I 期重建提供了有力论证。胸肌前假体置入可减轻扩张过程中胸肌牵张痛，减少远期臂外展无力和疼痛[46,54]。另有报道指出，高风险患者如皮瓣薄、BMI 高、循环障碍、有既往放疗者不宜采用该技术。Becker 等认为胸肌前术式更具优势，可降低血运障碍和创面愈合的风险。他们提出分阶段注入不同量空气达到预期愈合及美学效果后再置换为生理盐水的技术。在对 25 例患者长达 1 年的研究中，3 例接受辅助放疗，5 例有放疗史。仅 1 例有既往放疗史者发生内置物外露需取出。该方法采用近乎空置的扩张器使次优皮瓣血供恢复正常，避免了缺血并发症。与 Wagner 等不同，该术式未使用 ADM。该研究仅纳入由同一位术者施治的 25 例患者，需开展多中心研究以验证其成果是否适用于更广泛患者群体及术者。

19.6 扩张器类型与放疗

2016 年，基于 XPAND 试验结果，AeroForm 装置获得 FDA 批准，该试验将 AeroForm 与盐水扩张器进行了比较[55]，试验组患者每天通过充注 CO_2 实现 10mL 增量、最高可达 30mL 的组织扩张，对照组则由医生定期注入生理盐水。研究表明，CO_2 扩张器在总体不良事件发生率与盐水扩张器相当的同时，提供了更为便捷的扩张方式。

Tran 等指出，射束射出位置的实测剂量与计算剂量存在显著差异。鉴于该装置数据有限，目前建议放疗患者谨慎使用。虽然可将气体替换为盐水，但金属端口对剂量测定的影响仍需警惕[56]。CT 技术可通过在治疗计划扫描中扣除金属密度来克服此问题。此外，方便患者自行调节容积的装置存在放疗剂量重复的问题：完成模拟定位并基于 CT 生成放疗计划后，必须保持解剖结构稳定，内置物容积改变将导致预设剂量无法精确施照。

随着技术发展，肿瘤放疗专家倾向在治疗前清除扩张器内气体或二氧化碳。空气 / 二氧化碳界面处的剂量均匀性值得关注，该领域尚需进一步研究。

19.7 乳房切除类型与放疗时机

美国国立综合癌症网络（NCCN）指南建议，采用假体进行乳房重建者初始应选择扩张器重建。乳房切除术后重建与放疗的整合极为复杂，须与肿瘤科医生充分讨论以获得满意的肿瘤学与美学效果[57]。自体组织重建推荐于放疗结束后实施，避免纤维化影响外观美观。有研究比较了组织扩张器与置入永久内置物后放疗的并发症发生率，未见显著差异[58]。

在一项针对113例接受乳房切除术后放疗（PMRT）及乳房重建女性的回顾性研究中，先行放疗组并发症发生率为32%，先行乳房重建组为44%[59]。先行放疗组早期并发症更常见，而先行乳房重建组晚期并发症更普遍。Naoum等发表了1997年至2017年1 286例患者行1 814次乳房重建的回顾性研究[60]，根据重建类型及术后放疗应用将患者分为6组，排除术前接受化疗及因局部复发行乳房切除与重建者。主要研究终点为需手术干预的重建并发症（如感染、皮肤坏死及脂肪坏死），次要终点为比较组织扩张器组（TE）与直接置入组（DTI）的内置物相关并发症（如包膜挛缩、假体破裂、外露或失效）。多变量分析中，次要目标为对比即刻重建后放疗三种重建方式的差异。中位随访时间5.8年。41.1%患者接受术后放疗，非放疗组自体组织重建、DTI及TE重建并发症发生率分别为11.1%、12.6%及19.5%，术后放疗组5年发生率分别为15.1%、18.2%及36.8%。多变量分析显示，DTI组较TE/I组并发症风险更低，自体组织组与DTI组无显著差异。研究未发现保留乳头术式或腋窝淋巴结清扫对并发症的发生率有影响。

体重指数（BMI）和吸烟是需再次手术并发症的显著预测因子，而TE/I是重建失败的独立预测因素[61]。

皮瓣厚度是预测结局的最关键因素。乳房大小（可能与BMI相关）亦被报道为并发症的显著预测指标[62]。

术前化疗与辅助化疗相比、TE/I与内置物相比、BMI>30是总体失败率的显著预测因子，吸烟亦呈现显著趋势。乳房切除术后放疗的剂量、疗程或推量照射与重建失败或并发症无显著相关性。

荷兰8家医院开展了一项开放标签随机对照试验[63]。研究将女性随机分配接受ADM（Strattice, LifeCell, Branchburg, NJ, USA）辅助Ⅰ期置入物乳房重建（IBBR）或Ⅱ期IBBR。主要研究终点为安全性及生活质量相关不良结局发生率。2013至2015年共纳入142例患者，其中59例（91侧乳房）随机分入ADM联合直接置入组（DTI），62例（92侧乳房）分入组织扩张器/内置物组（TE/I）。结果显示，与Ⅱ期IBBR相比，ADM联合Ⅰ期IBBR组手术并发症（粗比值比3.81，95% CI：2.67~5.43，p<0.001）、再次手术（3.38，95% CI：2.10~5.45，p<0.001）及移除内置物/ADM或联合移除（8.80，95% CI：8.24~9.40，p<0.001）风险显著增高。ADM联合Ⅰ期IBBR组中，有26侧（29%）乳房发生3级不良事件，Ⅱ期IBBR组则为5侧（5%）。两组轻中度不良事件发生率相近。作者提示需谨慎应用Ⅰ期重建术式。但需注意，该试验DTI组纳入较多糖尿病患者、有吸烟史及接受术前化疗者。

重建与放疗的时序安排仍有争议。通常需待术后病理评估（一般于乳房切除术后3~5日完成）明确后方能决定是否需行PMRT。本院通过多学科肿瘤委员会对每位患者进行评估，但部分患者术前淋巴结阴性（cN0）而术后阳性（pN+），术前无法确定PMRT指征。此外，术前cN1

患者经新辅助化疗后可转为 pN0，可入组 NSABP B51 试验随机分配至不放疗组。

部分学者主张在乳房切除前行前哨淋巴结（SLN）活检[64]。若前哨淋巴结无肿瘤转移，则肿瘤 < 5cm 的患者需要术后放疗的可能性较低，此时可考虑即刻重建。这种方法需要患者接受 2 次麻醉。

内置物的位置和体积不仅会影响放疗剂量分布的均质性，还可能减少肺部受照体积。

有人认为，过度扩张的组织扩张器会影响皮肤完整性，从而可能损害血液灌注和最终美容效果。此外，由于放疗依赖组织氧合，血管生成不良也可能降低放疗疗效。

19.8 小结

虽然术后放疗的应用标准随着治疗倾向的变化而演变——从仅治疗 ≥ 4 枚淋巴结转移患者，逐步扩展至 1~3 枚淋巴结转移患者，未来或可能排除化疗后达到病理完全缓解的患者——但总会有部分患者从术后放疗中获益。这些女性中的多数将接受乳房重建。为获得最佳疗效，必须由多学科团队对这些患者进行评估与讨论（图 19.1，图 19.2）。数据显示，患者 BMI 及其他合并症等多种因素可能影响理想重建方案的选择。疾病范围将决定是否采用新辅助化疗、手术范围及术后放疗的必要性；对于更晚期的患者，可能还需考虑追加放疗。研究表明，胸壁追加照射会增加假体外露风险，并且在多数情况下可能无法改善局部控制，因此应避免。对于肿瘤较大或存在真皮浸润需考虑追加放疗的患者，胸肌前假体重建可能不利于美学效果及疾病控制。由于高风险组织包绕假体，电子

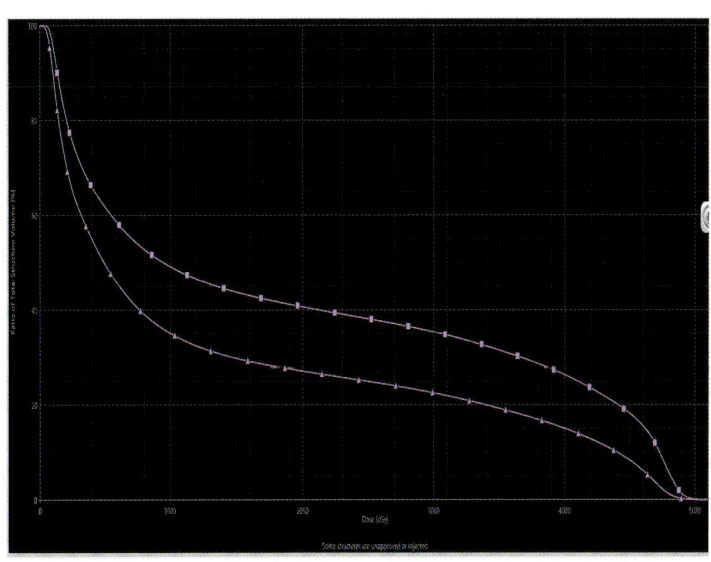

图 19.2　肺组织剂量体积直方图变化（扩张器未抽液时■与抽液后△）。容积缩小显著降低肺受照剂量体积，而照射体积与放射性肺炎风险相关。此案例证实多学科协作的重要性：通过缩小扩张器容积，可优化靶区剂量覆盖，同时保护正常组织

线追加照射将不可行，而光子线追加照射会增加左肺及左侧患者心脏的受照剂量。

存在不确定性时，最好使用组织扩张器或可调节假体以调整容积进行治疗。虽然 CO_2 扩张器提供了一种便利且可能更舒适的扩张方式，但患者自主控制扩张可能导致假体轮廓的不连续变化，进而影响放疗剂量及治疗结果，不推荐在此类扩张器在位时实施放疗。胸肌前与胸肌后放置方式应根据疾病范围、合并症、解剖结构及可用放疗技术综合判断，患者年龄亦会影响重建决策。整形外科医生可能更倾向为年轻患者选择美观效果最佳的重建方案，但放疗技术对此类患者同样重要，因她们更可能罹患侵袭性较高的病变，且长期心脏毒性及对侧乳腺癌发生风险更高。整形外科医生与肿瘤放疗专家的持续沟通至关重要，以期为患者提供最佳局部控制及生存机会，而重建术可改善其生活质量。在患者等待放疗期间，可调节扩张器/假体可使整形外科医生继续进行组织扩张及牵张。接受化疗的患者可在化疗期间保持扩张状态以充分牵张皮肤，但可能需在放疗前调减假体容积，从而优化靶区剂量投递并最大限度减少正常组织受照剂量及毒性反应（图 19.1，图 19.2）。

传统认为乳房切除术后随访仅行体格检查即可。于胸肌后置入假体时复发小病灶较易扪及，而胸肌前假体充填于胸肌与皮肤之间，该区域可能残存乳腺组织，恰为复发高危区域。因此，对高复发风险女性或许应避免使用胸肌前假体。若评估为高危患者但需行胸肌前假体置入，则应每年行 MRI 检查并定期体检以便早期发现复发。该领域尚需更多生活质量相关研究。

不断精进的放疗技术有助于进一步提升疗效并降低毒性，而整形外科界亦持续致力于改善患者美容效果——这对提升癌症幸存者的福祉至关重要[62]。

参考文献

1. O'Shaughnessy J. Extending survival with chemo¬therapy in metastatic breast cancer. Oncologist. 2005,10（Suppl 3）:20–9.

2. Cardoso F, Costa A, Senkus E, Aapro M, André F, Barrios CH, Bergh J, Bhattacharyya G, Biganzoli L, Cardoso MJ, Carey L, Corneliussen-James D, Curigliano G, Dieras V, El Saghir N, Eniu A, Fal¬lowfield L, Fenech D, Francis P, Gelmon K, Gennari A, Harbeck N, Hudis C, Kaufman B, Krop I, Mayer M, Meijer H, Mertz S, Ohno S, Pagani O, Papado¬poulos E, Peccatori F, Penault-Llorca F, Piccart MJ, Pierga JY, Rugo H, Shockney L, Sledge G, Swain S, Thomssen C, Tutt A, Vorobiof D, Xu B, Norton L, Winer E. 3rd ESO-ESMO international consensus guidelines for advanced breast cancer（ABC 3）. Ann On-col. 2017,28（12）:3111. https://doi.org/10.1093/annonc/mdx036. Erratum for: Ann Oncol. 2017 Jan 1;28（1）:16–33. PMID: 28327998; PM-CID: PMC5834023

3. Christiansen P, Carstensen SL, Ejlertsen B, Kro-man N, Offersen B, Bodilsen A, Jensen MB. Breast con¬serving surgery versus mastectomy: overall and rela¬tive survival-a population based study by the Danish breast cancer cooperative group（DBCG）. Acta Oncol. 2018,57(1):19–25. https://doi.org/10.1080/0284186X.2017.1403042. Epub 2017 Nov 23

4. Fisher B, Jeong J-H, Anderson S, Bryant J, Fisher ER, Wolmark N. Twenty-five-year follow-up of a random¬ized trial comparing radical mastectomy,

total mastec¬tomy, and total mastectomy followed by irradiation. N Engl J Med. 2002,347:567–75.

5. Fisher B, Bauer M, Margolese R, et al. Five-year results of a randomized clinical trial comparing total mastectomy and segmental mastectomy with or with¬out radiation in the treatment of breast cancer. N Engl J Med. 1985,312:665–73.

6. Early Breast Cancer Trialists' Collaborative Group. Effects of radiotherapy and surgery in early breast cancer: an overview of the randomized trials. N Engl J Med. 1995,333:1444–55.［Erratum, N Engl J Med 1996,334:1003.］

7. Veronesi U, Saccozzi R, Del Vecchio M, et al. Com¬paring radical mastectomy with quadrantectomy, axillary dissection, and radiotherapy in patients with small cancers of the breast. N Engl J Med. 1981,305:6–11.

8. NIH Consensus Conference. Treatment of early-stage breast cancer. JAMA. 1991,265:391–5.

9. Van Maaren MC, de Munck L, de Bock GH, Jobsen JJ, van Dalen T, Linn SC, Poortmans P, Strobbe LJA, Siesling S. 10 year survival after breast-conserving surgery plus radiotherapy compared with mastectomy in early breast cancer in The Netherlands: a population-based study. Lancet Oncol. 2016,17（8）:1158–70.

10. Pesce CE, Liederbach E, Czechura T, Winchester DJ, Yao K. Changing surgical trends in young patients with early stage breast cancer, 2003 to 2010: a report from the National Cancer Data Base. J Am Coll Surg. 2014,219（1）:19–28. https://doi.org/10.1016/j.jam-coll-surg.2014.03.043. Epub 2014 Apr 1

11. Sinnadurai S, Kwong A, Hartman M, Tan EY, Bhoo-Pathy NT, Dahlui M, See MH, Yip CH, Taib NA, Bhoo-Pathy N. Breast-conserving surgery versus mastectomy in young women with breast cancer in Asian settings. BJS Open. 2018,3（1）:48–55. https://doi.org/10.1002/bjs5.50111. PMID: 30734015; PMCID: PMC6354186

12. Mahmood U, Hanlon AL, Koshy M, Buras R, Chum¬sri S, Tkaczuk KH, Cheston SB, Regine WF, Feigen¬berg SJ. Increasing national mastectomy rates for the treatment of early stage breast cancer. Ann Surg Oncol. 2013:20（5）:1436–43. https://doi.org/10.1245/s10434–012–2732–5.Epub 2012 Nov 8

13. Yang B, Ren G, Song E, Pan D, Zhang J, Wang YLiao N, Tang J, Wang X, Cui S, Jin F, Geng C, SunO, Li H, Fan Z,Cao X, Wang H, Wang S, Shao ZWu J. Current status and factors influencing surgical options for breast cancer in China: a nationwidecross-sectional survey of 110 hospitals. Oncologist. 2020,25（10）:e1473–80. https://doi.org/10.1634theoncologist.2020–0001. Epub 2020 May 13.PMID:32333626:PMCID: PMC7543333

14. Kummerow KL, Du L, Penson DF, Shyr Y, Hooks14.MA. Nationwide trends in mastectomy for early-stagebreast cancer. JAMA Surg. 2015:150:9–16.

15. 15.Lagendijk M,van Maaren MC,Saadatmand SStrobbe LJA, Poortmans PMP, Koppert LB, TilanusLinthorst MMA, Siesling S. Breast conserving therapy and mastectomy revisited: breast cancer-specifdsurvival and the infuence of prognostic factors in129,692 patients. Int] Cancer. 2018,142（1）:165–75https://doi.org/10.1002/ijc.31034. Epub 2017 Sep

16. Garcia-Etienne CA, Tomatis M, Heil J, Danaei M6.Rageth CI, Marotti L, Rosselli Del Turco M, PontiA.Fluctuating mastectomy rates across time andgeography. Ann Surg Oncol. 2013:20（7）:2114–6https://doi.org/10.1245/s10434–013–2982-x.

17. Albornoz CR, Matros E, Lee CN, et al. Bilateral mastectomy versus breast-conserving surgery for early-stage breast cancer: the role of breast reconstruction. Plast Reconstr Surg. 2015,135:1518–26.

18. EBCTCG（Early Breast Cancer Trialists' Collaborative Group）, McGale P, Taylor C, Correa C, Cutter D, Duane F, Ewertz M, Gray R, Mannu G, Peto R, Whelan T, Wang Y, Wang Z, Darby S. Effect of radiotherapy after mastectomy and ax-

illary surgery on 10-year recurrence and 20-year breast cancer mortality: meta-analysis of individual patient data for 8135 women in 22 randomized trials. Lancet. 2014,383（9935）:2127–35. https://doi.org/10.1016/S0140-6736（14）60488-8. Epub 2014 Mar 19. Erratum in: Lancet. 2014 Nov 22;384（9957）:1848. PMID: 24656685; PMCID: PMC5015598

19. Donker M, Slaets L, van Tienhoven G, Rutgers EJ. Okselklierdissectie versus okselbestraling bij borstkankerpatiënten met een positieve schildwachtklier: de EORTC 10981 AMAROS-studie [Axillary lymph node dissection versus axillary radiotherapy in patients with a positive sentinel node: the AMAROS trial]. Ned Tijdschr Geneeskd. 2015,159:A9302. Dutch

20. Bernstein-Molho R, Laitman Y, Galper S, Jacobson G, Boursi B, Gal-Yam EN, Kaufman B, Friedman E, Kaidar-Person O. Locoregional treatments and ipsilateral breast cancer recurrence rates in BRCA1/2 mutation carriers. Int J Radiat Oncol Biol Phys. 2021,109(5):1332–40. https://doi.org/10.1016/j.ijrobp.2020.11.058. Epub 2020 Nov 28

21. Kaidar-Person O, Vrou Offersen B, Hol S, Arenas M, Aristei C, Bourgier C, Cardoso MJ, Chua B, Coles CE, Engberg Damsgaard T, Gabrys D, Jagsi R, Jimenez R, Kirby AM, Kirkove C, Kirova Y, Kouloulias V, Marinko T, Meattini I, Mjaaland I, Nader Marta G, Witt Nystrom P, Senkus E, Skyttä T, Tvedskov TF, Verhoeven K, Poortmans P. ESTRO ACROP consensus guideline for target volume delineation in the setting of post mastectomy radiation therapy after implant-based immediate reconstruction for early stage breast cancer. Radiother Oncol. 2019,137:159–66. https://doi.org/10.1016/j.radonc.2019.04.010. Epub 2019 May 17

22. Ragaz J, Jackson SM, Le N, Plenderleith IH, Spinelli JJ, Basco VE, Wilson KS, Knowling MA, Coppin CM, Paradis M, Coldman AJ, Olivotto IA. Adjuvant radiotherapy and chemotherapy in node-positive premenopausal women with breast cancer. N Engl J Med. 1997,337（14）:956–62. https://doi.org/10.1056/NEJM199710023371402.

23. Overgaard M, Hansen PS, Overgaard J, Rose C, Andersson M, Bach F, Kjaer M, Gadeberg CC, Mouridsen HT, Jensen MB, Zedeler K. Postoperative radiotherapy in high-risk premenopausal women with breast cancer who receive adjuvant chemotherapy. Danish breast cancer cooperative group 82b trial. N Engl J Med. 1997,337（14）:949–55. https://doi.org/10.1056/NEJM199710023371401.

24. Poortmans PM, Weltens C, Fortpied C, Kirkove C, Peignaux-Casasnovas K, Budach V, van der Leij F, Vonk E, Weidner N, Rivera S, van Tienhoven G, Fourquet A, Noel G, Valli M, Guckenberger M, Koiter E, Racadot S, Abdah-Bortnyak R, Van Limbergen EF, Engelen A, De Brouwer P, Struikmans H, Bartelink H, European Organisation for Research and Treatment of Cancer Radiation Oncology and Breast Cancer Groups. Internal mammary and medial supraclavicular lymph node chain irradiation in stage I-III breast cancer （EORTC 22922/10925）: 15-year results of a randomized, phase 3 trial. Lancet Oncol. 2020,21（12）:1602–10. https://doi.org/10.1016/S1470-2045（20）30472-1. Epub 2020 Nov 2. Erratum in: Lancet Oncol. 2021 Jan;22（1）:e5

25. Thorsen LBJ, Overgaard J, Matthiessen LW, Berg M, Stenbygaard L, Pedersen AN, Nielsen MH, Overgaard M, Offersen BV, DBCG Radiotherapy Committee. Internal mammary node irradiation in patients with node-positive early breast cancer: fifteen-year results from the Danish breast cancer group internal mammary node study. J Clin Oncol. 2022,40（36）:4198–206. https://doi.org/10.1200/JCO.22.00044. Epub 2022 Apr 8

26. Cuzick J, Stewart H, Peto R, et al. Overview of randomized trials of postoperative adjuvant radiotherapy in breast cancer. Cancer Treat Rep. 1987,71（1）:15–29.

27. Henson KE, et al. Radiation-related mortality from heart disease and lung cancer more than 20 years after radiotherapy for breast cancer. Br J Cancer. 2013,108:179–82.

28. Darby SC. Risk of ischemic heart disease in women after radiotherapy for breast cancer. NEJM. 2013,368:987–98.

29. Abi Jaouadi J, de Azambuja E, Maki M, Tamim H, Thayil A, Geara F, Piccart M, Poortmans P, Zeidan YH. Post-mastectomy radiation therapy in human epidermal growth factor receptor 2 positive breast cancer patients: analysis of the HERA trial. Int J Radiat Oncol Biol Phys. 2020,106（3）:503–10. https://doi.org/10.1016/j.ijrobp.2019.10.022. Epub 2019 Oct 22

30. Mamounas EP, Bandos H, White JR, et al. NRG Oncology/NSABP B-51/RTOG 1304: Phase III trial to determine if chest wall and regional nodal radiotherapy（CWRNRT）post mastectomy（Mx）or the addition of RNRT to breast RT post breast-conserving surgery（BCS）reduces invasive breast cancer recurrence free interval（IBCRFI）in patients（pts）with positive axillary（PAx）nodes who are ypN0 after neoadjuvant chemotherapy（NC）. J Clin Oncol. 2019, 2019:37.

31. Zucali R. Early breast cancer: evaluation of the prognostic role of the site the primary tumor. J Clin Oncol. 1998,16:1363–6.

32. Giuliano AE, Ballman K, McCall L, Beitsch P, Whitworth PW, Blumencranz P, Leitch AM, Saha S, Morrow M, Hunt KK. Locoregional recurrence after sentinel lymph node dissection with or without axillary dissection in patients with sentinel lymph node metastases: long-term follow-up from the American College of Surgeons oncology group（Alliance）ACOSOG Z0011 randomized trial. Ann Surg. 2016,264（3）:413–20. https://doi.org/10.1097/SLA.0000000000001863. PMID: 27513155; PMCID: PMC5070540

33. Donker M, van Tienhoven G, Straver ME, Meijnen P, van de Velde CJ, Mansel RE, Cataliotti L, Westenberg AH, Klinkenbijl JH, Orzalesi L, Bouma WH, van der Mijle HC, Nieuwenhuijzen GA, Veltkamp SC, Slaets L, Duez NJ, de Graaf PW, van Dalen T, Marinelli A, Rijna H, Snoj M, Bundred NJ, Merkus JW, Belkacemi Y, Petignat P, Schinagl DA, Coens C, Messina CG, Bogaerts J, Rutgers EJ. Radiotherapy or surgery of the axilla after a positive sentinel node in breast cancer（EORTC 10981–22023 AMAROS）: a randomized, multicentre, open-label, phase 3 non-inferiority trial. Lancet Oncol. 2014,15（12）:1303–10. https://doi.org/10.1016/S1470-2045（14）70460-7. Epub 2014 Oct 15. PMID: 25439688; PMCID: PMC4291166

34. Morrow M, Van Zee KJ, Patil S, Petruolo O, Mamtani A, Barrio AV, Capko D, El-Tamer M, Gemignani ML, Heerdt AS, Kirstein L, Pilewskie M, Plitas G, Sacchini VS, Sclafani LM, Ho A, Cody HS. Axillary dissection and nodal irradiation can be avoided for Most node-positive Z0011-eligible breast cancers: a prospective validation study of 793 patients. Ann Surg. 2017,266（3）:457–62. https://doi.org/10.1097/SLA.0000000000002354. PMID: 28650355; PMCID: PMC5649371

35. Naoum GE. Single stage direct to implant breast reconstruction has lower complication rates than tissue expander and implant and comparable rates to autologous reconstruction in patients receiving post mastectomy radiation. Int J Radiat Oncol Biol Phys. 2020,106:514–24.

36. Albert A, et al. The impact of a post mastectomy chest wall scar boost on local recurrence-free survival in high-risk patients. Clin Breast Cancer. 2019,19（5）:363–9.

37. Marta GN, Coles C, Kaidar-Person O, Meattini I, Hijal T, Zissiadis Y, Pignol JP, Ramiah D, Ho AY, Cheng SH, Sancho G, Offersen BV, Poortmans P. The use of moderately hypofractionated post-operative radiation therapy for breast cancer in clinical practice: a critical review. Crit Rev Oncol Hematol. 2020,156:103090.

38. Haviland JS, Owen JR, Dewar JA, Agrawal

RK, Barrett J, Barrett-Lee PJ, Dobbs HJ, Hopwood P, Lawton PA, Magee BJ, Mills J, Simmons S, Sydenham MA, Venables K, Bliss JM, Yarnold JR. The UK standardization of breast radiotherapy（START）trials of radiotherapy hypofractionation for treatment of early breast cancer: 10-year follow-up results of two randomized controlled trials. Lancet Oncol. 2013,14（11）:1086–94.

39. Chen JS. Influence of radiation dose to reconstructive breast following mastectomy and complication in breast cancer patients undergoing 2 stage prosthetic breast reconstruction. Front Oncol. 2019,9:243.

40. Offersen B, Nielsen HM, Jacobsen EH, et al. Hypovs normofractionated radiation of early breast cancer in the randomized DBCG HYPO trial. Radiother Oncol. 2018,127:S312.

41. Wang SL, Fang H, Song YW, et al. Hypofractionated versus conventional fractionated post mastectomy radiotherapy for patients with high-risk breast cancer: a randomized, non-inferiority, open-label, phase 3 trial. Lancet Oncol. 2019,20:352–60.

42. Snyderman RK, Guthrie RH. Reconstruction of the female breast following radical mastectomy. Plast Reconstr Surg. 1971 Jun;47（6）:565–7. https://doi.org/10.1097/00006534–197106000–00008.

43. Wagner RD, Braun TL, Zhu H, Winocour S. A systematic review of complications in prepectoral breast reconstruction. J Plast Reconstr Aesthet Surg. 2019,72（7）:1051–9.

44. Bernini M. Subcutaneous direct-to-implant breast reconstruction: surgical, functional, and aesthetic results after long-term follow-up. Plast Reconstr Surg Glob Open. 2016,3（12）:e574.

45. Nahabedian MY, Cocilovo C. Two-stage prosthetic breast reconstruction: a comparison between prepectoral and partial subpectoral techniques, plastic and reconstructive surgery. Plast Reconstr Surg. 2017,140（6S）:22S–30S.

46. Walia GS, Aston J, Bello R, et al. Prepectoral versus subpectoral tissue expander placement: a clinical and quality of life outcomes study. Plast Reconstr Surg Glob Open. 2018,6（4）:e1731.

47. Sigalove S. Prepectoral implant-based breast reconstruction and post mastectomy radiotherapy: short-term outcomes. Plast Reconstr Surg Glob Open. 2017:1–7.

48. Sbitany H, Gomez-Sanchez C, Piper M, Lentz R. Prepectoral breast reconstruction in the setting of post mastectomy radiation therapy: an assessment of clinical outcomes and benefits. Plast Reconstr Surg. 2019,143（1）:10–20.

49. Sigalove S, Maxwell GP, Sigalove NM, et al. Prepectoral implant-based breast reconstruction and postmastectomy radiotherapy: short-term outcomes. Plast Reconstr Surg Glob Open. 2017,5(12):e1631.

50. Sinnott CJ, Persing SM, Pronovost M, Hodyl C, McConnell D, Ott YA. Impact of postmastectomy radiation therapy in prepectoral versus subpectoral implant-based breast reconstruction. Ann Surg Oncol. 2018,25(10):2899–908.

51. Kaidar-Person O, Vrou Offersen B, Hol S, et al. ESTRO ACROP consensus guideline for target volume delineation in the setting of postmastectomy radiation therapy after implant-based immediate reconstruction for early stage breast cancer. Radiother Oncol. 2019,137:159–66.

52. Becker H, et al. Immediate prepectoral breast reconstruction in suboptimal patients using an air-filled spacer. Plast Reconstr Surg Glob Open. 2019,7:e2470.

53. Becker H, et al. Tissue contraction---a new paradigm in breast reconstruction. Plast Reconstr Surg Glob Open. 2018,6:e1865.

54. Sigalove S, Maxwell GP, Sigalove NM, et al. Prepectoral implant-based breast reconstruction: rationale, indications, and preliminary results. Plast Reconstr Surg. 2017,139:287–94.

55. Ascherman JA, Zeidler K, Morrison KA, et al. Carbon dioxide-based versus saline tissue expansion for breast reconstruction: results of the XPAND prospective, randomized clinical trial.

Plast Reconstr Surg. 2016,138(6):1161–70.
56. Moni J, Saleeby J, Bannon E, Lo Y-C, Fitzgerald TJ. Dosimetric impact of the AeroForm tissue expander in postmastectomy radiation therapy: an ex vivo analysis. Pract Radiat Oncol. 2015,5(1):e1–8.
57. Ho AY, Hu ZI, Mehrara BJ, Wilkins EG. Radiotherapy in the setting of breast reconstruction: types, techniques, and timing. Lancet Oncol. 2017,18(12):e742–53. https://doi.org/10.1016/S1470-2045(17)30617-4.
58. Santosa KB. Postmastectomy radiation therapy and two-stage implant-based breast reconstruction: is there a better time to irradiate? Plast Reconstr Surg. 2016,138:761–9.
59. Adesiyun TA, Lee BT, Yueh JH, et al. Impact of sequencing of postmastectomy radiotherapy and breast reconstruction on timing and rate of complications and patient satisfaction. Int J Radiat Oncol Biol Phys. 2011,80(2):392–7.
60. Naoum GE. The impact of chest wall boost on reconstruction complications and local control in patients treated for breast cancer. Int J Radiat Oncol Biol Phys. 2019,105:155–64.
61. Manyam M, et al. Comparing 10 year outcomes in radiated patients with breast autologous reconstruction or tissue expander/implant based reconstruction. Int J Radiat Oncol Biol Phys. 2018,102:S45.
62. Negenborn VL. Quality of life and patient satisfaction after one-stage implant-based breast reconstruction with an acellular dermal matrix versus two-stage breast reconstruction (BRIOS): primary outcome of a randomized, controlled trial. Lancet. 2018,19:1205–14.
63. Dikmans REG, et al. Two-stage implant-based breast reconstruction compared with immediate one-stage implant-based breast reconstruction augmented with an acellular dermal matrix: an open-label, phase 4, multicentre, randomized, controlled trial. Lancet Oncol. 2017,18:251–8.
64. Schrenk P, et al. The use of sentinel node biopsy in breast cancer patients undergoing skin sparing mastectomy and immediate autologous reconstruction. Plast Reconstr Surg. 2005,116(5):1278.

20 预期放疗时的胸肌前重建方案

编者：Yoav Gronovich, Merav Ben-David, Michael Scheflan

译者：张思浩　张　梅

20.1 引言

假体重建是最常见的乳房重建形式。随着技术的进步和对各种乳腺肿瘤病理生理学机制认识的深入，需要将放疗纳入乳腺癌整体治疗方案的患者数量有所增加。许多情况下，放疗紧随乳腺肿瘤切除术之后进行，并为复发性癌症的乳房切除术和后续重建留下空间。而在其他许多情况下，辅助放疗在乳房切除即刻假体置入式乳房重建后进行。过去通常避免在受照射组织或未来可能接受放疗的患者中进行假体重建。随着重建技术的进步，包括脱细胞真皮基质（ADM）的应用、胸肌前假体置入和自体脂肪移植（AFT），目前已能在不增加并发症风险的前提下拓宽假体置入式乳房重建的适应证。尽管在受照射组织中进行假体置入式重建的并发症发生率较高，并且部分患者重建效果欠佳或较差，但在乳房切除术后放疗或既往有乳腺肿瘤切除术后放疗史的情况下，假体置入式乳房重建仍是最常见的选择。

20.2 放疗（XRT）

20.2.1 必要性

放疗被视为多种肿瘤综合治疗的重要组成部分。对于乳腺癌，放疗已被证实对浸润性导管癌、小叶癌、导管原位癌（DCIS）及其他亚型具有显著疗效。对淋巴结阳性的乳腺癌患者而言，乳房切除术后放疗可降低复发风险并提高总体生存率[1]。

乳房切除术后放疗（PMRT）的适应证正在逐步扩展。美国放射学会目前建议

放疗用于直径 > 5cm 的肿瘤或 > 4 枚淋巴结转移的患者。然而，鉴于 PMRT 在预防局部复发方面的获益[2-4]，其通常的应用范围更为宽泛。尤其当采纳美国国立综合癌症网络的推荐意见——将乳房切除术后放疗的适应证范围扩展至肿瘤直径为 5cm 或更小，或存在 1~3 枚阳性淋巴结的患者时[5]，这一趋势更为明显。由于乳房切除术后放疗的适应证已从局部进展期扩展至中早期，因此接受即刻乳房重建后行术后放疗的患者比例持续增高[6-10]。需要指出的是，不同医疗机构的放疗方案存在显著差异，主要体现在分次数、单次剂量及总照射剂量等方面，导致机构间的横向比较变得复杂，因为放射效应的生物学影响呈现高度剂量/方案依赖性[11]。

20.2.2 放疗技术的进步

与过去数十年相比，目前对乳房切除术后放疗相关不良事件的担忧有所减轻，这是由于放疗技术的进步提高了治疗的耐受性[12]。文献数据强有力地佐证了疗效改善与放疗技术更新的因果关系。近年来放疗实践的演变，主要体现在认识到分割剂量、分割次数、总剂量及总治疗时间对肿瘤与正常组织反应的重要性，以及保乳疗法的引入[13]。不同医疗机构采用的乳房放疗方案及剂量存在显著差异，甚至在常规放疗方案中因肿瘤特性及已实施的新辅助治疗不同，放疗时机的选择也存在差异[14]。放射肿瘤学持续发展的方向包括：开展临床试验，采用更为精准的照射技术替代单纯全乳照射等[15]。为简化乳房切除术后放疗（PMRT）背景下的重建流程，许多机构遵循标准化操作流程[16-19]。

20.2.3 组织损伤的分类

明确影响放射性损伤风险的内在（细胞）放射敏感性差异及外部因素至关重要，目前尚不明确是细胞固有放射敏感性还是外部因素在损伤表现的个体差异性中起主导作用[20-23]。现有研究显示，在良好控制条件下，已知影响正常组织反应的因素仅能解释 30% 的乳腺癌患者个体差异，进而推测大部分并发症严重程度的差异源于遗传或表观遗传机制决定的细胞放射敏感性差异[20,23]。阐明放射敏感性差异的成因，对肿瘤治疗具有重要指导价值。特定遗传综合征中细胞/组织放射敏感性增强的报道[24]，以及同一个体不同型正常细胞类放射敏感性相关的证据[25]，均提示此类差异性可能存在遗传学基础。这些证据亦证实细胞放射敏感性与组织反应密切相关。当前放射生物学研究聚焦于：识别具有放射性敏感异常（放疗急性及晚期不良反应高危）的患者[26,27]，以及探索可增强放疗抗瘤效应的分子标志物[28]。放射暴露可导致皮肤及皮下组织纤维化、弹性组织变性及血管内膜增厚。放疗诱导的组织损伤可分为急性或早期损伤慢性或晚期损伤[29]。急性损伤包括红斑、水肿、脱屑、色素沉着及溃疡[30]，严重程度从轻度到重度不等。如红斑、脱屑等早期效应通常于放疗期间或放疗完成后即刻显现。急性Ⅰ级放射性皮炎可见于多达 85% 的接受放疗的乳腺癌患者[30]。慢性损伤包括皮肤萎缩、干燥、毛细血管扩张、色素异常及肤色改变[31]。在乳房区域，可致皮肤和皮下组织的慢性纤维化[11]。射线所致慢性改变的全部表现可能需要数月乃至数年方能完全显现[32]。放射性后遗症的病程遵循独特的临床模式。接受照射的患者的皮肤可在暴露数小时内出现红斑样皮疹，并可持续或缓慢加重直至放疗结束。此种情况具有一过性特征。严重且罕见病例中可出现表皮下水疱和溃疡。多数损伤在末次放疗后10~20天内愈合。晚期损伤通常呈现进行性加重且多不可逆转[33]。周围组织的损伤可依据严重程度进行分级，不仅包括皮肤表观，还包括以放疗肿瘤学组/欧洲癌症研究与治疗组织提出的绝对不良反应量表制定的评分体系进行评估的表皮下组织弹性及柔韧性[22]，或参照Burnet等提出的替代分级系统[34]。对于接受假体重建的患者，放疗可导致瘢痕增生、包膜挛缩、感染及皮肤坏死风险增高、切口延迟愈合以及疼痛[35-39]。自体组织移植重建术在经历放射暴露时亦会面临放疗相关性并发症，包括皮瓣萎缩挛缩、纤维化及脂肪坏死等[35, 40, 41]。然而，从患者角度分析，研究显示放疗对接受假体重建者的满意度有负面影响，但对自体组织移植者无此效应[42, 43]。放射暴露与重建失败风险的显著上升有关，增幅可高达未放疗者的3倍[44]。目前整形外科与放射肿瘤学领域的协作研究，将深化对放疗如何影响重建后转归的理解[45]。

20.2.4　重建前放疗

尽管不同机构报告的发病率差异较大，但既往放疗显著增加即刻或延期假体重建失败及并发症风险。汇总分析显示重建失败发生率约为14%[11]。应用背阔肌联合假体可显著降低既往放射野的重建失败发生率（风险降低72%）[46]。曾接受放疗且需重建的患者大致可分为两类：需行乳房切除并行即刻乳房重建的保乳治疗失败患者，或乳房切除后接受辅助放疗的延期重建患者[11]。关于既往保乳治疗联合放疗对后续重建影响的评估性研究较少。研究表明，自体组织重建术后患者满意度稳定且并发症发生率低，但也有研究指出即刻假体乳房重建术前存在乳腺放疗史者较未行放疗者更易出现严重并发症及失败事件[47]，此发现与假体重建受照乳腺的其他研究结果一致[35-39]。针对曾行放疗者开展保留乳头的乳房切除即刻重建的研究表明，与未行放疗者相比，其并发症发生率更高，但多数重建仍获成功[48]。关于即刻假体重建术前放疗与乳房切除术后放疗的并发症发生率的系列对比研究显示，两者无显著差异，但保乳治疗后行乳房切除重建者的并发症发生率呈下降趋势。采用保留皮肤乳房切除即刻组织扩张器或假体重建的研究提示，两组在放疗后重建失败率方面无显著差异[49, 50]。关于患者满意度和报告的结局指标的研究结果存在不一致。部分研究报道放疗会对乳房重建患者报告的结局产生负面影响[42, 51, 52]，亦有研究表明完成保乳治疗联合放疗与未放疗者在即刻假体重建术后 2 年患者报告结局无显著差异[50]。相反，与有保乳治疗史或无放疗史者相比，乳房切除假体重建放疗的患者报告的结局更差[50]。

放疗技术的改进以及脱细胞真皮基质、自体脂肪移植（AFT）技术的进步，改变了传统延迟乳房重建的模式，使得对于已接受放疗者亦可实施包含Ⅰ期组织扩张器置入的两阶段重建或直接假体重建。自体脂肪移植可于假体置入前作为改善组织质量的预备阶段实施，或如第一作者（Y.G.）所描述的那样[53]（图 20.1），作为同期联合手术的辅助手段。Ⅱ期假体置入后采用自体脂肪移植完成重建，亦是改善组织质量、矫正畸形及补充体积的常用选择。笔者推荐对既往接受放疗者应用脱细胞真皮基质实施胸肌前假体置入式乳房重建。根据作者经验，放疗所致组织损伤程度（色素沉着、硬化、毛细血管扩张及萎缩）是拟定乳房重建方案的核心依据。若组织顺应性良好、柔软且富弹性，同时且皮肤损伤征象轻微（见于大多数病例），则实施胸肌前乳房重建是安全的。

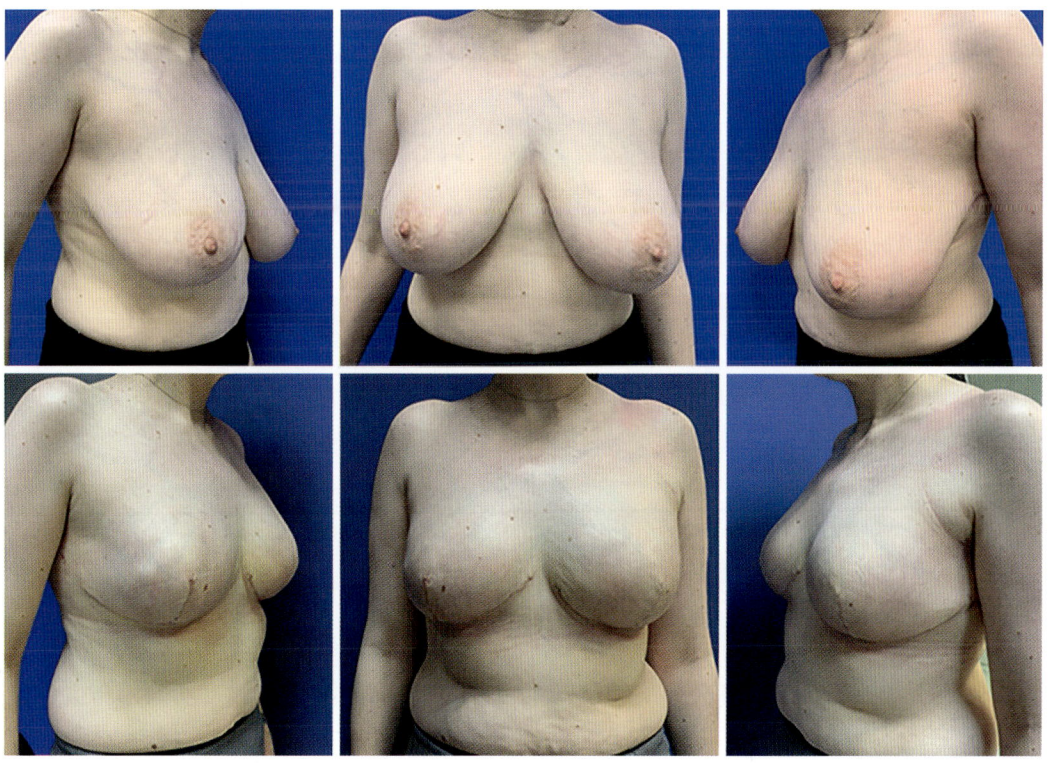

图 20.1　重建前（上）与 SSM（Wise 术）和即刻胸肌前假体重建（使用 Mentor CPG 322 475mL 假体及 8cm×16cm 加 6cm×12cm；Alloderm 真皮基质，联合每侧乳房 60mL 自体脂肪移植）术后 12 个月（下）

20.3 重建前放疗条件下的胸肌前重建

20.3.1 适应证分析

胸肌前重建术近年迅速流行，主要归因于其操作简单、非劣效性以及患者与术者的满意度高。根据笔者经验，无论采取何种胸肌前重建术式，均建议采用脱细胞真皮基质（ADM）至少覆盖假体前表面。胸肌前重建可缩短手术时间，促进患者康复，减少麻醉药物需求，美学效果与部分肌下重建相当。该术式禁忌证包括：乳腺肿瘤距胸大肌≤5mm，BMI＞30、吸烟、糖化血红蛋白水平＞7.5的糖尿病或免疫抑制状态。通过临床评估或先进技术检测手段证实乳房切除存在明显灌注不良时亦不宜采用。尽管较厚的皮下脂肪层是必要因素，但灌注质量比脂肪厚度更重要。即使皮下脂肪厚度仅0.5cm的菲薄皮瓣，只要外观健康、血供良好且无创伤，仍可行胸肌前即刻重建。对于皮下脂肪层极薄者，建议采用两阶段组织扩张器策略而非直接假体置入方案。

20.3.2 胸肌前重建的优势

首先，采用胸肌前重建时，胸肌后重建潜在的美学缺陷，如双囊畸形、动态畸形或假体上移等问题均可消除。对于不愿接受对侧乳房悬吊术的乳房下垂患者，胸肌前重建可获得胸肌后重建难以实现的良好对称形态（图20.2）。

建议要求延期重建的放疗患者于放疗结束后等待4~6个月，使炎症消退。此类患者在放疗完成后2个月内的炎症期可行脂肪移植，以减轻纤维化阶段瘢痕形成。组织质量参数包括肤色、捏持感、弹性与厚度，会影响最终重建时机与术式的选择。若组织存在色素沉着、硬化、毛细血管扩张及萎缩等临床损伤征象，推荐行自体组织重建；或可在置入组织扩张器（TE）或假体前，开展自体脂肪移植（AFT）预备性独立阶段。第一作者（Y.G.）建议术前使用外部扩张装置（BRAVA；图20.3）。经数次BRAVA联合AFT治疗且组织质量改善后，可视患者意愿完成胸肌前假体重建。

若其他患者放疗后组织质量尚可且满足重建条件，则可在组织扩张器与永久假体间进行选择。对胸部脂肪层较薄者，建议采用两阶段方案：于胸肌前置入组织扩张器并以ADM覆盖，第二阶段置换为永久假体（图20.4）。对于软组织松弛、延展性佳者（较罕见），初次手术即可采用永久假体完成乳房重建（DTI）。第三作者（M.S.）主张对所有曾接受放疗的延期重建患者，无论组织状态如何，均应在置入扩张器或永久假体前3~4个月行自体脂肪移植。

作者处理方法总结详见下方流程图。

对于既往接受过肿瘤切除术与放疗且面临同侧乳腺癌复发者，须在行乳房切除术前评估确认是否适合进行假体重建，应特别关注如吸烟、肥胖、乳房巨大且下垂、皮纹、皮肤菲薄及皮下脂肪层过厚等危险因素。对重建条件欠佳者，应建议减少危

20 预期放疗时的胸肌前重建方案

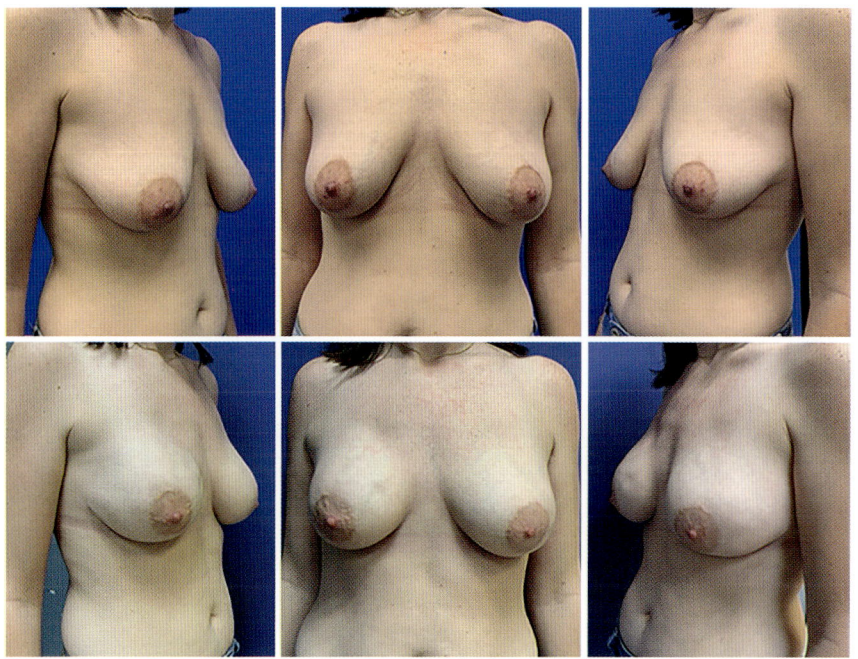

图 20.2 双侧乳房重建前（上图），行保留乳头 – 乳晕乳房切除（IMF 切口）胸肌前直接假体置入术（使用 Mentor CPG323 型 390mL 假体）及异体真皮基质补片（8cm×16 cm 加 6cm×12 cm；Alloderm）即刻重建术后 3 个月（下图）

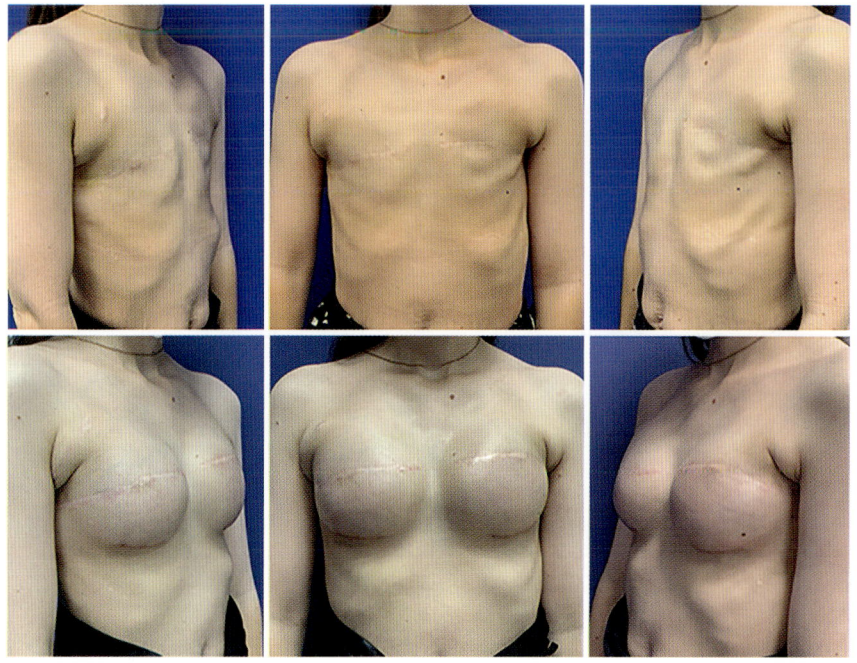

图 20.3 双侧乳房切除术后及左侧乳房切除术后放疗（6 年）（上图），与胸肌前扩张器（Mentor CPX4 型 250mL 扩张器）联合异体真皮基质补片（8cm×16 cm 加 6cm×12 cm；Alloderm）重建术后 3 个月（IMF 切口）（下图）

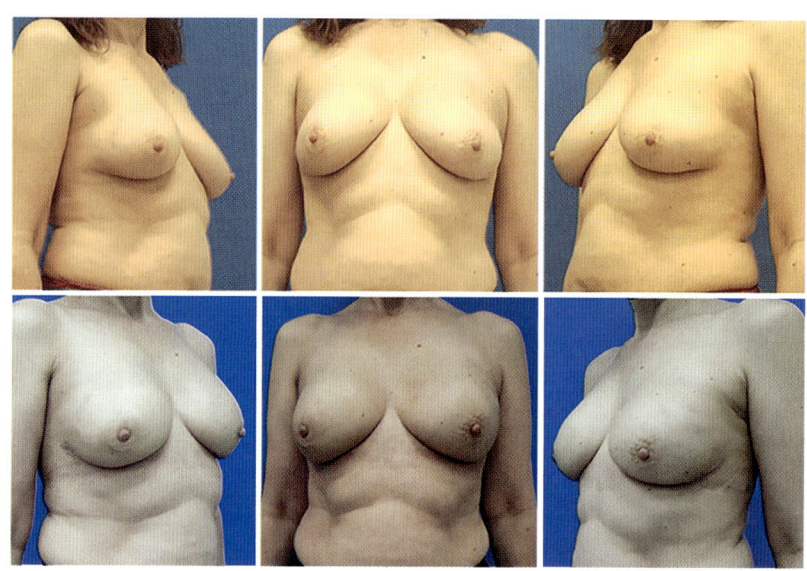

图 20.4 双侧乳房肿瘤切除术及放疗后（3 年）（上图），保留乳头-乳晕乳房切除（IMF 切口）胸肌前直接假体置入（Mentor CPG321 型 280mL 假体）及异体真皮基质补片（8cm×16 cm 加 6cm×12 cm；Alloderm）即刻重建术后 6 个月（下图）

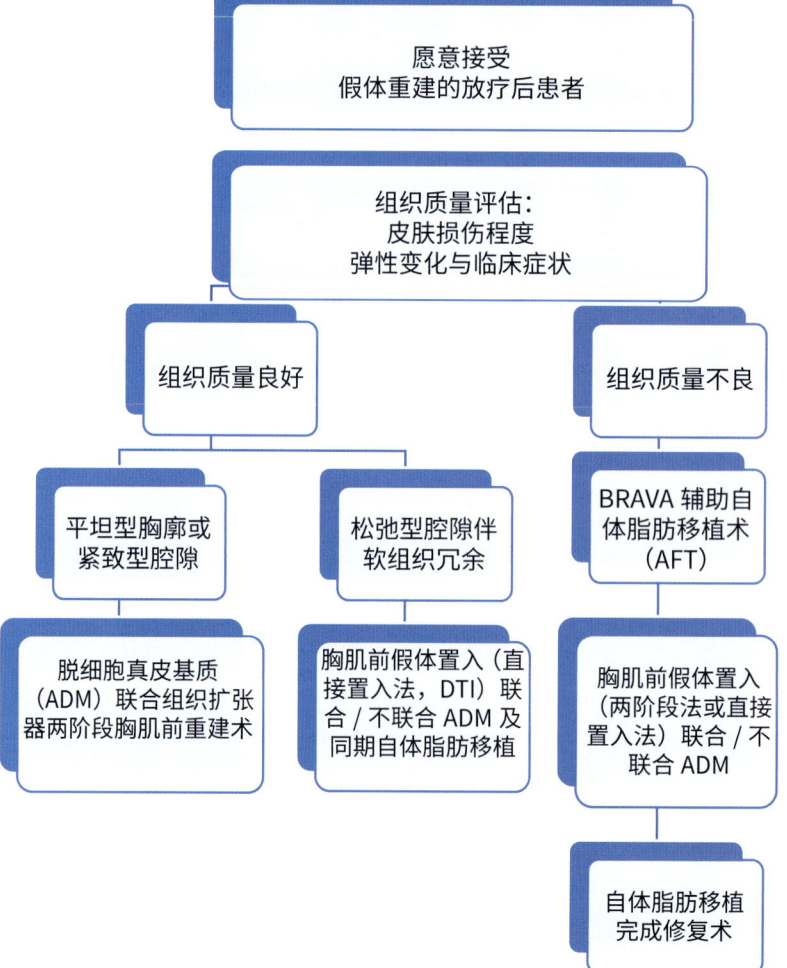

险因素或考虑行自体组织重建。对于无明显放射损伤临床证据者，需待乳房切除术完成后进一步评估。优良的重建始于规范的乳房切除术（避免组织损伤，确保皮瓣血运充分）。皮瓣质量应通过临床评估或专用仪器检测。若皮瓣条件不良，建议终止即刻胸肌前重建转为延迟Ⅰ期或两阶段胸肌后重建术式；若评估皮瓣质量良好，则推荐胸肌前重建，根据术者操作习惯及患者对乳房容积的诉求，选择直接假体重建（DTI）或两阶段术式（图20.5）。

作者处理策略的总结详见下方流程图。

20.3.3 重建术后放疗

进行乳房重建时，需考虑约35%患者可能接受过乳房切除术后放疗（PMRT）。在部分病例中，PMRT的明确适应证需待淋巴结及乳房标本的永久病理学报告出具后方可确定。即刻假体重建术后放疗可分为两个时间节点——组织扩张器置入后、永久假体置换前，或完成最终假体置换术后。荟萃分析和最新前瞻性研究显示不同治疗时机的疗效无显著差异，但仍存在多项相互矛盾的研究结论[11]。尽管术后放疗会使假体丢失风险超过单纯辅助化疗的2倍，但对于多数患者，与费用更高且需延期进行的皮瓣重建相比，假体乳房重建仍为可行选择[54]。

20.3.4 对组织的影响

放疗也会对组织造成损伤。射线可导致从皮肤至骨的所有被覆软组织损伤：皮肤可能发生轻度至中度皮炎，表现为色素沉着改变，少数情况下会因胶原纤维损伤导致组织硬化及弹性受限；肌肉组织可出现纤维化而引发纤维挛缩及活动受限；骨组织（肋骨）也会因成骨细胞功能受损发生损伤，但罕有临床表现。当假体位于照射区域内时，其周围包膜同样会受到辐射损伤，促进包膜挛缩的发生。基于以上原因，乳房切除术后放疗（PMRT）已被证

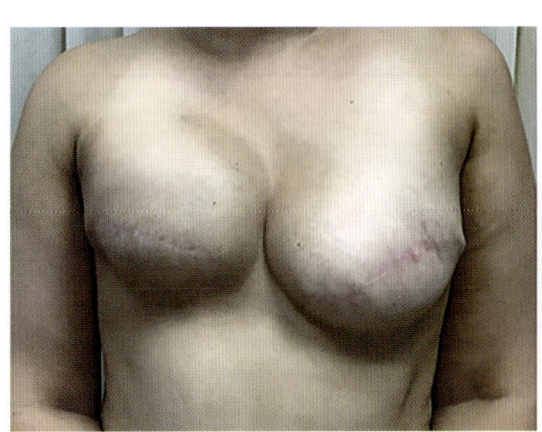 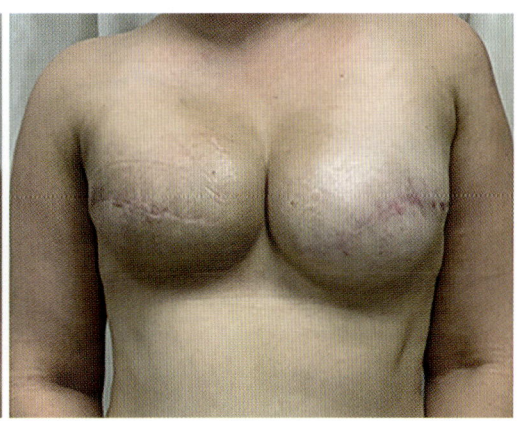

图20.5 （左）胸肌后假体重建术后放疗，使用Allergan 410MF 420g假体及8cm×16cm Alloderm脱细胞真皮基质；（右）更换为胸肌前假体术后放疗

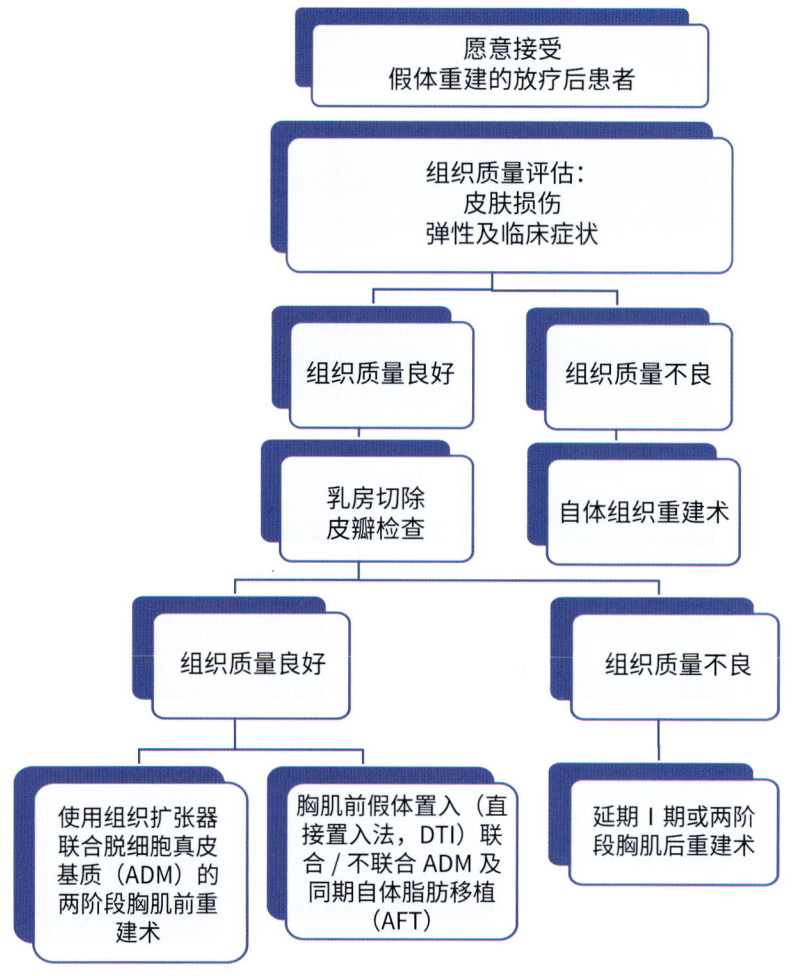

实会增加假体重建术的并发症发生率，因此许多医生对计划行 PMRT 的患者调整了原定术式决策，避免行直接即刻假体重建（DTI）。他们会根据患者情况选择 II 期重建方式——即在放疗期间暂停扩张器注水，并于放疗结束经评估后继续后续治疗；或直接选择自体组织重建术式。根据笔者经验，针对计划行 PMRT 的患者，胸肌前直接假体重建是具有短期恢复快、长期效果稳定等优点的安全替代方案；而从肿瘤学角度来看，此方式使得放疗与手术的时间间隔较短（通常为 6 周），可避免治疗延迟。

20.3.5 预期重建术后放疗下的胸肌前重建术

根据笔者经验，对于接受放疗的患者来说，胸肌后重建的主要缺陷有：

1. 照射导致胸大肌纤维化，引发假体向侧上方移位。
2. 放射损伤及所致的包膜挛缩。

胸肌后假体置入可导致欠美观的动

态畸形及肌肉痉挛。上述缺陷与并发症在胸肌前重建中均被最小化。若初始选择胸肌后术式，现有研究表明将假体改为胸肌前置入后上述缺陷均获得改善[55-57]，此亦为本研究团队的临床实践方案（图20.6）。

胸肌前假体乳房重建术放疗后的远期效果已获评估。该术式的优势包括外观自然、手术时间短、术后疼痛轻及非劣效的美学效果，均与将胸大肌保留于解剖位置直接相关[58]。胸肌前乳房重建术可消除动态畸形并具有较高的患者满意度[59-61]。关于胸肌后与胸肌前扩张器置入的对比研究显示，后者可减轻疼痛及包膜挛缩程度，提升扩张效率并改善美学效果[62,63]。目前，关于胸肌前假体、假体周围包膜及胸肌受照射影响的数据仍有限[62,63]。尽管多数研究表明胸肌前假体重建术后即使接受 PMRT 仍能维持稳定的美学效果，但与未放疗乳房相比，其总体并发症发生率略高（差异无统计学意义），最显著的差异为放疗乳房的手术部位感染率较高[58]。无论是否行放疗，应用 ADM 均有助于降低包膜挛缩发生率，作用包括支撑假体以减轻假体造成的软组织负荷增加，通过真皮层整合增厚强化皮肤屏障；与全肌下重

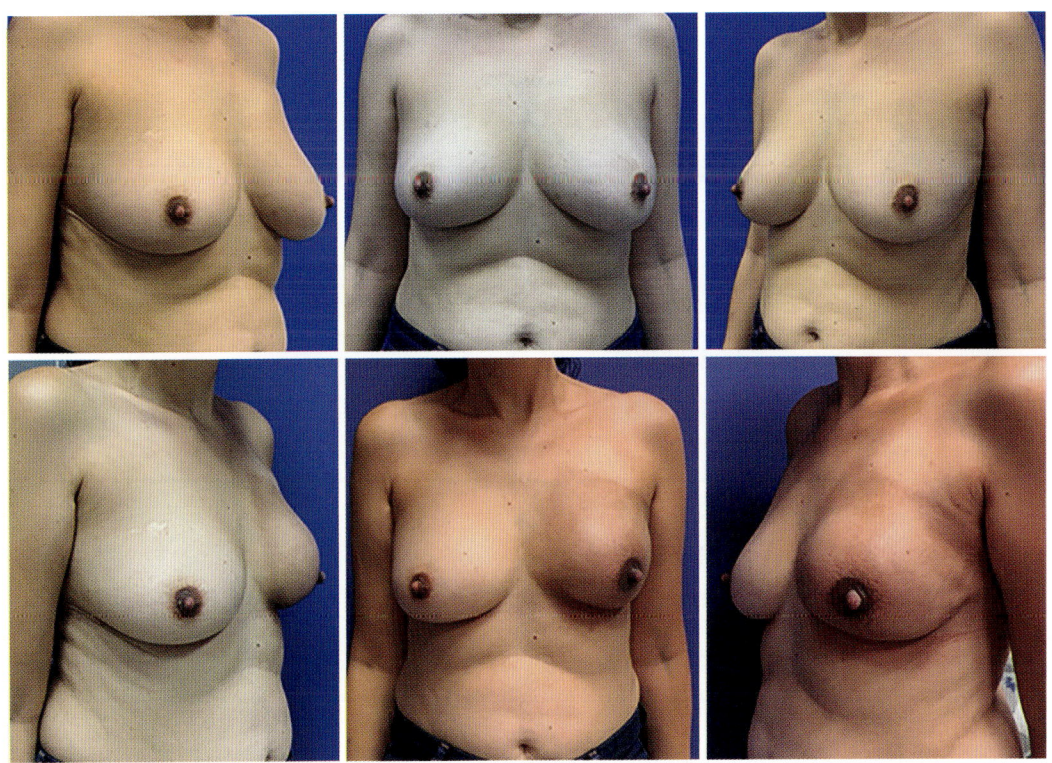

图 20.6　左乳重建术前（上图）及保留乳头 - 乳晕乳房切除（乳房下皱襞切口）术后 6 个月行胸肌前假体重建术（DTI）：置入 Mentor 光滑圆形中高凸度 400mL 假体，联合应用 Alloderm 8cm×16cm 及 6cm×12cm 补片并行 80mL 自体脂肪移植（AFT）；左乳术后放疗（PMRT）后 3 个月并行 120mL 自体脂肪移植（下图）

建术相比，具有降低假体外露及包膜化风险的效应[64-66]。此外，ADM 可作为吸收部分射线的屏障，从而减轻包膜、假体及深层组织的损伤。研究证实，经射线处理的 ADM、未经射线处理的 ADM 及自然包膜具有相似的血管密度；但与放疗后的自然包膜相比，经射线处理的 ADM 可减轻假体周围炎性反应及非血管性 α-平滑肌肌动蛋白表达[67]。最新研究表明，胸肌前重建对于拟行乳房切除术后放疗的患者是有效术式，其并发症发生率与全肌下及双平面假体重建术后放疗者相当[51]。目前，尚无法确认包裹补片的效果是否优于仅覆盖假体前方的补片。

20.3.6 两阶段重建与 I 期重建

研究证实，在行乳房切除术后放疗的情况下，采用组织扩张器的两阶段重建术式比置入永久假体后放疗更易引发重建失败。潜在原因可能与放疗引起的微血管或细胞水平的结构及超结构改变相关，包括成纤维细胞及成纤维干细胞的损伤，此时重复手术步骤可能加剧局部损伤[12]。基于上述原因，笔者建议对于需行乳房切除术后放疗（PMRT）且乳房切除皮瓣条件适宜的患者，优选胸肌前直接假体重建术（DTI）。多数放疗乳房的修复效果可通过后期脂肪移植得到显著改善。对于接受乳房切除术后放疗的胸肌前假体重建患者，脂肪移植可减轻放射诱导的纤维化效应，软化并增厚软组织覆盖层及乳房切除皮瓣[66]。因此，笔者建议在完成术后放疗后的两阶段假体置换术之前或术中同期实施脂肪移植。尽管接受放疗的胸肌前重建患者因皮肤受照射会出现收紧效应而不存在放疗后相同程度的假体皱褶风险，但脂肪移植对于改善皮肤厚度、柔软度及延展性仍具同等重要性[54]。笔者推荐方案见下方流程图。

20.4 小结

假体重建是目前最常见的乳房重建方式。尽管既往在预期术后行放疗时存在争议，但随着放疗技术的升级及 ADM 与脂肪移植技术的应用，胸肌前 I 期/ II 期假体重建手术已成为放疗背景下安全的重建方案。对既往接受过放疗但要求重建的患者，需通过详细评估组织放射性损伤的临床表现来判断可否行假体重建。在脂肪移植的背景下，即使组织受放疗损伤的患者也可通过先行脂肪移植对组织进行修复，再置入假体或组织扩张器实现重建。

20.5 最新文献回顾与诊疗要点

20.5.1 诊疗要点

对重建前已行放疗（XRT）的患者：
- 若组织受损：推荐自体组织重建。意向接受自体脂肪移植重建的患者，术前需使用外部扩张装置进行预处理。
- 若皮瓣顺应性良好、柔软且弹性正常（符合大多数病例），可安全进行胸肌前重建。
- 在准备阶段可先行自体脂肪移植（AFT）

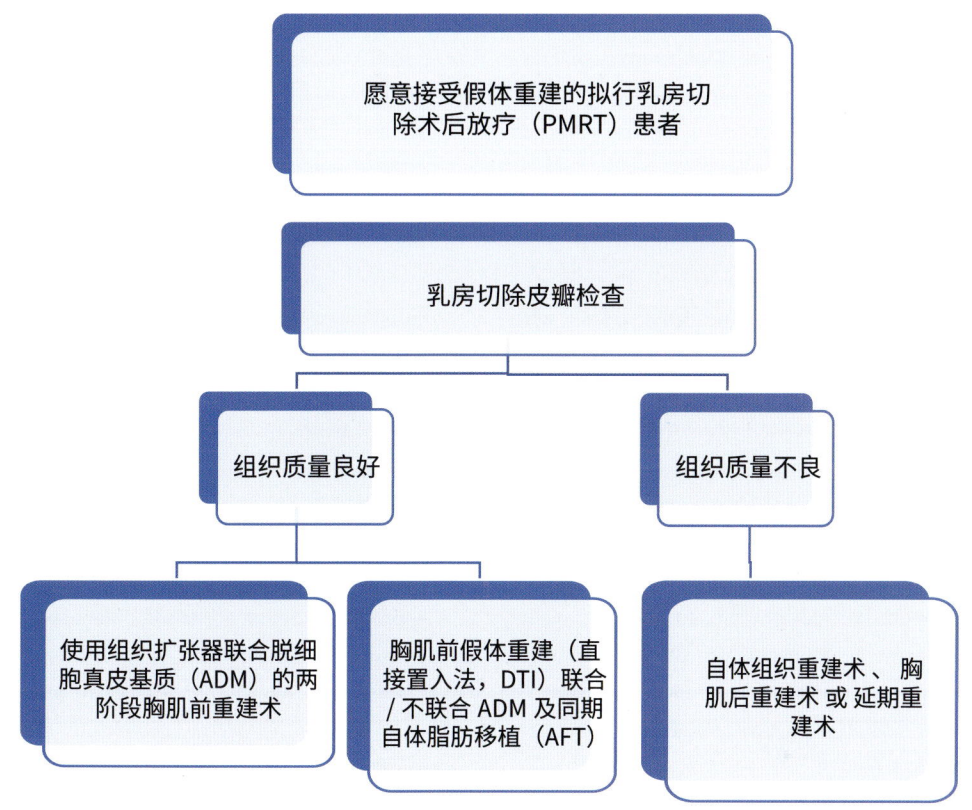

来改善组织质量。
- 自体脂肪移植（AFT）可同期作为重建术的辅助步骤。
- 假体置入后可追加自体脂肪移植（AFT）完成重建。

对重建后需行放疗（XRT）的患者：
- 推荐全乳切除术后接受 PMRT 者优先选择胸肌前假体重建（DTI）（需确保皮瓣条件优良）。
- 建议在完成术后放疗后、Ⅱ期置换手术前或术中追加自体脂肪移植（AFT）。

参考文献

1. Recht A, Comen EA, Fine RE, et al. post mastectomy radiotherapy: an American Society of Clinical Oncology, American Society for Radiation Oncology, and Society of Surgical Oncology Focused Guideline Update. Ann Surg Oncol. 2017,24:38–51.
2. Taylor ME, Haffty BG, Rabinovitch R, et al. ACR appropriateness criteria on post mastectomy radiotherapy expert panel on radiation oncology-breast. Int J Radiat Oncol Biol Phys. 2009,73:997–1002.
3. Horst KC, Haffty BG, Harris EE, et al. Expert panel on radiation oncology—breast. ACR Appropriateness Criteria® post mastectomy Radiotherapy. Reston: American College of Radiology（ACR）; 2012.
4. Clarke M, Collins R, Darby S, et al. Early

Breast Cancer Trialists' Collaborative Group (EBCTCG). Effects of radiotherapy and of differences in the extent of surgery for early breast cancer on local recurrence and 15-year survival: an overview of the randomized trials. Lancet. 2005,366:2087–106.

5. Overgaard M, Hansen PS, Overgaard J, et al. Postoperative radiotherapy in high-risk premenopausal women with breast cancer who receive adjuvant chemotherapy: Danish Breast Cancer Cooperative Group 82b Trial. N EnglJMed.1997,337:949–55.https://www.nccn.org/store/login/login.aspx?ReturnURL=https://www.nccn.org/professionals/physician_gls/pdf/breast.pdf.

6. Overgaard M, Jensen MB, Overgaard J, et al. Postoperative radiotherapy in high-risk postmenopausal breast-cancer patients given adjuvant tamoxifen: Danish Breast Cancer Cooperative Group DBCG 82c randomized trial. Lancet. 1999,353:1641–8.

7. Ragaz J, Jackson SM, Le N, et al. Adjuvant radiotherapy and chemotherapy in node-positive premenopausal women with breast cancer. N Engl J Med. 1997,337:956–62.

8. McGale P, Taylor C, Correa C, et al. Effect of radiotherapy after mastectomy and axillary surgery on 10-year recurrence and 20-year breast cancer mortality: meta-analysis of individual patient data for 8135 women in 22 randomized trials. Lancet. 2014,383:2127–35.

9. Kummerow KL, Du L, Penson DF, Shyr Y, Hooks MA. Nationwide trends in mastectomy for early-stage breast cancer. JAMA Surg. 2015,150:9–16.

10. Nelson JA, Disa JJ. Breast reconstruction and radiation therapy: an update. Plast Reconstr Surg. 2017,140:60s–8s.

11. Dicuonzo S, Leonardi MC, Radice D, et al. Longterm results and reconstruction failure in patients receiving post mastectomy radiation therapy with a temporary expander or permanent implant in place. Plast Reconstr Surg. 2020,145:317–27.

12. López E, Guerrero R, Núñez MI, et al. Early and late skin reactions to radiotherapy for breast cancer and their correlation with radiation-induced DNA damage in lymphocytes. Breast Cancer Res. 2005,7:690–8.

13. Muresan H, Lam G, Cooper BT, et al. Impact of evolving radiation therapy techniques on implant based breast reconstruction. Plast Reconstr Surg. 2017,139:1232e–9e.

14. Speers C, Pierce LJ. Postoperative radiotherapy after breast conserving surgery for early-stage breast cancer: a review. JAMA Oncol. 2016,2:1075–82.

15. El-Sabawi B, Carey JN, Hagopian TM, et al. Radiation and breast reconstruction: algorithmic approach and evidence based outcomes. J Surg Oncol. 2016,113:906–12.

16. Patel KM, Albino F, Fan KL, et al. Microvascular autologous breast reconstruction in the context of radiation therapy: comparing two reconstructive algorithms. Plast Reconstr Surg. 2013,132:251–7.

17. Cordeiro PG, Albornoz CR, McCormick B, et al. The impact of post mastectomy radiotherapy on two-stage implant breast reconstruction: an analysis of long-term surgical outcomes, aesthetic results, and satisfaction over 13 years. Plast Reconstr Surg. 2014,134:588–95.

18. Ben-David MA, Granot H, Gelernter I, Schefan M. Immediate breast reconstruction with anatomical implants following mastectomy: the radiation perspective. Med Dosim. 2016,41（2）:142–7.

19. Turesson I, Nyman J, Holmberg E, Oden A. Prognostic factors for acute and late skin reactions in radiotherapy patients. Int J Radiat Oncol Biol Phys. 1996,36:1065–75.

20. Barber JB, Burrill W, Spreadborough AR, Levine E, Warren C, Kiltie AE, Roberts SA, Scott D. Relationship between in vitro chromosomal radio sensitivity of peripheral blood lymphocytes and the expression of normal tissue damage fol-

lowing radiotherapy for breast cancer. Radiother Oncol. 2000,55:179–86.
21. López E, Núñez MI, Guerrero MR, del Moral R, de Dios Luna J, del Mar Rodríguez MM, Valenzuela MT, Villalobos M, Ruiz de Almodóvar JM. Breast cancer acute morbidity evaluated by different scoring systems. Breast Cancer Res Treat. 2002,73:127–34.
22. Peacock JH, Ashton A, Bliss J, Bush C, Eady J, Jackson C, Owen R, Regan J, Yarnold J. Cellular radio sensitivity and complication risk after curative radiotherapy. Radiother Oncol. 2000,55:173–8.
23. Gatti RA. The inherited basis of human radio sensitivity. Acta Oncol. 2001,40:702–11.
24. Núñez MI, Guerrero R, López E, del Moral R, Valenzuela MT, Siles E, Villalobos M, Pedraza V, Peacock JH, Ruiz de Almodóvar JM. DNA damage and prediction of radiation response in lymphocytes and epidermal skin cells. Int J Cancer. 1998,76:354–61.
25. Ruiz de Almodóvar JM, Guirado D, Núñez MI, López E, Guerrero R, Valenzuela MT, Villalobos M, Ruiz de Almodóvar JM. Individualization of radiotherapy in breast cancer patients: possible usefulness of a DNA damage assay to measure normal cell radio sensitivity. Radiother Oncol. 2002,62:327–33.
26. Carlomagno F, Burnet NG, Turesson I, Nyman J, Peacock JH, Dunning AH, Ponder BA, Jackson SP. Comparison of DNA repair protein expression and activities between human fibroblast cell lines with different radio sensitivities. Int J Cancer. 2000,85:845–9.
27. Krause M, Hessel F, Szips D, Hilberg F, Baumann M. Adjuvant inhibition of the epidermal growth factor receptor after fractionated irradiation of FaDu human squamous cell carcinoma. Radiother Oncol. 2004,72:95–101.
28. Haubner F, Ohmann E, Pohl F, et al. Wound healing after radiation therapy: review of the literature. Radiat Oncol. 2012,7:162.
29. Salvo N, Barnes E, van Draanen J, et al. Prophylaxis and management of acute radiation-induced skin reactions: a systematic review of the literature. Curr Oncol. 2010,17:94–112.
30. El-Sabawi B, Carey JN, Hagopian TM, et al. Radiation and breast reconstruction: algorithmic approach and evidenced based outcomes. J Surg Oncol. 2016,113:906–12.
31. Bentzen SM, Thames HD, Overgaard M. Latent-time estimation for late cutaneous and subcutaneous radiation reactions in a single-follow-up clinical study. Radiother Oncol. 1989,15:267–74.
32. Johansson S, Svensson H, Denenkamp J. Timescale of evolution of late radiation injury after postoperative radiotherapy of breast cancer patients. Int J Radiat Oncol Biol Phys. 2000,48:745–50.
33. Burnet NG, Johansen J, Turesson I, Nyman J, Peacock JH. Describing patients' normal tissue reactions: concerning the possibility of individualizing radiotherapy dose prescriptions based on potential predictive assays of normal tissue radio sensitivity. Steering Committee of the BioMed 2 European Union Concerted Action Program on the Development of Predictive Tests of Normal Tissue Response to Radiation Therapy. Int J Cancer. 1998,79:606–13.
34. Jagsi R, Jiang J, Momoh AO, et al. Complications after mastectomy and immediate breast reconstruction for breast cancer: a claims-based analysis. Ann Surg. 2016,263:219–27.
35. Krueger EA, Wilkins EG, Strawderman M, et al. Complications and patient satisfaction following expander/implant breast reconstruction with and without radiotherapy. Int J Radiat Oncol Biol Phys. 2001,49:713–21.
36. Contant CM, van Geel AN, van der Holt B, Griep C, Tjong Joe Wai R, Wiggers T. Morbidity of immediate breast reconstruction (IBR) after mastectomy by a sub pectorally placed silicone prosthesis: the adverse effect of radiotherapy. Eur J Surg Oncol. 2000,26:344–50.
37. Tallet AV, Salem N, Moutardier V, et al. Radio-

therapy and immediate two-stage breast reconstruction with a tissue expander and implant: complications and esthetic results. Int J Radiat Oncol Biol Phys. 2003,57:136–42.

38. Ascherman JA, Hanasono MM, Newman MI, Hughes DB. Implant reconstruction in breast cancer patients treated with radiation therapy. Plast Reconstr Surg. 2006,117:359–65.

39. Williams JK, Carlson GW, Bostwick J III, Bried JT, Mackay G. The effects of radiation treatment after TRAM fap breast reconstruction. Plast Reconstr Surg. 1997,100:1153–60.

40. Rogers NE, Allen RJ. Radiation effects on breast reconstruction with the deep inferior epigastric perforator fap. Plast Reconstr Surg. 2002,109:1919–24; discussion 1925–6.

41. Chetta MD, Aliu O, Zhong L, et al. Reconstruction of the irradiated breast: a national claims-based assessment of postoperative morbidity. Plast Reconstr Surg. 2017,139:783–92.

42. Hu ES, Pusic AL, Waljee JF, et al. Patient-reported aesthetic satisfaction with breast reconstruction during the long-term survivorship period. Plast Reconstr Surg. 2009,124:1–8.

43. Ho AY, Hu ZI, Mehrara BJ, Wilkins EG. Radiotherapy in the setting of breast reconstruction: types, techniques, and timing. Lancet Oncol. 2017,18:e742–53.

44. Muresan H, Lam G, Cooper BT, et al. Impact of evolving radiation therapy techniques on implant-based breast reconstruction. Plast Reconstr Surg. 2017,139:1232–9.

45. Lee KT, Mun GH. Prosthetic breast reconstruction in previously irradiated breasts: a meta-analysis. J Surg Oncol. 2015,112:468–75.

46. Khansa I, Colakoglu S, Curtis MS, et al. post mastectomy breast reconstruction after previous lumpectomy and radiation therapy: analysis of complications and satisfaction. Ann Plast Surg. 2011,66:444–51.

47. Reish RG, Lin A, Phillips NA, et al. Breast reconstruction outcomes after nipple sparing mastectomy and radiation therapy. Plast Reconstr Surg. 2015,135:959–66.

48. Peled AW, Sears M, Wang F, et al. Complications after total skin-sparing mastectomy and expander implant reconstruction: effects of radiation therapy on the stages of reconstruction. Ann Plast Surg. 2018,80:10–3.

49. Olinger TA, Berlin NL, Qi J, et al. Outcomes of immediate implant-based mastectomy reconstruction in women with previous breast radiotherapy. Plast Reconstr Surg. 2020,145:1029–35.

50. Albornoz CR, Matros E, McCarthy CM, et al. Implant breast reconstruction and radiation: a multicenter analysis of long-term health-related quality of life and satisfaction. Ann Surg Oncol. 2014,21:2159–64.

51. Behranwala KA, Dua RS, Ross GM, Ward A, A'hern R, Gui GP. The infuence of radiotherapy on capsule formation and aesthetic outcome after immediate breast reconstruction using biodimensional anatomical expander implants. J Plast Reconstr Aesthet Surg. 2006,59:1043–51.

52. Lam TC, Borotkanics R, Hsieh F, et al. Immediate two-stage prosthetic breast reconstruction failure: radiation is not the only culprit. Plast Reconstr Surg. 2018,141:1315–24.

53. Gronovich Y, Winder G, Maisel-Lotan A, et al. Hybrid Prepectoral Direct-to-Implant and Autologous Fat Graft Simultaneously in Immediate Breast Reconstruction: A Single Surgeon's Experience with 25 Breasts in 15 Consecutive Cases. Plast Reconstr Surg. 2022,149（3）:386–91.

54. Sigalove S, Maxwell GP, Sigalove NM, et al. Prepectoral implant-based breast reconstruction: rationale, indications, and preliminary results. Plast Reconstr Surg. 2017,139:287–94.

55. Spear SL, Schwartz J, Dayan JH, Clemens MW. Outcome assessment of breast distortion following submuscular breast augmentation. Aesthet Plast Surg. 2009,33:44–8.

56. Hammond DC, Schmitt WP, O'Connor EA. Treatment of breast animation deformity in implant-based reconstruction with pocket change to the subcutaneous position. Plast Reconstr Surg.

2015,135:1540–4.
57. Elswick SM, Harless CA, Bishop SN. Prepectoral implant-based breast reconstruction with post mastectomy radiation therapy. Plast Reconstr Surg. 2018,142:1–12.
58. Sbitany H. Important considerations for performing prepectoral breast reconstruction. Plast Reconstr Surg. 2017,140（6S Prepectoral Breast Reconstruction）:7S–13S.
59. Gabriel A, Maxwell GP. Prepectoral breast reconstruction in challenging patients. Plast Reconstr Surg. 2017,140（6S Prepectoral Breast Reconstruction）:14S–21S.
60. Nahabedian MY, Cocilovo C. Two-stage prosthetic breast reconstruction: a comparison between prepectoral and partial subpectoral techniques. Plast Reconstr Surg. 2017,140（6S Prepectoral Breast Reconstruction）:22S–30S.
61. Zhu L, Mohan AT, Abdelsattar JM, et al. Comparison of subcutaneous versus submuscular expander placement in the first stage of immediate breast reconstruction. J Plast Reconstr Aesthet Surg. 2016,69:e77–86.
62. Bernini M, Calabrese C, Cecconi L, et al. Subcutaneous direct-to-implant breast reconstruction: surgical, functional, and aesthetic results after long-term follow-up. Plast Reconstr Surg Glob Open. 2015,3:e574.
63. Sbitany H, Wang F, Peled AW, et al. Immediate implant based breast reconstruction following total skin-sparing mastectomy: defning the risk of preoperative and postoperative radiation therapy for surgical outcomes. Plast Reconstr Surg. 2014,134:396–404.
64. Seth AK, Hirsch EM, Fine NA, Kim JY. Utility of acellular dermis-assisted breast reconstruction in the setting of radiation: a comparative analysis. Plast Reconstr Surg. 2012,130:750–8.
65. Spear SL, Seruya M, Rao SS, et al. Two-stage prosthetic breast reconstruction using AlloDerm including outcomes of different timings of radiotherapy. Plast Reconstr Surg. 2012,130:1–9.
66. Moyer HR, Pinell-White X, Losken A. The effect of radiation on acellular dermal matrix and capsule formation in breast reconstruction: clinical out comes and histologic analysis. Plast Reconstr Surg. 2014,133:214–21.
67. Sbitany H, Gomez-Sanchez C, Piper M, et al. Prepectoral breast reconstruction in the setting of post mastectomy radiation therapy: an assessment of clinical outcomes and benefts. Plast Reconstr Surg. 2019,143:10–20.

21 胸肌前假体重建术中的脂肪移植增容

编者：William R. Moritz, Halley Darrach, Hayden Schott, Michael Finnan, Sarah Chiang, Annahita Fotouhi, Franca Kraenzlin, Nima Khavanin, Karan Chopra, Justin M. Sacks

译者：陈晓洁

21.1 概述

假体乳房重建仍是乳房切除术后的主要重建方式[1]，但具体术式存在差异。重建时机可选择即刻或延期，假体可置于胸大肌与前锯肌构成的肌层下方或前方。美国目前的主流方式是延期重建[2]。

自20世纪60年代硅胶假体问世以来，假体置入平面随外科技术进步不断演变。早期假体常置于胸大肌浅层的皮下平面[3]，但由于软组织支撑不足导致皮瓣坏死、包膜挛缩及假体移位等并发症发生率显著升高[4,5]。为降低并发症，转而将假体置于胸大肌下的平面[4]，但可能引发肩关节活动受限[6]、慢性疼痛[7]及动态畸形等[8]。2001年，脱细胞真皮基质的引入有效解决了胸肌无法覆盖假体下极的问题[9]，随着皮瓣灌注评估技术的进步，胸肌前假体置入已成为假体乳房重建的常规术式。

当前数据显示，采用脱细胞真皮基质后，胸肌前与胸肌后假体置入术在皮瓣坏死率和假体取出率方面相近[10]，胸肌前重建在肩关节功能保留、术后疼痛控制和乳房形态满意度等方面优势显著[6]，但也面临新挑战——与肌下或部分胸肌后重建相比，胸肌前重建中的假体与胸壁易形成明显台阶感，尤其在乳房上极区会出现"泪滴"样形态缺失。同时，较薄的皮瓣对假体边缘显现及褶皱的遮盖能力有限[8]，使得脂肪移植成为形态缺陷矫正的主要手段。在2016年全美3万余例乳房重建术中，

W. R. Moritz · H. Schott · M. Finnan · S. Chiang ·
A. Fotouhi · J. M. Sacks (✉)
Division of Plastic and Reconstructive Surgery,
Department of Surgery, School of Medicine,
Washington University, St. Louis, MO, USA
e-mail: moritzwr@wustl.edu; jmsacks@wustl.edu

H. Darrach · F. Kraenzlin · N. Khavanin · K. Chopra
Department of Plastic and Reconstructive Surgery,
The Johns Hopkins University School of Medicine,
Baltimore, MD, USA

© The Author(s), under exclusive license to Springer Nature Switzerland AG 2023
R. Vidya, H. Becker (eds.), *Prepectoral Breast Reconstruction*,
https://doi.org/10.1007/978-3-031-15590-1_21

30% 采用了自体脂肪移植[11]。

尽管脂肪移植操作简便且应用广泛，但高吸收率（小容量移植 140 天体积保持率 25%、大容量 50%[14]）、油性囊肿形成及脂肪坏死/钙化等并发症不容忽视[12]。Losken 等[13]发现，假体乳房重建术后的脂肪移植并发症显著高于其他术式。此外，受供区脂肪量限制（尤其消瘦者[15]），开展胸肌前假体乳房重建时必须严格进行术前评估和手术规划。

21.2 手术技术

自体脂肪移植需实现三重目标：修正乳房切除术后的轮廓畸形，掩盖较薄皮瓣下显露的假体褶皱，以及通过体积增容塑造自然的乳房形态（图 21.1）。鉴于脂肪存活率有限，术前必须告知患者可能需多次手术方能达到满意效果。临床经验显示，胸肌前重建所需脂肪移植量常大于胸肌后或部分胸肌后重建，术前应充分沟通多次治疗的必要性。

脂肪移植时机选择是首要考量：虽可在初次组织扩张器置入时实施，但更推荐推迟至最终体积确定后与永久假体置入同期操作。此策略具多重优势：可确保手术切缘阴性及明确患者后续治疗方案；待永久假体就位后，更易暴露需修正的轮廓缺陷与皮瓣薄弱区；可避免因脂肪移植加大皮瓣张力。本机构常规在永久假体置入的同时实施首次脂肪填充，优先矫正上极轮廓异常，Ⅱ 期处理假体褶皱（图 21.2），亦有学者主张更晚干预[16]。

术前评估应于站立位完成，该体位能直观显现轮廓缺陷。与胸肌后重建相比，胸肌前重建者上极体积需求更为显著（需重点标记）。美学设计应遵从患者意愿，可采集额外脂肪用于塑形（如加深乳沟或

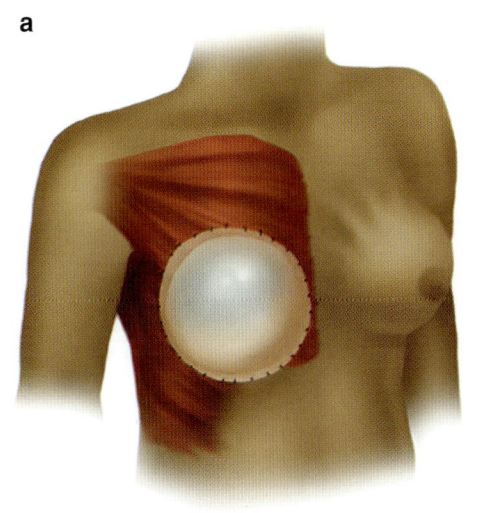 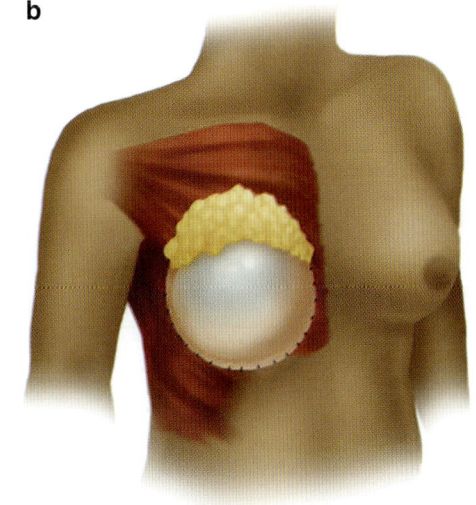

图 21.1 （a）胸肌前假体置入后出现褶皱；（b）上极脂肪移植可矫正褶皱畸形[60]（AME 出版社授权使用）

优化乳头区凸度），但假体褶皱矫正通常安排至Ⅱ期手术。

吸脂部位选择须权衡供区美观性。研究证实不同部位脂肪的细胞活性无显著差异[17-19]，但大腿脂肪结构完整性较高，腹部脂肪血管化更优[18]，常规选择侧腹部、腹部及大腿（避免重复采集同一区域）。操作中应避免过量抽取浅层脂肪，并且需注意规避易出现供区凹陷的高风险区（如髋外侧凹陷、臀沟、股后远端、股内侧中部及髂胫束下外侧区[20]）。

胸肌前重建因皮瓣菲薄，须防范锐性操作损伤假体。推荐采用手部遮挡技术保护假体，同时严格控制填充量。过量填充可能引发皮瓣压力性坏死（归咎于受压或血供超负荷），并导致脂肪移植物整体失活[21]。

脂肪获取与处理方式是近年研究热点，直接影响细胞活性。研究表明，注射器抽吸、负压辅助吸脂及超声辅助吸脂术对细胞存活率影响各异[22-28]。提升基质血管成分细胞与脂肪干细胞含量或可改善移植物存活情况[29]。动物实验提示，Telfa纱布过滤法较离心法可能更优[30]，但大容量脂肪处理可行性不足且尚未经人体试验证实[22, 29, 31, 32]。掺入富血小板血浆的临床效果研究结果存在分歧：Salgarello等[33]发现该技术未显著改善乳房重建效果，而Gentile等[34]报道其可提升术后1年乳廓形态与体积稳定性。

21.3 讨论

胸肌前假体乳房重建因优势显著已成为胸肌后重建的优选替代方案[5, 35-38]。该术式术程短、创伤小[39]，并且因未扰动胸大肌而术后疼痛轻、肌痉挛少[7, 38, 39]，同时保留胸肌于解剖位可规避肩关节功能障碍[6]与动态畸形[40]。

胸肌前重建并非新技术——早期直接将假体置于皮下，因缺乏软组织支撑导致包膜挛缩、皮瓣坏死及假体移位等并发症高发。脱细胞真皮基质、新型组织扩张器及术中皮瓣灌注评估技术的联合应用，使

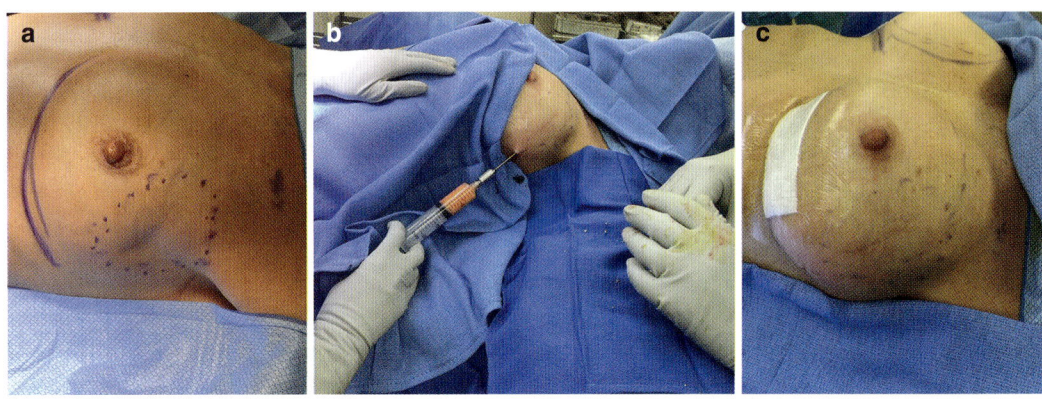

图 21.2 （a）永久假体置入时患者乳房轮廓异常；（b，c）腹部取脂后填充上极区，矫正畸形并形成自然乳房形态

该术式焕发新生[39, 41-45]。

脂肪移植作为重要辅助手段，在胸肌前重建中尤为重要[37, 46]。脱细胞真皮基质多作为内置支架（本机构常规仅覆盖假体下极，以控制成本并降低包膜挛缩风险[47]）使用，但其对胸肌前假体上缘及胸壁衔接区的修饰能力有限，加之假体褶皱暴露率高（前间隙重建者对此不满率显著高于肌下重建[48]），使脂肪移植成为必要补充。

本机构常规于更换永久假体时同步实施脂肪移植（一次性手术占85%~82%[12, 37, 44]），既可验证切缘状态，又能精准定位永久假体就位后的薄弱区域。需要注意的是，胸肌前皮瓣厚度限制了单次脂肪移植量，并且有放疗史者常需二次干预[13]，故术前须充分沟通多次手术可能。

降低假体褶皱的技术策略包括：适度欠充组织扩张器以构建紧致囊袋[49]，依据乳房基底径精选假体并满注[35]，选用形态稳定型凝胶假体[35, 50-53]或超量充注盐水假体[49]。即使无褶皱显现，多数患者仍需补充上极体积以实现自然形态。

既往脂肪移植用于异体材料乳房重建，因可能干扰肿瘤复发的早期诊断备受争议[54]，但近期研究支持其安全性。Petit等[12]证实，脂肪填充术不影响乳腺癌影像学检出；Delay等[55]对734例患者10年随访亦得出相同结论。Seth等[16]长期随访发现，脂肪移植组与未移植组的肿瘤复发率及总体生存率无显著差异。然而，该技术可能诱发脂肪坏死或油性囊肿而需要二次手术[12, 16, 55]，尤其在区域放疗后更易发生[56]。

脂肪移植可明确提升乳房重建术后美观度与患者满意度。de Blacam等[57]报道术后平均10.8个月随访显示，乳房体积、轮廓、位置及内上象限饱满度均有改善。脂肪高吸收特性制约其效果持久性——Choi等[14]指出，140天后大、小容量移植体积保持率分别为52%、27%，提示需长期随访评估最终疗效。目前关于胸肌前重建中脂肪移植远期效果的研究仍然有限[35, 37-40, 43, 44, 47, 58]。现有数据显示，术后1~3.5年脂肪移植可显著改善假体褶皱[53]；在平均42个月随访中，移植组患者心理社会适应性与性健康评分更优[59]。现有研究尚未阐明胸肌前薄层皮瓣对脂肪存活率、囊肿及坏死发生率的影响，但不可否认脂肪移植是实现最佳美学效果的关键环节。

21.4 小结

- 胸肌前乳房重建中，脂肪移植可矫正轮廓畸形，掩盖假体褶皱并重塑自然乳房形态。
- 术后140天小、大容量脂肪移植体积保持率分别为25%、50%，往往需多次手术方能取得理想美学效果。
- 推荐在永久假体置入的同时进行脂肪移植。
- 术前评估应取站立位以凸显轮廓缺陷。
- 优先矫正上极形态缺陷，Ⅱ期手术处理假体褶皱，塑造乳沟及加强乳头凸度。
- 优选侧腹、腹部、大腿为吸脂部位，禁忌区域包括髋外侧凹陷、臀沟、股后远端、股内侧中部及髂胫束下外侧区。避免重复采集及浅层过量抽吸。
- 假体表面采用手部遮挡技术预防穿刺损伤。
- 避免过量填充所致的皮瓣压力性坏死风险。
- 脂肪处理方式尚存争议，联合应用富血小板血浆或有助于提升体积稳定性。
- 仍需长期随访研究评估脂肪移植远期美学效果及并发症发生率。

参考文献

1. Albornoz CR, Bach PB, Mehrara BJ, et al. A paradigm shift in U.S. Breast reconstruction: increasing implant rates. Plast Reconstr Surg. 2013,131（1）:15– 23. https://doi.org/10.1097/PRS.0b013e3182729cde.
2. American Society of Plastics Surgeons. Plastic surgery statistics report. American Society of Plastic Surgeons; 2020. Published online 2020:1– 26. http:// scholar.google.com/scholar?hl=en&btnG=Search&q =intitle:Plastic+Surgery+Statistics+Report#1.
3. Nahabedian MY, Glasberg SB, Maxwell GP. Introduction to "prepectoral breast reconstruction". Plast Reconstr Surg. 2017,140（6S）:4S–5S. https://doi.org/10.1097/PRS.0000000000004066.
4. Gruber RP, Kahn RA, Lash H, Master MR, Apfelberg D, Laub DR. Breast reconstruction following mastectomy: a comparison of submuscular and subcutaneous techniques. Plast Reconstr Surg. 1981,67（3）:312–7.
5. Highton L, Johnson R, Kirwan C, Murphy J. Prepectoral implant-based breast reconstruction. Plast Reconstr Surg Glob Open. 2017,5（9）:1–9. https://doi.org/10.1097/GOX.0000000000001488.
6. Caputo GG, Zingaretti N, Kiprianidis I, et al. Quality of life and early functional evaluation in direct-to-implant breast reconstruction after mastectomy: a comparative study between prepectoral versus dual-plane reconstruction. Clin Breast Cancer. 2021,21（4）:344–51. https://doi.org/10.1016/j.clbc.2020.11.013.
7. Wallace MS, Wallace AM, Lee J, Dobke MK. Pain after breast surgery: a survey of 282 women. Pain. 1996,66（2）:195–205. https://journals.lww.com/pain/ Fulltext/1996/08000/Pain_after_breast_surgery__a_ survey_of_282_women.12.aspx. 8. King CA, Bartholomew AJ, Sosin M, et al. A critical appraisal of late complications of prepectoral versus subpectoral breast reconstruction following nipple-sparing mastectomy. Ann Surg Oncol. 2021,28（13）:9150–8. https://doi.org/10.1245/ s1043402110085z.
9. Basu CB, Leong M, Hicks MJ. Acellular cadaveric dermis decreases the inflammatory response in capsule formation in reconstructive breast surgery. Plast Reconstr Surg. 2010,126（6）:1842–7. https://doi. org/10.1097/PRS.0b013e3181f44674.
10. Manrique OJ, Banuelos J, Abu-Ghname A, et al. Surgical outcomes of prepectoral versus subpectoral implant-based breast reconstruction in young women. Plast Reconstr Surg Glob Open. 2019,7（3）:1–5. https://doi.org/10.1097/GOX.0000000000002119.
11. American Society of Plastic Surgeons. Plastic surgery statistics report. American Society of Plastic Surgeons; 2016. Published online 2016:1–25. https://www. plasticsurgery.org/documents/News/Statistics/2016/ plasticsurgerystatisticsfullreport2016.pdf.
12. Petit JY, Lohsiriwat V, Clough KB, et al. The oncologic outcome and immediate surgical complications of lipoflling in breast cancer patients: a multicenter study-Milan-Paris-Lyon experience of 646 lipoflling procedures. Plastic Surgery Complete: The Clinical Masters of PRS-Breast Reconstruction. Published online 2015:14–19. https://doi.org/10.1097/PRS.0b013e31821e713c.

13. Losken A, Pinell XA, Sikoro K, Yezhelyev MV, Anderson E, Carlson GW. Autologous fat grafting in secondary breast reconstruction. Ann Plast Surg. 2011,66（5）:518–22. https://doi.org/10.1097/ SAP.0b013e3181fe9334.
14. Choi M, Small K, Levovitz C, Lee C, Fadl A, Karp NS. The volumetric analysis of fat graft survival in breast reconstruction. Plast Reconstr Surg. 2013,131（2）:185–91. https://doi.org/10.1097/ PRS.0b013e3182789b13.
15. Weichman KE, Broer PN, Thanik VD, et al. Patient-reported satisfaction and quality of life following breast reconstruction in thin patients: a comparison between microsurgical and prosthetic implant recipients. Plast Reconstr Surg. 2015,136（2）:213–20. https://doi.org/10.1097/ PRS.0000000000001418. W. R. Moritz et al.257
16. Seth AK, Hirsch EM, Kim JYS, Fine NA. Long-term outcomes following fat grafting in prosthetic breast reconstruction: a comparative analysis. Plast Reconstr Surg. 2012,130（5）:984–90. https://doi.org/10.1097/ PRS.0b013e318267d34d.
17. Small K, Choi M, Petruolo O, Lee C, Karp N. Is there an ideal donor site of fat for secondary breast reconstruction? Aesthet Surg J. 2014,34（4）:545–50. https:// doi.org/10.1177/1090820X14526751.
18. Ullmann Y, Shoshani O, Fodor A, et al. Searching for the favorable donor site for fat injection: in vivo study using the nude mice model. Dermatol Surg. 2005,31（10）:1304–7. https://doi.org/10.1097/00042728200510000000007.
19. Li K, Gao J, Zhang Z, et al. Selection of donor site for fat grafting and cell isolation. Aesthet Plast Surg. 2013,37（1）:153–8. https://doi.org/10.1007/ s0026601299911.
20. Rohrich RJ, Smith PD, Marcantonio DR, Kenkel JM. The zones of adherence: role in minimizing and preventing contour deformities in liposuction. Plast Reconstr Surg. 2001,107（6）:1562.
21. del Vecchio DA, del Vecchio SJ. The graft-to-capacity ratio: volumetric planning in large-volume fat transplantation. Plast Reconstr Surg. 2014,133（3）:561–9. https://doi.org/10.1097/01.prs.0000438471.23249.6e.
22. Fisher C, Grahovac TL, Schafer ME, Shippert RD, Marra KG, Peter RJ. Comparison of harvest and processing techniques for fat grafting and adipose stem cell isolation. Plast Reconstr Surg. 2013,132（2）:351– 61. https://doi.org/10.1097/ PRS.0b013e3182958796.
23. Smith P, Adams WP, Lipschitz AH, et al. Autologous human fat grafting: effect of harvesting and preparation techniques on adipocyte graft survival. Plast Reconstr Surg. 2006,117（6）:1836–44. https://doi.org/10.1097/01. prs.0000218825.77014.78.
24. Keck M, Kober J, Riedl O, et al. Power assisted liposuction to obtain adipose-derived stem cells: impact on viability and differentiation to adipocytes in comparison to manual aspiration. J Plast Reconstr Aesthet Surg. 2014,67（1）:e1. https://doi.org/10.1016/j. bjps.2013.08.019.
25. Lee JH, Kirkham JC, McCormack MC, Nicholls AM, Randolph MA, Austen WG. The effect of pressure and shear on autologous fat grafting. Plast Reconstr Surg. 2013,131（5）:1125– 36. https://doi.org/10.1097/ PRS.0b013e-3182879f4a.
26. Pu LLQ, Coleman SR, Cui X, Ferguson REH, Vasconez HC. Autologous fat grafts harvested and refined by the Coleman technique: a comparative study. Plast Reconstr Surg. 2008,122（3）:932–7. https://doi.org/10.1097/ PRS.0b013e3181811ff0.
27. Ochoa O, Robinson J, Beran SJ. Cosmetic comparative lipoplasty analysis of in vivo-treated adipose tissue. Plast Reconstr Surg. 2000,105:2152–8.
28. Crawford JL, Hubbard BA, Colbert SH, Puckett CL. Fine tuning lipoaspirate viability for fat grafting. Plast Reconstr Surg. 2010,126（4）:1342–8. https://doi.org/10.1097/ PRS.0b013e3181ea44a9.
29. Strong AL, Cederna PS, Rubin JP, Coleman SR,

Levi B. The current state of fat grafting. Plast Reconstr Surg. 2015,136（4）:897–912. https://doi.org/10.1097/ prs.0000000000001590.

30. Canizares O, Thomson JE, Allen RJ, et al. The effect of processing technique on fat graft survival. Plast Reconstr Surg. 2017,140（5）:933–43. https://doi. org/10.1097/PRS.0000000000003812.

31. Tuin AJ, Domerchie PN, Schepers RH, et al. What is the current optimal fat grafting processing technique? A systematic review. J Craniomaxillofac Surg. 2016,44（1）:45–55. https://doi.org/10.1016/j. jcms.2015.10.021.

32. Cleveland EC, Albano NJ, Hazen A. Roll, spin, wash, or filter? Processing of lipoaspirate for autologous fat grafting: an updated, evidence-based review of the literature. Plast Reconstr Surg. 2015,136（4）:706–13. https://doi.org/10.1097/PRS.0000000000001581.

33. Salgarello M, Visconti G, Rusciani A. Breast fat grafting with platelet-rich plasma: a comparative clinical study and current state of the art. Plast Reconstr Surg. 2011,127（6）:2176–85. https://doi.org/10.1097/ PRS.0b013e3182139fe7.

34. Gentile P, di Pasquali C, Bocchini I, et al. Breast reconstruction with autologous fat graft mixed with platelet-rich plasma. Surg Innov. 2013,20（4）:370–6. https://doi.org/10.1177/1553350612458544.

35. Sbitany H. Important considerations for performing prepectoral breast reconstruction. Plast Reconstr Surg. 2017,140（6S）:7S–13S. https://doi.org/10.1097/PRS.0000000000004045.

36. Snyderman RK, Guthrie RH. Reconstruction of the female breast following radical mastectomy. Plast Reconstr Surg. 1971,47（6）:565–7.

37. Sbitany H, Piper M, Lentz R. Prepectoral breast reconstruction: a safe alternative to submuscular prosthetic reconstruction following nipple-sparing mastectomy. Plast Reconstr Surg. 2017,140（3）:432–43. https://doi.org/10.1097/PRS.0000000000003627.

38. ter Louw RP, Nahabedian MY. Prepectoral breast reconstruction. Plast Reconstr Surg. 2017,140（5S）:51S–9S. https://doi.org/10.1097/PRS.0000000000003942.

39. Sigalove S, Maxwell GP, Sigalove NM, et al. Prepectoral implant-based breast reconstruction: rationale, indications, and preliminary results. Plast Reconstr Surg. 2017,139（2）:287–94. https://doi. org/10.1097/PRS.0000000000002950.

40. Jones G, Yoo A, King V, et al. Prepectoral immediate direct-to-implant breast reconstruction with anterior AlloDerm coverage. Plast Reconstr Surg. 2017,140（6S）:31S–8S. https://doi.org/10.1097/PRS.0000000000004048.

41. Nahabedian MY. What are the long-term aesthetic issues in prepectoral breast reconstruction? Aesthet Surg J. 2020,40:S29–37. https://doi.org/10.1093/ASJ/SJAA164.

42. Wagner RD, Braun TL, Zhu H, Winocour S. A systematic review of complications in prepectoral 21 Fat Grafting for Volume Augmentation in Prepectoral Breast Reconstruction258 breast reconstruction. J Plast Reconstr Aesthet Surg. 2019,72（7）:1051–9. https://doi.org/10.1016/j.bjps.2019.04.005.

43. Khavanin N, Gust MJ, Grant DW, Nguyen KT, Kim JYS. Tabbed tissue expanders improve breast symmetry scores in breast reconstruction. Arch Plast Surg. 2014,41（1）:57–62. https://doi.org/10.5999/ aps.2014.41.1.57.

44. Elswick SM, Harless CA, Bishop SN, et al. Prepectoral implant-based breast reconstruction with post mastectomy radiation therapy. Plast Reconstr Surg. 2018,142（1）:1–12. https://doi.org/10.1097/PRS.0000000000004453.

45. Jordan SW, Khavanin N, Fine NA, Kim JYS. An algorithmic approach for selective acellular dermal matrix use in immediate two-stage breast reconstruction: indications and outcomes. Plast Reconstr Surg. 2014,134（2）:178–88. https://doi.org/10.1097/PRS.0000000000000366.

46. Delay E, Guerid S. The role of fat grafting in breast reconstruction. Clin Plast Surg. 2015,42

47. Reitsamer R, Peintinger F. Prepectoral implant placement and complete coverage with porcine acellular dermal matrix: a new technique for direct-to-implant breast reconstruction after nipple-sparing mastectomy. J Plast Reconstr Aesthet Surg. 2015,68（2）:162–7. https://doi.org/10.1016/j.bjps.2014.10.012.
48. Baker BG, Irri R, Maccallum V, Chattopadhyay R, Murphy J, Harvey JR. A prospective comparison of short-term outcomes of subpectoral and prepectoral Strattice-based immediate breast reconstruction. Plast Reconstr Surg. 2018,141（5）:1077–84. https://doi. org/10.1097/PRS.0000000000004270.
49. Graziano FD, Henderson PW, Jacobs J, Salzberg CA, Sbitany H. How to optimize prepectoral breast reconstruction. Aesthet Surg J. 2020,40:S22–8. https://doi. org/10.1093/asj/sjaa214.
50. Panettiere P, Marchetti L, Accorsi D. Soft cohesive silicone gel breast prostheses: a comparative prospective study of aesthetic results versus lower cohesivity silicone gel prostheses. J Plast Reconstr Aesthet Surg. 2007,60（5）:482–9. https://doi.org/10.1016/j. bjps.2006.04.020.
51. Brown MH, Shenker R, Silver SA. Cohesive silicone gel breast implants in aesthetic and reconstructive breast surgery. Plast Reconstr Surg. 2005,116（3）:768–79. https://doi.org/10.1097/01. prs.0000176259.66948.e7.
52. Cordeiro PG, McGuire P, Murphy DK. Natrelle 410 extra-full projection silicone breast implants: 2-year results from two prospective studies. Plast Reconstr Surg. 2015,136（4）:638–46. https://doi.org/10.1097/ PRS.0000000000001636.
53. Belmonte BM, Campbell CA. Safety profile and predictors of aesthetic outcomes after prepectoral breast reconstruction with meshed acellular dermal matrix. Ann Plast Surg. 2021,86（6S Suppl 5）:S585–92. https://doi.org/10.1097/SAP.0000000000002764.
54. Riggio E, Bordoni D, Nava MB. Oncologic surveillance of breast cancer patients after lipofilling. Aesthet Plast Surg. 2013,37（4）:728–35. https://doi. org/10.1007/s0026601301665.
55. Delay E, Garson S, Tousson G, Sinna R. Fat injection to the breast: technique, results, and indications based on 880 procedures over 10 years. Aesthet Surg J. 2009,29（5）:360–76. https://doi.org/10.1016/j. asj.2009.08.010.
56. Rietjens M, de Lorenzi F, Rossetto F, et al. Safety of fat grafting in secondary breast reconstruction after cancer. J Plast Reconstr Aesthet Surg. 2011,64（4）:477–83. https://doi.org/10.1016/j.bjps.2010.06.024.
57. de Blacam C, Momoh AO, Colakoglu S, Tobias AM, Lee BT. Evaluation of clinical outcomes and aesthetic results after autologous fat grafting for contour deformities of the reconstructed breast. Plast Reconstr Surg. 2011,128（5）:411–8. https://doi.org/10.1097/PRS.0b013e318226669f.
58. Hudson DA. Optimizing aesthetics with prosthetic prepectoral breast reconstruction. Plast Reconstr Surg. 2018,141（4）:611e–2e. https://doi.org/10.1097/ PRS.0000000000004206.
59. Le NK, Persing S, Dinis J, et al. A comparison of BREAST-Q scores between prepectoral and subpectoral direct-to-implant breast reconstruction. Plast Reconstr Surg. 2021,148（5）:708e–14e. https://doi. org/10.1097/prs.0000000000008410.
60. Darrach H, Kraenzlin F, Khavanin N, Chopra K, Sacks JM. The role of fat grafting in prepectoral breast reconstruction. Gland Surg. 2019,8（1）:61–6. https://doi.org/10.21037/gs.2018.10.09.

22 LOTUS 胸肌前乳房重建术

编者：M. Asher Schusterman II and Robert D. Rehnke
译者：范杰后

22.1 引言

乳房重建是整形外科医师的核心能力之一。在过去 50 年里，乳房重建方式历经演变，从硅胶假体重建转向自体皮瓣移植（带蒂或游离组织移植），随后又回归以假体为主的策略。这一回归趋势源于医疗资源限制及乳房切除术向保留乳头-乳晕复合体与软组织包膜的微创化发展。乳房切除术的革新显著提升了胸肌前平面假体重建的效果。25 年来，本团队致力于浅筋膜系统（superficial fascia system, SFS）的解剖研究[1]。SFS 构成乳腺体边界，以其为标志引导乳房切除术，旨在彻底清除外胚层起源的小叶与导管组织（乳腺癌发生部位），在确保切缘阴性的同时尽可能保留皮肤包膜及 SFS 结构。现代辅助治疗（如放疗、内分泌治疗、细胞毒性化疗及靶向治疗）的进步，使精准乳房切除术更趋安全。本领域的关键突破在于乳房切除术后即刻采用内荷包缝合法重建环状乳房韧带（circummammary ligament, CML）。该技术显著减少了需替代组织的体积，使单纯自体脂肪移植 I 期重建成为可能。即刻脂肪移植受限于乳腺体切除遗留的无效腔，且单纯脂肪移植难以塑造乳房凸度。为此，本团队开发了用可吸收网片构建的三维支架，可充填空腔并抵抗挛缩/瘢痕收缩。术后数周至数月内，生物网片将与患者的细胞与细胞外基质修复系统整合。组织学观察显示，网片形成高细胞密度工程化筋膜层，包含成纤维细胞、巨噬细胞、致密胶原及毛细血管（图 22.1），成为支持脂肪生成及组织长入的结构性支架与血供来源（需多次脂肪移植，图 22.2）。2020 年本团队提出的可吸收网片内置物（命名为 LOTUS）[2]可提供表面积与凸度，

M. Asher Schusterman II
Institute for Reconstructive Surgery, Houston
Methodist Willowbrook Hospital, Houston, TX, USA
e-mail: maschustermanii@houstonmethodist.org

R. D. Rehnke (✉)
Private Practice Plastic Surgery,
St. Petersburg, FL, USA

The Center for Surgical Excellence,
St. Petersburg, FL, USA

© The Author(s), under exclusive license to Springer Nature Switzerland AG 2023
R. Vidya, H. Becker (eds.), *Prepectoral Breast Reconstruction*,
https://doi.org/10.1007/978-3-031-15590-1_22

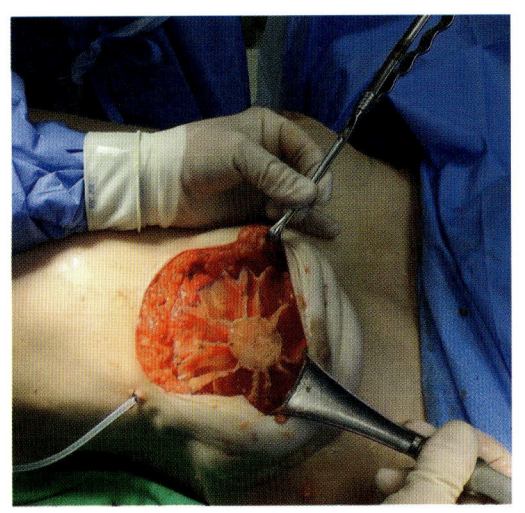

图 22.1 三维可吸收网片支架在保留皮肤和乳头全乳切除即刻重建中的应用。用该内置物充填乳腺体切除后的死腔，在逐步转化为"工程化筋膜"为重建乳房提供凸度的同时，为脂肪移植提供基质界面

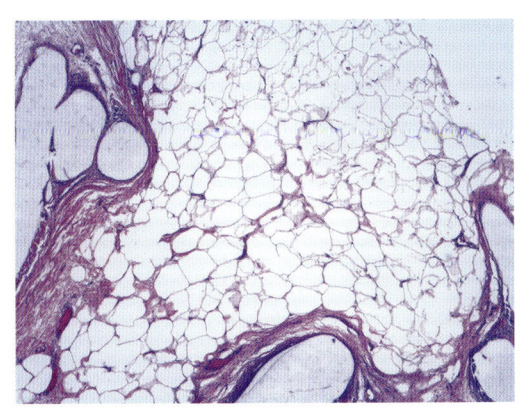

图 22.2 假体置入后 10 个月的苏木精-伊红（H&E）染色活检标本，可见 P4HB 单丝周围成纤维细胞、胶原纤维及毛细血管结构重建，网片间隔内形成成熟脂肪组织

维持低组织张力空间，创建拟合体内多维几何工程化腔室的生物工程区域。此类腔室为人体自身 SFS 小叶脂肪单元的改造变体（图 22.3），其概念最早由 Doldere 等[3]于 2011 年提出。

过去 6 年里 118 例临床应用显示，该技术兼具自体重建的优良效果与假体重建的简便性/低风险性，有望使乳房重建重新成为整形外科普适性术式，推动高质量医疗广泛可及。

22.1.1 微创乳房切除术

本团队由普外科与整形外科医师协作开展即刻乳房重建的历史已有 25 年以上。起初施行保留皮肤乳房切除术，手术边界为浅筋膜与胸壁深筋膜融合处（即环状乳房韧带；图 22.4）。乳腺体（含乳腺癌起源的小叶与导管结构）位于前、后浅筋膜层之间的中层结构——乳房中层膜内。青春期乳腺发育使乳腺体扩展，乳房中层膜被压缩为乳腺体前囊与后囊。在腺体周围，乳房中层膜与前、后筋膜层融合，于环状乳房韧带处变为二维筋膜结构。近五年半来，本团队改良了解剖导向乳房切除术技术：在保留周围浅筋膜系统的前提下，整体切除具有完整包膜的乳腺体。

该技术（称为微创乳房切除术）将乳房切除分两阶段实施：第一阶段切除肿瘤涉及的亚象限区域（占全乳的 12.5%~25%），确保切缘阴性（如肿瘤表浅者可切除表面皮肤，深在者可能需切除部分下方肌肉，周边肿瘤可切除部分环状乳房韧带）；第二阶段切除剩余 75%~87.5% 的乳腺组织，保留皮肤、肌肉、乳头及浅筋膜系统。

三维乳腺 X 线摄影、超声及 MRI 等术前影像对定位原发肿瘤亚象限及排除其他可疑病灶至关重要。本团队采用

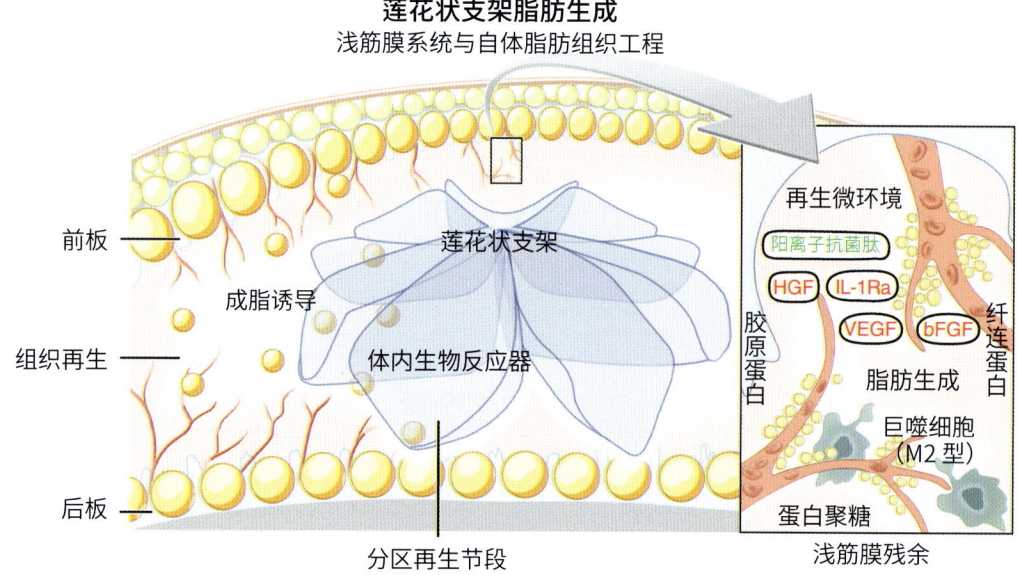

图 22.3 LOTUS 内置物示意图——多节段开放组织工程腔室呈放射状排列。内置物置于乳房切除后的空腔内，与浅筋膜残端接触（该区域毛细血管末端为成脂活性区）。插图示网片周围液体中已鉴定的生长因子

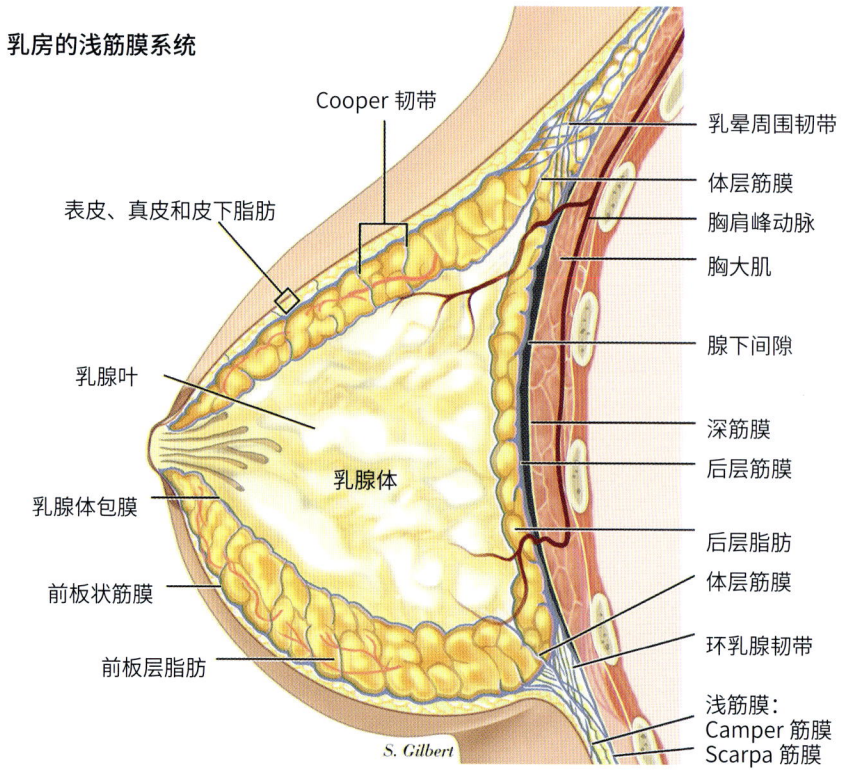

图 22.4 乳房矢状面观：浅筋膜层与深筋膜及胸壁在特定融合区（即"乳腺周围韧带"）紧密连接，构成乳房边界

Salibian 所述技术[4]，术中切除 Cooper 韧带基底。标本前表面可见由 Stiles[5] 描述的"汹涌海面波浪"样外周锥状突起（图 22.5）。此术式的根本原则是实现肿瘤切缘阴性与精准解剖切除。

22.1.2　LOTUS 乳房重建术

2015 年初，本团队开始应用生物可吸收网片支架替代硅胶假体，于微创乳房切除术后行胸肌前即刻乳房重建。2 年后首次开展硅胶假体取出后延迟 LOTUS 乳房重建术。可吸收网片由市售二维网片材料剪裁，在无菌条件下于术中行三维塑形（患者入室前完成），成为避免硅胶使用、以脂肪移植为主要重建模式的关键。完成乳房切除（保留皮肤或乳头）后，使用聚丙烯倒刺缝线行环形 CML 荷包缝合，以重建乳房基底径线（图 22.6）。该缝合形成的浅筋膜"巢"用于放置 LOTUS 支架，支架通过缝合固定于浅筋膜，可沿基底修

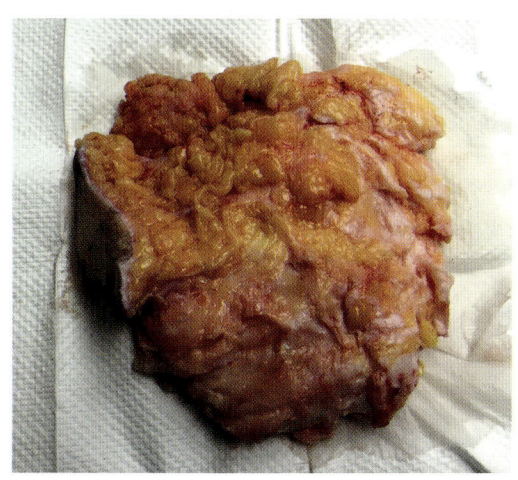

图 22.5　乳头保留全乳切除术标本前视图（覆盖肿瘤的乳房外上象限皮肤）。注意表面锥形突起为垂直支持带（Cooper 韧带）

剪以贴合胸壁。与无法整合的硅胶假体相比，LOTUS 支架在术后 1~2 个月内即可实现与细胞的完全整合。初期网片质地较硬，随时间溶解逐渐软化，3 年后通常难以触及。

支架由 4~5 张 15cm×20cm 可吸收网片（根据个体化设计）组装而成。目前，本团队使用过三种产品：TIGR 外科网片（新加坡 Novus Scientific 公司）、SERI 外科支架（美国 Allergan 公司）及 Phasix 网片（美国 C.R. Bard/Davol 公司，成分为基因工程大肠杆菌生物发酵产物聚 4-羟基丁酸酯[P4HB]）。前 3 例患者采用 TIGR 与 SERI 网片，后续病例均选用 P4HB 产品（因更优操作特性与生物相容性）[1]。支架构建前需评估乳腺体置换体积、基底径及凸度。

三维褶皱网片结构以中央核心缝合固定，各网片分支呈钟表 12 点位放射状排列，外周固定于环形基底网片（直径与乳房基底匹配）。顶端环形网片支撑放射状分支，置于乳头 - 乳晕复合体下方。术中采用双极电凝刀（盐水浴环境）熔合相邻网片子段，形成张力性网泡结构（类似气泡膜）。该张力网络与脂肪填充间隙，构成经典张 - 拉整体系统，模拟天然浅筋膜系统的生物力学特性。术后首月可见成纤维细胞快速长入，形成胶原纤维、巨噬细胞、淋巴细胞及毛细血管网络（类似天然筋膜）。网片子段间隙的脂肪组织增生源自微创切除术中保留的浅筋膜脂肪供血末梢[6]。自体脂肪移植可加速该过程（图 22.7）。网片子段形成围绕核心放射排列的部分开放

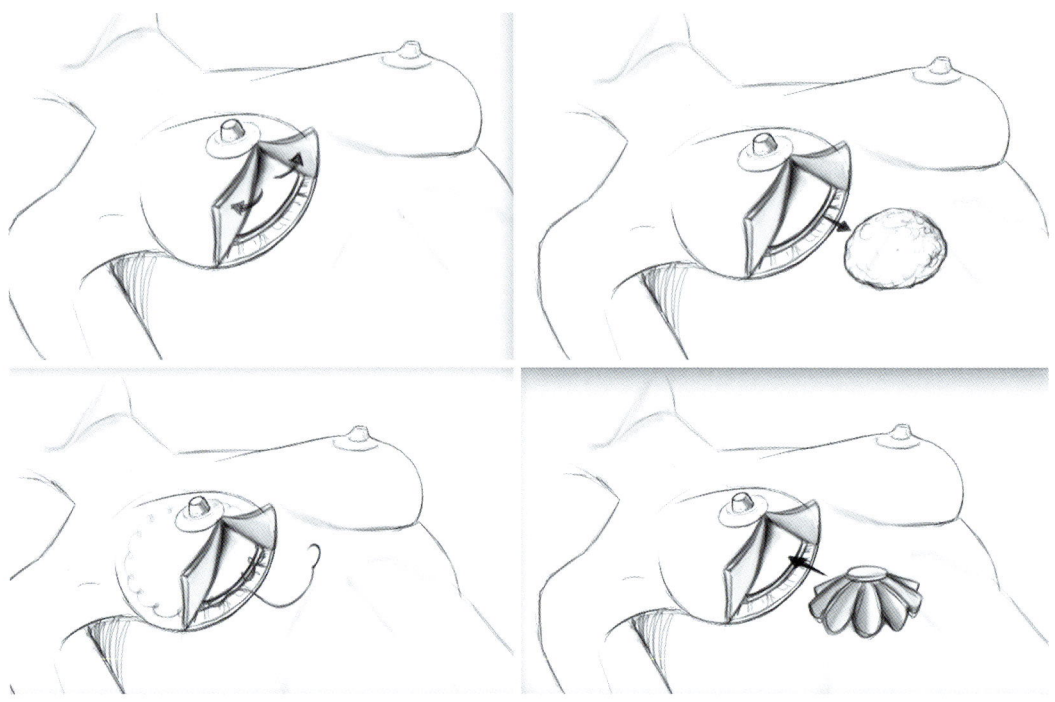

图 22.6　LOTUS 即刻乳房重建：经倒"T"形或乳房下皱襞切口行保留乳头全乳切除术→环乳韧带荷包缝合收紧→长效可吸收网片支架置入

组织工程腔室，其容积可通过半球体积公式估算。

$$\text{sphere:}\ \dfrac{\frac{4}{3}\pi r^3}{2}.$$

自体脂肪移植术始于 LOTUS 支架置入 3~4 周后（此时血管网络完成再生）。首次操作多采用小剂量脂肪立体注射，涉及皮下层、支架胸壁侧及假体各分段。后续每次增量移植间隔 3~4 个月，直至构建足够的健康组织体积。临床数据显示，多数患者除乳房切除术中置入 LOTUS 装置外，还需追加多次脂肪移植[2]。

治疗过程中需警惕皮肤包裹状态异常。LOTUS 型号选择不当致软组织过度收缩，将形成垂直向支持带纤维，阻

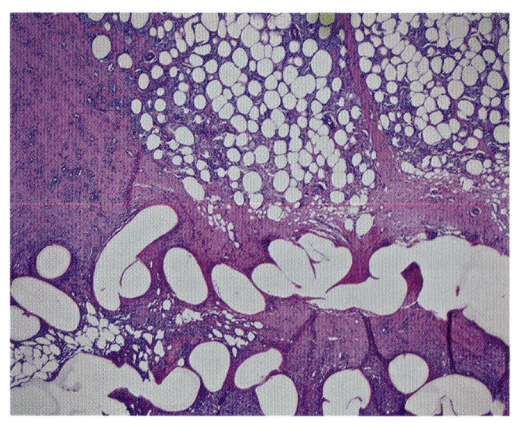

图 22.7　LOTUS 重建标本 H&E 染色显示，网片支架表面移植脂肪形成小叶结构，由细密筋膜间隔支撑

碍脂肪移植期间的组织扩张。此时可行 Rigottomy 松解术（用 14 号粗针经皮穿刺，松解束带结构），但松解过度可能导致出血及血清肿。合理选择支架规格并于术后

3~4 周内完成首次脂肪移植，可有效规避此类问题。而初始皮肤/筋膜包裹过紧者，则需更大的支架支撑创口防止挛缩，单纯依赖脂肪移植，难以实现稳定凸度。

22.2 结果

自 2015 年 2 月首例 LOTUS 可吸收网片重建术实施以来，共纳入 50 例乳腺癌全乳切除术后重建患者（37 例即刻重建，13 例延期重建）。其中，50 侧乳房为治疗性切除，19 侧为高风险预防性切除。50 例患者共行 69 侧 LOTUS 重建术，平均随访 26 个月。

严重不良事件包括 3 例术后皮下软组织复发（于门诊随访体检中发现），治疗性乳房切除组局部区域复发率为 6%（3/50），平均随访 2 年 2 个月。我院历史对照数据（2008—2015）显示，39 例治疗性保留皮肤/乳头的全乳切除硅胶假体重建未应用可吸收网片及脂肪移植组的局部区域复发率为 7.69%（平均随访 7 年）。2009 年，Gerber 报道的 60 例保留乳头全乳切除自体组织瓣重建复发率为 11.7%（平均随访 8.4 年）[7]。本组复发率较低与随访周期较短有关——3 例复发均见于未接受辅助治疗的高危癌患者（表 22.1）。

次重要不良事件为术后触及性肿块：11 侧乳房体检发现实质性团块［6 例（8.7%）为油性囊肿，5 例（7.2%）为脂肪坏死］，影像学检查另检出 16 个无临床症状油性囊肿（23.2%）及 7 处影像学脂肪坏死病灶（10.1%）。所有病灶均为良性，共行 10 次活检（门诊开放切除活检 6 次，影像引导下穿刺活检 4 次），活检率为 14.5%，结果均为阴性。4 例（5.8%）触及多个厘米级油性囊肿合并坏死灶（其中 3 例为放疗后或硅胶重建失败修复病

表 22.1 局部复发辅助治疗

病例编号	复发时间（年）	分期	肿瘤特征	化疗史	激素治疗	放疗史	乳头复发	备注信息
5	1	IA 期（T1Nx）	浸润性导管癌（IDC），Her2 阳性	–	–	–	(–)	接受过双侧保乳术及放疗，未进行辅助化疗 复发前未使用赫赛汀（Herceptin）辅助治疗
23	1	IA 期（T1cNo）	浸润性导管癌（IDC），雌激素受体阳性（ER+），同步肿瘤	–	+/–	–	(–)	ASA 3 级，BMI 40，化疗尝试失败，复发前已停用激素治疗 存在化疗禁忌
38	0.5	IIB 期（T2N0）	浸润性导管癌（IDC），三阴性（ER-/PR-/Her2-），组织学分级 3 级	–	–	–	(–)	拒绝辅助化疗及放疗 家族史（侄女 30 余岁因同类癌症去世）

例）。其他术后肿块均需细致触诊方可发现。

其他事件包括8侧乳房术后积液（11.6%），其中4例发生于微创全乳切除LOTUS置入重建术后（3例未常规留置引流管），4例见于脂肪移植术后。积液培养显示6侧伴细菌定植（仅2侧伴蜂窝织炎临床表现），经口服抗生素治愈。另有1例脂肪注射点表浅感染（口服抗生素消退）。总体的轻症感染发生率为10%（7/69），无需住院或静脉用药的严重感染病例。

3例发生部分乳头-乳晕复合体缺失（2例因合并下垂矫正术致缺血坏死，1例因癌浸润切除），发生率为4.3%。6侧接受放疗乳房仅1例出现慢性毛细血管扩张。经验显示，放疗会增加脂肪移植难度（通常所需移植次数可能会加倍）。

未见血肿、网片移位、包膜挛缩、假体外露、皮瓣坏死、假体取出或慢性疼痛等并发症。

22.2.1 术后监测建议

在这项新型乳房重建技术的初期应用中，油性囊肿与脂肪坏死是常见并发症，但局部复发率仅为6%（均为体检发现并经切除活检确诊）。超声检查是诊断深部良性肿块（疑似油性囊肿或脂肪坏死）的首选方法。如前所述，4例影像学结果模棱两可的患者而需行穿刺活检。

22.2.2 重建效果评级

本机构近年方引入乳腺Q量表用于疗效评估，此前主要依赖主观评级：由熟悉LOTUS队列患者的4位办公室成员及术者对60侧已完成重建的乳房（1例失访、8例未完成）进行评价。评级标准如下：A级，术后乳房与健侧无异/双侧重建无手术痕迹；B级，效果优良但可觉察重建痕迹；C级，着衣效果良好而裸体形态欠自然；D级，效果差但可接受；F级，佩戴外置假体更佳。为避免自评偏差，将结果分为三类：优，A+B占比65%；良，C占比21%；差，D+F占比14%。近2/3病例获得优异效果，多数D/F级病例可通过追加脂肪移植改善评级。

22.2.3 小结

百年间乳腺癌术式向微创精准演进，推动重建技术进步和胸肌前乳房重建技术的复兴。脂肪移植技术的突破实现了无需组织瓣移植的自体重建，可吸收网片支架的应用使即刻乳房重建联合序贯脂肪移植（平均两次）获得自然形态成为可能。

本组病例未见严重并发症，局部复发均位于真皮下层且易于体检发现。油性囊肿与脂肪坏死为最常见并发症（多数经影像学评估为良性），疑诊者行微创穿刺活检即可。随着技术的规范化，有望进一步规避积液与感染等严重并发症。这项融合假体重建简便性与自体重建自然性的混合技术，展现了乳房重建新的发展方向。

参考文献

1. Rehnke RD, Groening RM, Van Buskirk ER,

Clarke JM. Anatomy of the superfcial fascia system of the breast. Plast Reconstr Surg. 2018,142（5）:1135–44.
2. Rehnke RD, Schusterman MA, Clarke JM, Price BC, Waheed U, Debski RE, Badylak SF, Rubin JP. Breast reconstruction using a three-dimensional absorbable mesh scaffold and autologous fat grafting. Plast Reconstr Surg. 2020,146（4）:409e–13e.
3. Doldere JH, Thompson EW, Slavin J, et al. Long-term stability of adipose tissue generated from a vascularized pedicle fat fap inside a chamber. Plast Reconstr Surg. 2011,127:2283–92.
4. Salibian A, Harness JK, Mowlds DS. Staged suprapectoral expander/implant reconstruction. Plast Reconstr Surg. 2017,139（1）:30–9. https://doi.org/10.1097/PRS.0000000002845.
5. Stiles H. The surgical anatomy of the breast and axillary lymphatic gland. Edinburgh: Oliver and Boyd; 1892. https://doi.org/10.1136/bmj.1.2007.1452.
6. Su X, Lyu Y, Wang W, et al. Fascia origin of adipose cells. Stem Cells. 2016,34:1407–19.
7. Gerber B, Krause A, Dieterich M, et al. The oncologic safety of skin sparing mastectomy with conservation of the nipple-areola complex and autologous reconstruction: an extended follow-up study. Ann Surg. 2009,249（3）:461–8. https://doi.org/10.1097/sla.0b013e31819a044f.

23 内镜辅助保留乳头和皮肤乳房切除术

编者：Hung-Wen Lai and Chi Wei Mok
译者：徐娜娜　霍志军

23.1 引言

微创或小切口乳房手术主要指借助内镜器械及近年发展起来的机器人手术平台实行的乳房手术[1]，技术核心在于通过隐蔽部位小切口（图23.1）实现肿瘤根治性切除，在保障手术安全性的同时提升美学效果，并可通过同一切口完成即刻乳房重建[2-4]。通过内镜器械的高清光学显像优化术野暴露，使小切口下的肿瘤根治性切除成为可能[5-7]。

内镜辅助乳房切除术最早在部分亚洲国家开展并推广[7-10]，显著优势在于：对于小乳房体积患者，保乳手术常面临切除范围不足或切缘阳性风险，并且美学效果欠佳；而该术式能显著改善此类患者的术后美观度。尽管多项研究已证实该技术的可行性、美学优势及安全性[7, 8, 11~15]，但其尚未成为乳腺癌治疗的主流方案，可能原因包括：缺乏长期随访数据以明确局部区域复发、远处转移及疾病生存结局的肿瘤学安全性；患者筛选及适应证把控也可能是限制其常规应用的重要因素。本章将系统阐述内镜辅助保留乳头-乳晕复合体或皮肤的乳房切除术（NSM）在乳腺癌治疗中的应用。图23.1展示了传统、内镜辅助及机器人辅助NSM的临床照片及示意图。

图 23.1 不同术式与切口设计对照（C-NSM，常规保留乳头乳房切除术；E-NSM，内镜辅助保留乳头乳房切除术；3D-E-NSM，单孔三维腔镜辅助保留乳头乳房切除术；R-NSM，机器人辅助保留乳头乳房切除术）

C-NSM

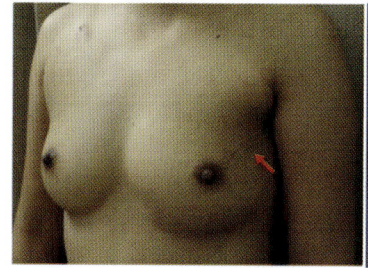
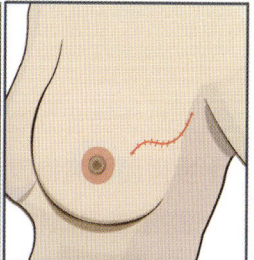

E-NSM（双切口）

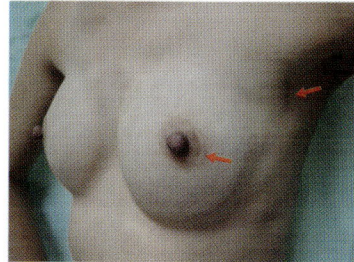
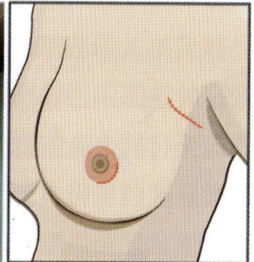

E-NSM（腋下单一切口）

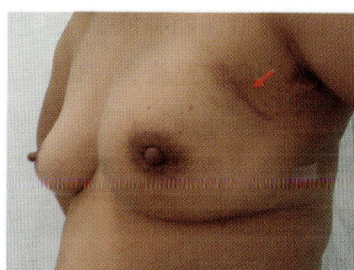
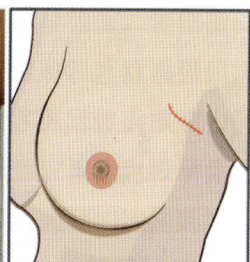

3D-E-NSM（腋下单一切口）

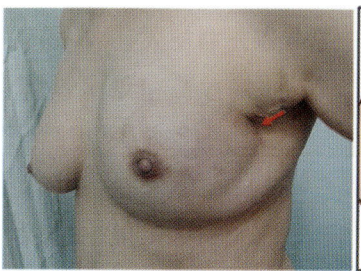
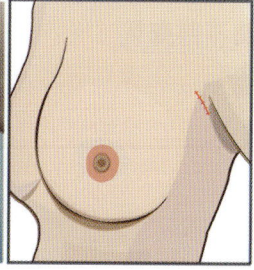

R-NSM（侧胸切口）

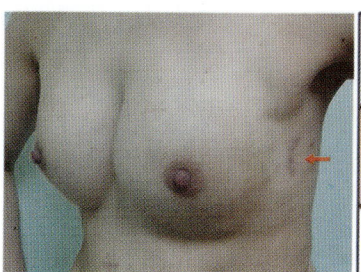
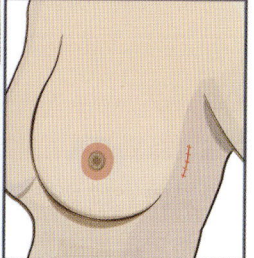

23.2 技术细节详解[16]

23.2.1 体位与前哨淋巴结活检

患者取仰卧位，术侧上肢外展90°置于托手板上。需行前哨淋巴结活检（SLNB）者，可采用单一或联合应用锝-99m（Tc99m）和/或亚甲蓝染料的双重示踪法。手术当日或术前一日于真皮层注射2~3mCi放射性核素Tc99m。注射亚甲蓝后，使用手持式γ探针定位热点区域并标记高摄取淋巴结位置。双重示踪法中，将稀释的1%亚甲基蓝溶液（德国默克公司）2~3mL等分后注入乳晕区真皮下层。

23.2.2 E-NSM皮肤切口设计

可选择腋窝或侧胸壁单/双切口，具体根据手术性质及腋窝分期需求决定。亦可采用腋窝-乳晕双切口或腋窝-乳房下皱襞双切口（图23.2）。切口通常长3~6cm，依据乳房体积调整。采用经腋窝切口，按需实施腋窝分期手术；若术中冰冻切片病理检查阳性，可在乳房切除前/后完成Ⅱ级腋窝淋巴结清扫（ALND）。

23.2.3 后平面解剖

腋窝分期操作完成后，自胸大肌外侧缘开始分离。明确胸大肌与乳腺体组织边界后，使用内镜专用超长静脉牵开器（Karl Storz或Johnson & Johnson KK，图23.3）将胸肌筋膜与乳腺体后部分离。用电凝或能量器械（双极电剪、超声刀）确保充分止血。为构建有效操作空间，可在内镜引导下用牵开器对抗牵引周围组织，并配合吸引器清除烟雾。图23.3展示内镜辅助乳房手术常用器械。

23.2.4 皮瓣剥离

以含0.05%利多卡因及1:1 000 000肾上腺素的混合溶液行全乳皮下注射，兼具镇痛、止血及辅助解剖分离作用。经腋窝或侧胸壁切口采用皮瓣隧道法构建厚3~5mm的皮瓣。若选择双切口入路，可依术者习惯行乳晕旁半环形切口或乳房下皱襞切口（3~4cm）。皮瓣隧道法可在内镜引导下用光学套管穿刺器Xcel（Johnson & Johnson，图23.3）完成，亦可采用Metzenbaum剪刀触诊引导。操作步骤见图23.4。

23.2.5 单孔气腔扩张法与牵拉法 E-NSM

行牵拉法E-NSM时，在内镜引导下用内镜剪、双极电剪或超声刀离断皮瓣与腺体间纤维隔。行气腔扩张法E-NSM时，则经腋窝或侧胸壁切口插入单孔套管，注入CO_2建立气腔（压力设定8~10mmHg，图23.5）。气腔扩张可提供更佳操作空间，尤其适用于NSM。三维内镜系统可增强术野立体感知，研究证实其在内镜辅助NSM中具有重要价值[16]。图23.5展示了单孔三维E-NSM关键步骤。

23.2.6 乳头下腺体活检

皮瓣剥离完成后，如拟行NSM，则需取乳头下腺体组织送冰冻切片病理检查

23 内镜辅助保留乳头和皮肤乳房切除术

图 23.2 内镜辅助保留乳头乳房切除术常见切口模式示意图

单腋窝切口

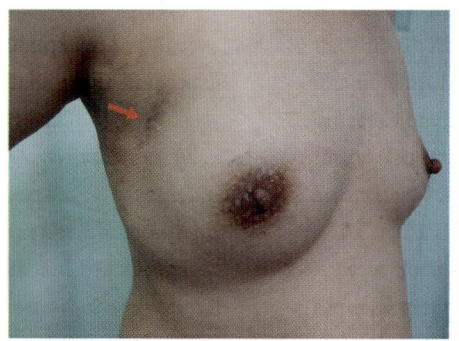
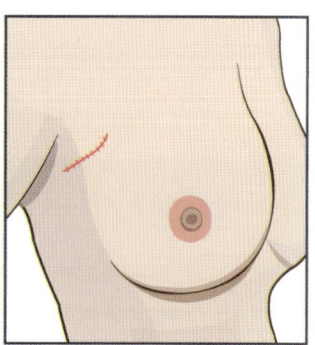

胸外侧切口

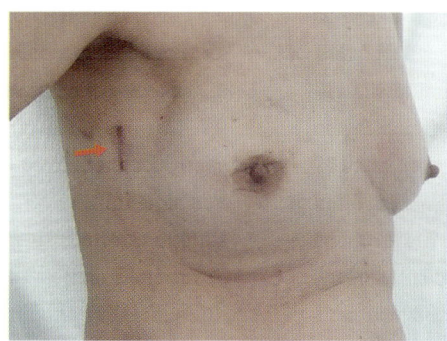
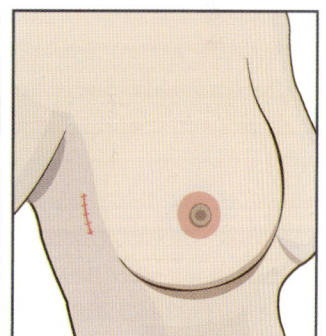

双腋窝 - 乳晕切口

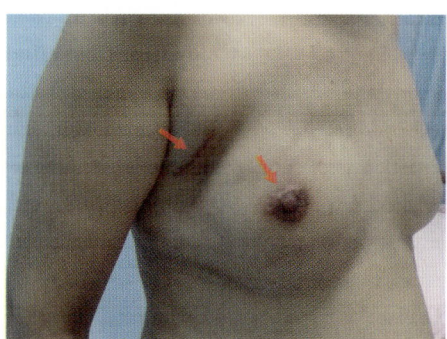
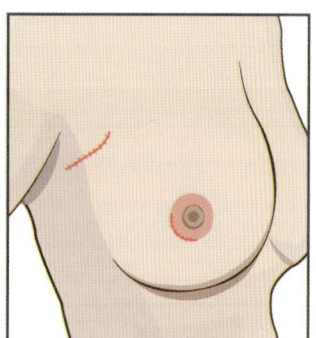

腋窝 - 乳房下切口

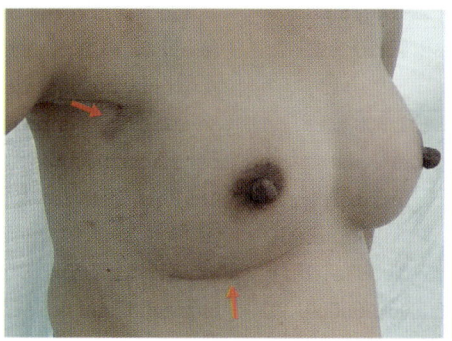
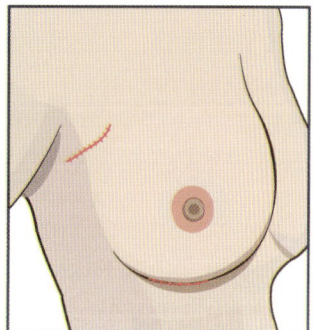

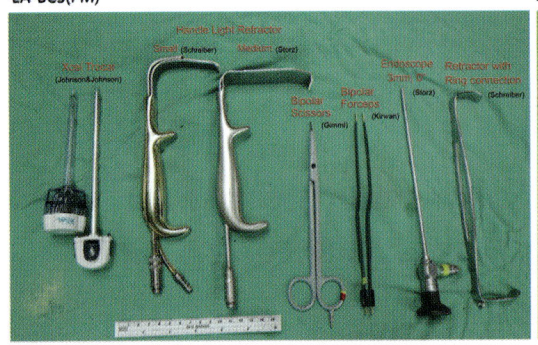 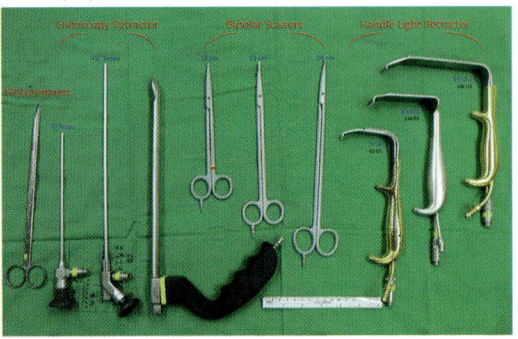

图 23.3　内镜辅助乳腺外科常用器械（EA-BCS，内镜辅助保乳术；PM，乳房部分切除术；EA-NSM，内镜辅助保留乳头乳房切除术；TM，全乳切除术）

（图 23.4）。若病理提示癌累及，则改为保留皮肤乳房切除术（SSM）。完整游离皮瓣并离断胸大肌筋膜及外周附着后，经腋窝或乳晕旁切口取出全乳标本（图 23.4）。

23.2.7　胸肌后假体重建

移除标本后，以生理盐水或聚维酮碘溶液充分冲洗术腔。随后，掀起胸大肌外侧缘在胸肌后平面进行分离，向内分离至胸骨旁，注意保护穿支血管；向下游离超过乳房下皱襞外侧部，在此水平以下松开肌肉，继续在皮下平面进行分离，可使假体被置于更自然的位置（图 23.4）。在外侧界，分离前锯肌浅筋膜至恰好容纳假体侧缘。置入假体后，于肌后平面及皮下分别放置引流管，并注意缝合外侧游离肌缘以确保假体充分覆盖。

23.3　内镜辅助保留乳头和皮肤的乳房切除术在适应证、技术与结局指标方面的现有证据（表 23.1）[17]

23.3.1　E-NSM 的适应证 [7, 15, 16]

E-NSM 的适应证包括早期乳腺癌，肿瘤大小不超过 5cm，无多发淋巴结转移证据，无皮肤或胸壁侵犯证据。禁忌证包括明显乳头-乳晕复合体受累，炎性乳腺癌，存在胸壁或皮肤侵犯的乳腺癌，局部进展期乳腺癌，伴广泛腋窝淋巴结转移的乳腺癌（ⅢB 期或更晚）以及合并严重基础疾病（如心脏病、肾衰竭、肝功能不全及全身状况差）的患者。

关于乳房大小与形态，理想适应人群为中小型乳房且无或仅有轻度下垂者。根据罩杯标准，建议选择 C 罩杯及以下病例。E 罩杯以上或乳房切除重量 >600g 并伴有乳房下垂者，由于技术难度及美学效果欠佳，不建议行 E-NSM 联合即刻假体重建。

23 内镜辅助保留乳头和皮肤乳房切除术

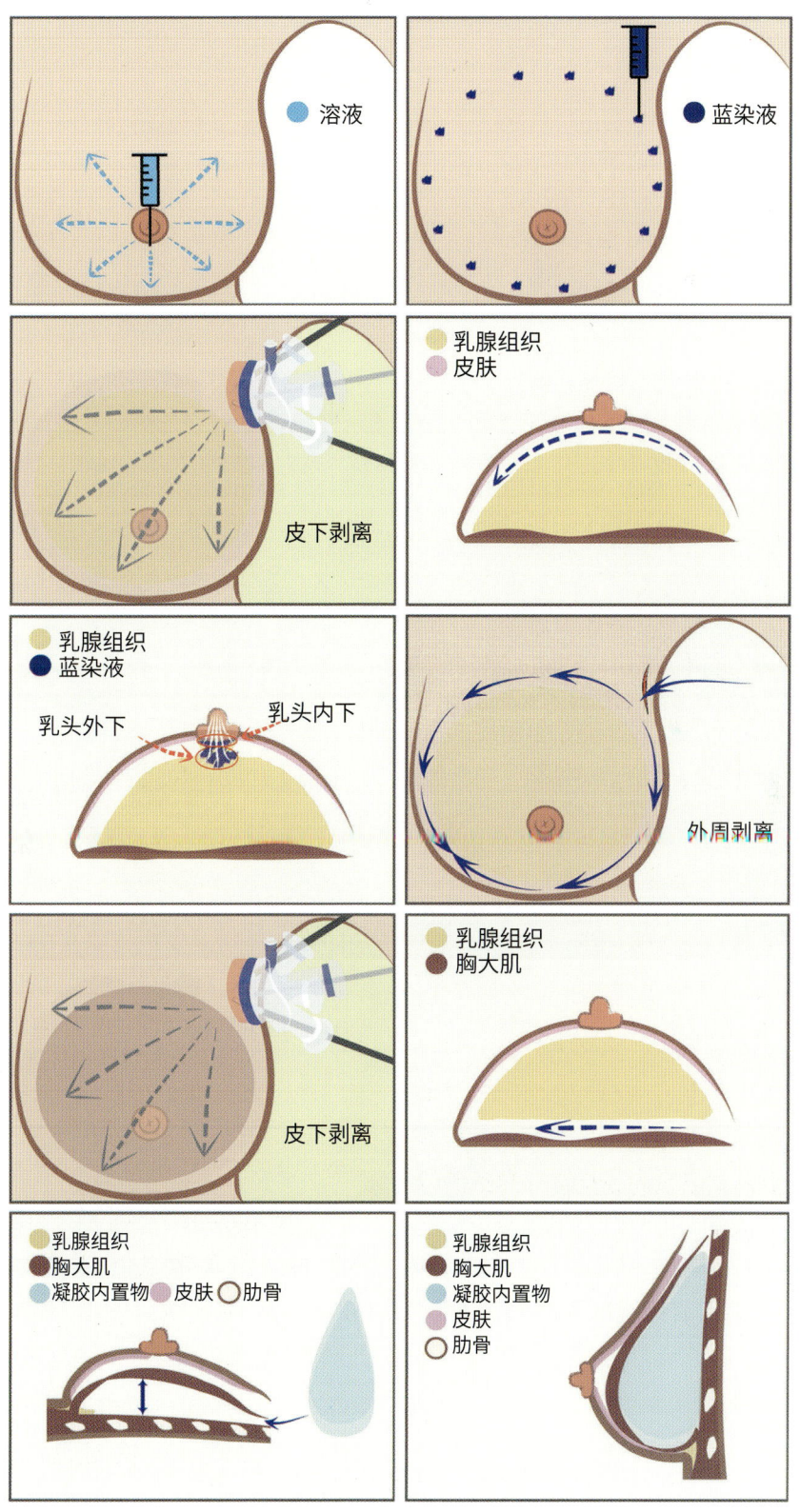

图 23.4　腋窝单切口内镜辅助保留乳头乳房切除联合假体即刻重建

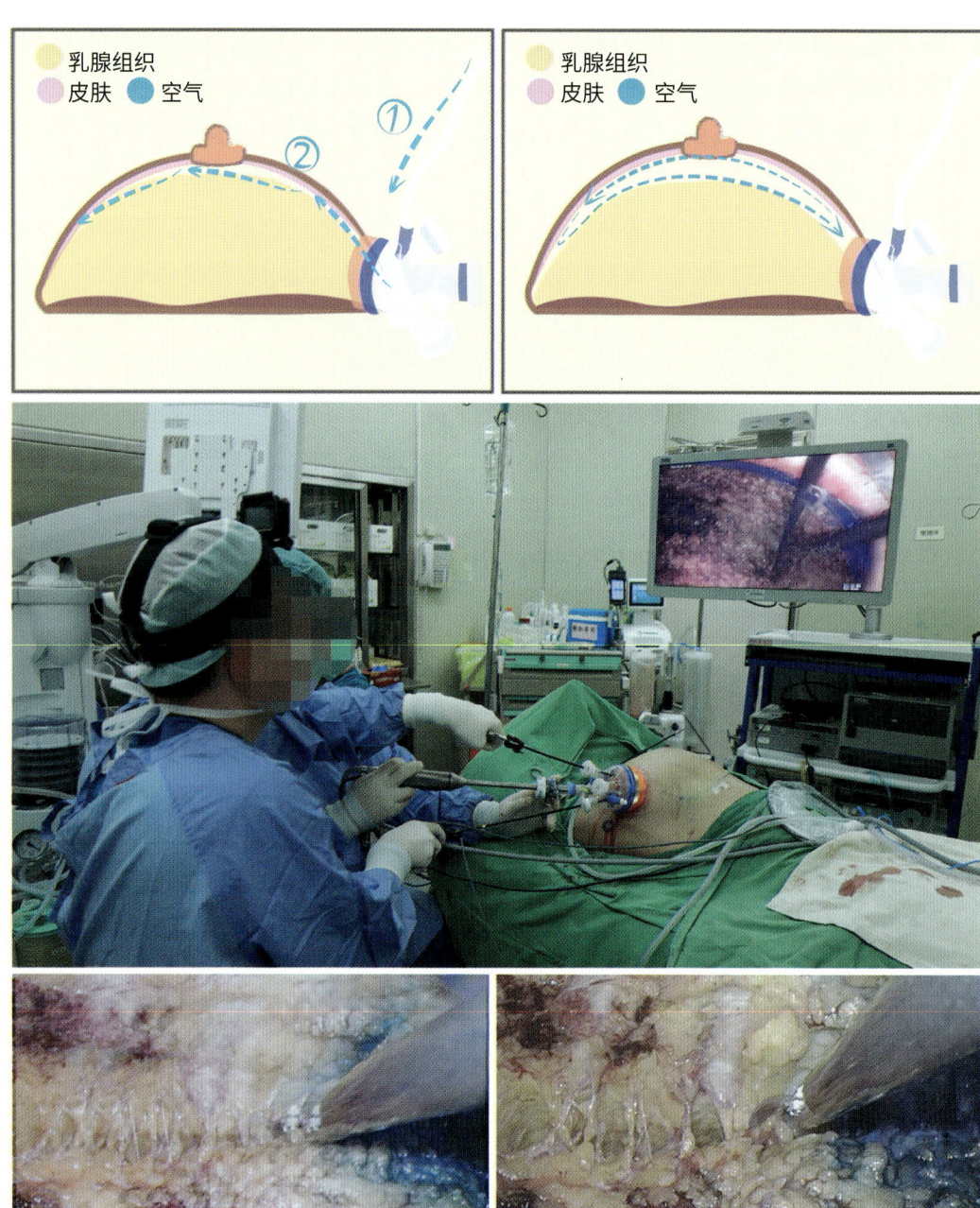

图 23.5　单孔三维腔镜系统辅助保留乳头乳房切除术（3D-E-NSM）操作理念与流程（解析见正文）

表 23.1 现有队列研究及精选病例系列研究的证据：内镜辅助与传统保留乳头乳房切除术的对比分析

序号	作者	发表年份	治疗患者/乳房数	手术方法	平均手术时间（分钟，范围或±标准差）	术中失血量（mL或g）	切缘阳性，n(%)	并发症，n(%)	随访时间（月）	局部复发	远处转移	死亡
1	Kitamura 等[11]	2002	20/21	内镜辅助保留乳头乳房切除术（E-NSM）	237±60	156±286g	1(4.8)	假体相关并发症：1(4.8)	19.2±9.8 (5.8-35.2)	无数据	无数据	0%
2	Fan 等[12]	2009	24/25	传统保留乳头乳房切除术（C-NSM）	176±32	189±72g	2(8.0)	假体相关并发症：3(12.0)	无数据	无数据	无数据	0%
			43	内镜辅助保留乳头乳房切除术（E-NSM）	168±32	15±44	0%	乳头或皮瓣坏死：5(11.6)	16.9±11.2	0%	0%	0%
			54	传统保乳手术（C-BCS）	139±37	102±48	0%	血清肿：6(11.1)	20.1±11.9	5.9%	0%	1.9%
3	Wang 等[8]	2016	24	内镜辅助保留乳头乳房切除术（E-NSM）	保乳手术+前哨淋巴结活检：102.38±28.8 保乳手术+腋窝清扫：122.49±40.5	无数据	10.6% (85/681)	无数据	12	0.3% (2/681)	无数据	无数据
			25	传统保留乳头乳房切除术（C-NSM）	69[55-104]	~5[10-80]	28.3% (17/60)	补片感染：11.7%(7/60)	无数据	无数据	无数据	无数据
4	Wang 等[13]	2017	30	内镜辅助保留乳头乳房切除术（E-NSM/E-SSM）		无数据	无数据	无数据	27.77±20.43	无数据	无数据	无数据
			30	传统保留乳头乳房切除术（C-NSM）		无数据	无数据	无数据	43.22±19.80	无数据	无数据	无数据
5	Du 等[14]	2017	157	内镜辅助保留乳头乳房切除术（E-NSM）	197	≤5mL	无数据	感染：5(3.18)；皮瓣坏死：11(7.01)；淋巴水肿：15(9.55)	74(52-111)	0%	4.5%	3.2%
			189	传统保乳手术（C-BCS）	165	≤3mL	无数据	感染：8(8.46)；皮缘坏死：16(8.46)；淋巴水肿：23(12.16)	无数据	3.2%	1.6%	3.2%
6	Lai 等[15]	2016	269	内镜辅助保留乳头/皮肤乳房切除术（E-NSM/E-SSM）	282±161 (65-1310)	104.5±74.9 (20-650)	1.1% (3/269)	总体并发症：15.2%(48/315)	26.8(3.3-68.6)	1.1% (3/269)	无数据	0.4% (1/269)
7	Lai 等[16]	2018	50	内镜辅助保留乳头乳房切除术（E-NSM）	244.3±82.8 (138-425)	74.5±47.7 (25-250)	0%	6%(3/50：乳头部分缺血2%，血清肿4%)	21.6±11.3 (1-42.4)	0%	0%	0%

E-NSM，内镜辅助保留乳头乳房切除术；E-SSM，内镜辅助保留皮肤乳房切除术；C-NSM，传统保留乳头乳房切除术；C-BCS，传统保乳手术；BCS，保乳手术；SNB，前哨淋巴结活检；Ax，腋窝淋巴结清扫

23.3.2 E-NSM 技术优化

近年来，多项技术改进（图 23.1~23.5），包括采用充气法替代牵引法以改善视野，保留乳晕周围切口而转为单一腋窝切口实施 E-NSM，有效降低了乳头-乳晕复合体缺血/坏死的发生率。

多年研究[7, 8, 14, 18]证实了 E-NSM 与传统术式具有等效的技术可行性[19]。如表 23.1 所示，E-NSM 手术时间延长未导致并发症增加，并且突破学习曲线后操作时间可缩短，术中出血量无临床或统计学显著差异；常见并发症（如皮瓣或乳头坏死）与传统术式相似，可能与皮瓣厚度及血供（尤其真皮层暴露的病例）相关。使用肿胀液处理皮瓣的研究显示其有助于提高解剖便利性并维持适当皮瓣厚度。

23.3.3 美学效果

在美学效果及患者满意度评估方面，多数患者对瘢痕位置及切口长度的美观度表示满意（图 23.1，图 23.2）。现有评估多集中于术后 3~6 个月，建议在术后 2~3 年（当乳腺实质重塑完成且完成必要辅助放疗后）进行二次评估。关于复发率、中转手术率及并发症率的具体数据已另文详述[20]。

23.4 讨论

23.4.1 双切口技术

自 2001 年首例报道以来[2]，内镜乳房手术历经了 20 来年技术革新。传统内镜辅助保留乳头乳房切除术（E-NSM）采用腋窝及乳晕周围双切口（图 23.2）进行：腋窝切口用于腋窝分期手术，通过内镜静脉拉钩完成乳腺实质与胸肌筋膜的剥离；乳晕周围小切口则用于分离乳腺实质与皮瓣间的隔。标本切除后可经任一切口取出，瘢痕通常隐蔽于腋窝或乳晕区域。乳晕切口的常见并发症——乳头-乳晕复合体（NAC）缺血或坏死可能造成严重后果，尤其在假体重建病例中可能引发感染，甚至需要取出内置物。

23.4.2 腋窝单切口混合式 E-NSM[15]

为降低 NAC 缺血/坏死风险，本团队首创腋窝单切口技术（图 23.2，图 23.4），显著改善了预后，开创了单切口内镜乳房切除术新趋势。该技术优选肿瘤位于外上象限且与皮肤保持足够距离者，以确保切缘阴性。对于大而下垂乳房，建议采用腋窝-乳房下皱襞（IMF）双切口（图 23.2），瘢痕可隐藏于 IMF 内。本术式推荐用于中小型乳房、轻度下垂、早期临床淋巴结阴性需行乳房切除的患者。

23.4.3 充气技术[6, 15, 16]

腋窝单切口混合式 E-NSM 虽可降低 NAC 坏死风险，但操作空间受限。基于无气内镜手术经验，本团队引入充气技术（图 23.5），通过扩张手术空间显著改善手术视野，同时促进解剖平面的分离与止血，成为技术发展的里程碑。

23.4.4 三维成像技术[16]

三维成像技术通过增强立体视感为内镜手术带来了革新。本团队采用单孔充气系统与 3D 内镜（图 23.5），有效降低了传统 2D 单切口 E-NSM 的技术难度。初步应用显示其美学效果优异且学习曲线短，展现了良好应用前景。

23.4.5 内镜辅助乳房手术的其他进展：机器人辅助保留乳头乳房切除术

除三维成像技术外，另一项具有变革性潜力的进展是机器人辅助乳房切除术。机器人手术整合三维成像系统，借助灵活机械臂及高自由度器械，已在多个外科领域得到应用。机器人辅助保留乳头的乳房切除术（R-NSM）通过达·芬奇手术平台经小腋窝切口行 NSM（联合/不联合即刻假体重建；图 23.6），研究显示其可克服 E-NSM 技术限制并改善美学效果[21-24]。另有研究探索了机器人平台在即刻自体乳房重建中的应用[24-26]，优势包括三维光学系统增强术野清晰度，器械高自由度提升操作舒适性，主要局限为手术时间长、费用高昂及机器人平台可及性不足[27,28]。近期机器人乳腺手术先驱发布共识声明[29]，明确了 R-NSM 的适应证、禁忌证及操作注意事项。

23.4.6 内镜辅助乳房切除假体重建：胸肌后与胸肌前

内镜辅助乳房切除术的即刻重建方式多采用假体置入，胸肌后假体置入（图 23.4，23.6）仍为主流术式，常联合脱细胞真皮基质（ADM）加强假体外下象限覆盖。近年来，对胸肌前假体置入联合 ADM/合成网片全包裹技术的研究逐渐增多[30,31]，潜在优势在于显著缩短手术时间，并且当发生皮瓣坏死时假体暴露/感染风险较低。因 E-NSM 或 R-NSM 单腋窝/侧胸切口可降低皮瓣及 NAC 缺血/坏死率，二者具备开展胸肌前假体重建的条件。胸肌前假体置入将成为微创乳房切除术的下一步发展方向[32-34]。

23.5 小结

随着技术进步与术式优化，微创/小切口乳房切除术未来十年将持续发展，技术完善与效果提升有望推动其成为乳腺癌外科治疗标准方案。未来需加强国际多中心协作，构建内镜/机器人辅助手术规范化培训体系，同时亟待开展长期肿瘤学结局评估及成本效益分析，以进一步确立内镜辅助技术在乳腺癌外科治疗中的地位。

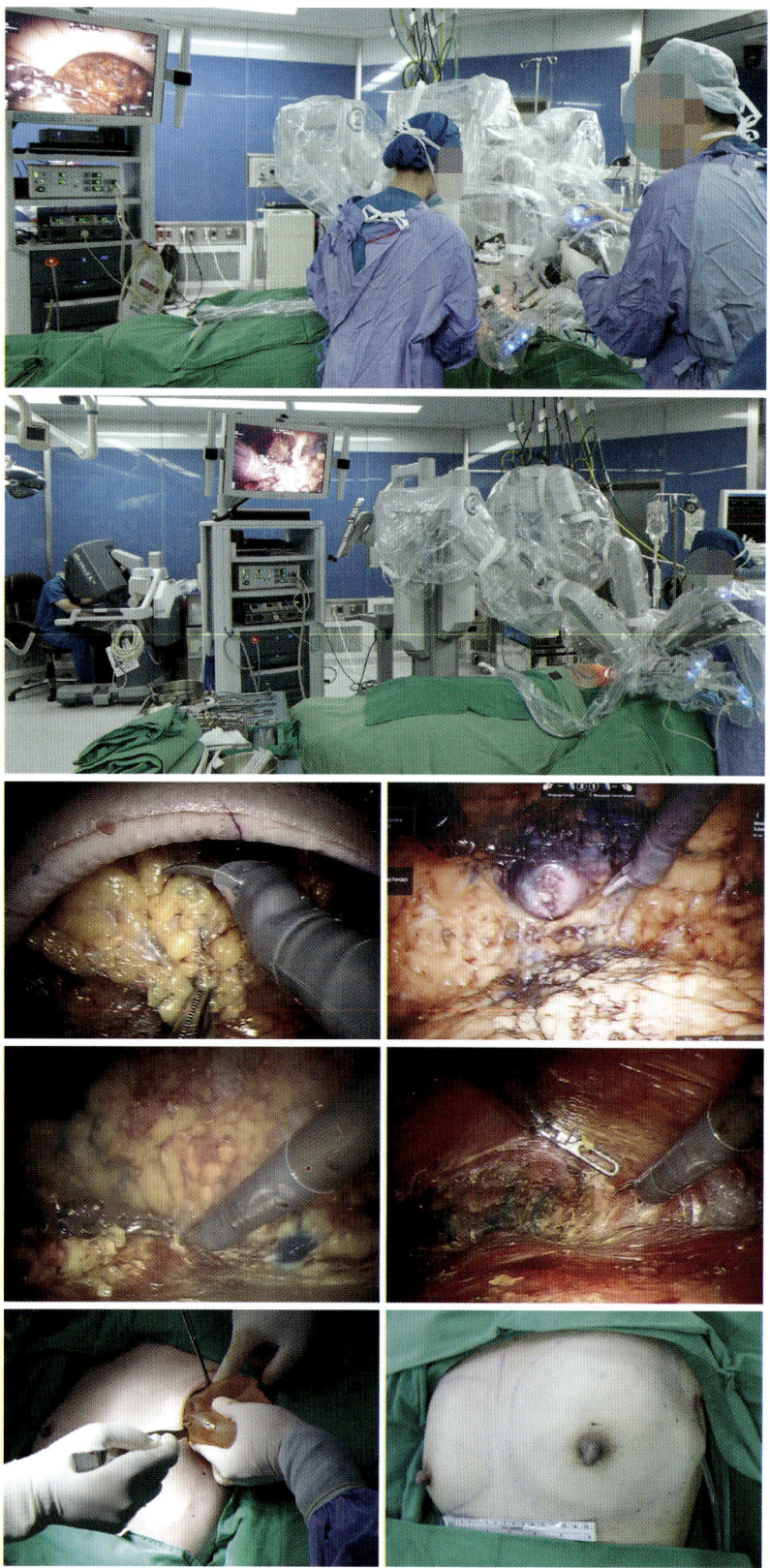

图 23.6 达·芬奇 Si 机器人系统辅助乳腺癌保留乳头乳房切除术（R-NSM）操作实景图（同期行假体即刻重建）

参考文献

1. Mok CW, Lai HW. Evolution of minimal access breast surgery. Gland Surg. 2019,8（6）:784–93. https://doi.org/10.21037/gs.2019.11.16. PMID: 32042687; PMCID: PMC6989909.
2. Tamaki Y, Sakita I, Miyoshi Y, Sekimoto M, Takiguchi S, Monden M, Noguchi S. Transareolar endoscopy-assisted partial mastectomy: a pre-liminary report of six cases. Surg Laparosc Endosc Percutan Tech. 2001,11（6）:356–62. https://doi.org/10.1097/00129689-200112000-00003. PMID: 11822858.
3. Ozaki S, Ohara M, Shigematsu H, Sasada T, Emi A, Masumoto N, Kadoya T, Murakami S, Kataoka T, Fujii M, Arihiro K, Okada M. Technical feasibility and cosmetic advantage of hybrid endoscopy-assisted breast-conserving surgery for breast cancer patients. J Laparoendosc Adv Surg Tech A. 2013,23（2）:91–9. https://doi.org/10.1089/lap.2012.0224. Epub 2012 Dec 28. PMID: 23272727.
4. Leff DR, Vashisht R, Yongue G, Keshtgar M, Yang GZ, Darzi A. Endoscopic breast surgery: where are we now and what might the future hold for video-assisted breast surgery? Breast Cancer Res Treat. 2011,125（3）:607–25. https://doi.org/10.1007/s10549-010-1258-4. Epub 2010 Dec 3. PMID: 21128113.
5. Fukuma E.［Endoscopic breast surgery for breast can-cer］. Nihon Geka Gakkai Zasshi. 2006,107（2）:64–8. Japanese. PMID: 16613205.
6. Tukenmez M, Ozden BC, Agcaoglu O, Kecer M, Ozmen V, Muslumanoglu M, Igci A. Videoendoscopic single-port nipple-sparing mastectomy and imme-diate reconstruction. J Laparoendosc Adv Surg Tech A. 2014,24（2）:77–82. https://doi.org/10.1089/lap.2013.0172. Epub 2014 Jan 8. PMID: 24401140; PMCID: PMC3935461.
7. Lai HW, Chen ST, Chen DR, Chen SL, Chang TW, Kuo SJ, Kuo YL, Hung CS. Current trends in and indications for endoscopy-assisted breast surgery for breast cancer: results from a six-year study conducted by the Taiwan endoscopic breast surgery coopera-tive group. PLoS One. 2016,11（3）:e0150310. https://doi.org/10.1371/journal.pone.0150310. PMID: 26950469; PMCID: PMC4780808.
8. Wang ZH, Qu X, Teng CS, Ge ZC, Zhang HM, Yuan Z, Gao YG, Lu C, Yu JA, Zhang ZT. Preliminary results for treatment of early stage breast cancer with endoscopic subcutaneous mastectomy com-bined with endoscopic sentinel lymph node biopsy in China. J Surg Oncol. 2016,113（6）:616–20. https://doi.org/10.1002/jso.24199. Epub 2016 Apr 4. PMID: 27040619.
9. Ho WS, Ying SY, Chan AC. Endoscopic-assisted sub-cutaneous mastectomy and axillary dissection with immediate mammary prosthesis reconstruction for early breast cancer. Surg Endosc. 2002,16（2）:302–6. https://doi.org/10.1007/s004640000203. Epub 2001 Nov 16. PMID: 11967683.
10. Nakajima H, Sakaguchi K, Mizuta N, Hachimine T, Ohe S, Sawai K. Video-assisted total glandectomy and immediate reconstruction for breast cancer. Biomed Pharmacother. 2002,56（Suppl 1）:205s–8s. https://doi.org/10.1016/s0753-3322（02）00281-0. PMID: 12487283.
11. Kitamura K, Ishida M, Inoue H, Kinoshita J, Hashizume M, Sugimachi K. Early results of an endoscope-assisted subcutaneous mastectomy and reconstruction for breast cancer. Surgery. 2002,131（1 Suppl）:S324–9. https://doi.org/10.1067/msy.2002.120120. PMID: 11821832.
12. Fan LJ, Jiang J, Yang XH, Zhang Y, Li XG, Chen XC, Zhong L. A prospective study comparing endoscopic subcutaneous mastectomy plus immediate reconstruc-tion with implants and breast conserving surgery for breast cancer. Chin Med J（Engl）. 2009,122（24）:2945–50. PMID: 20137479.
13. Wang Y, Wu JX, Guan S. A technique of endoscopic nipple-sparing mastectomy for breast cancer. JSLS. 2017,21（2）:e2017.00028. https://

14. Du J, Liang Q, Qi X, Ming J, Liu J, Zhong L, Fan L, Jiang J. Endoscopic nipple sparing mastectomy with immediate implant-based reconstruction versus breast conserving surgery: a long-term study. Sci Rep. 2017,7:45636. https://doi.org/10.1038/srep45636. PMID: 28361955; PMCID: PMC5374499.

15. Lai HW, Lin SL, Chen ST, Kuok KM, Chen SL, Lin YL, Chen DR, Kuo SJ. Single-axillary-incision endo¬scopic-assisted hybrid technique for nipple-sparing 2mastectomy: technique, preliminary results, and patient-reported cosmetic outcome from preliminary 50 procedures. Ann Surg Oncol. 2018,25(5):1340–9. https://doi.org/10.1245/s10434-018- 6383- z. Epub 2018 Feb 26. PMID: 29484564.

16. Lai HW, Mok CW. Endoscopic mastectomy with immediate implant reconstruction. In: Minimally invasive (endoscopic & robotic) breast surgery. Elsevier; 2020. p. 79–112. https://doi.org/10.1016/b978-0- 323- 73405- 9.00005- 4.

17. Mok CW, Lai HW. Endoscopic-assisted surgery in the management of breast cancer: 20 years review of trend, techniques and outcomes. Breast. 2019,46:144–56.https://doi.org/10.1016/j.breast.2019.05.013. Epub 2019 May 20. PMID: 31176887.

18. Lai HW, Chen ST, Mok CW, Lin SL, Tai CM, Chen DR, Kuo SJ. Single-port 3-dimensional videoscope-assisted endoscopic nipple-sparing mastectomy in the management of breast cancer. Plast Reconstr Surg Glob Open. 2019,7(8):e2367. https://doi.org/10.1097/GOX.0000000000002367. PMID: 31592384; PMCID: PMC6756665.

19. Sakamoto N, Fukuma E, Higa K, Ozaki S, Sakamoto M, Abe S, Kurihara T, Tozaki M. Early results of an endoscopic nipple-sparing mastectomy for breast cancer. Ann Surg Oncol. 2009,16(12):3406–13. https://doi.org/10.1245/s10434-009- 0661- 8. PMID: 19662457.

20. Frey JD, Salibian AA, Lee J, Harris K, Axelrod DM, Guth AA, Shapiro RL, Schnabel FR, Karp NS, Choi M. Oncologic trends, outcomes, and risk factors for locoregional recurrence: an analysis of tumor-to-nipple distance and critical factors in therapeutic nipple-sparing mastectomy. Plast Reconstr Surg. 2019,143(6):1575–85. https://doi.org/10.1097/PRS.0000000000005600. PMID: 30907805.

21. Toesca A, Peradze N, Manconi A, Galimberti V, Intra M, Colleoni M, Bonanni B, Curigliano G, Rietjens M, Viale G, Sacchini V, Veronesi P. Robotic nipple-sparing mastectomy for the treatment of breast cancer: feasibility and safety study. Breast. 2017,31:51–6. https://doi.org/10.1016/j.breast.2016.10.009. Epub 2016 Nov 2. PMID: 27810700; PMCID: PMC5278881.

22. Sarfati B, Struk S, Leymarie N, Honart JF, Alkhashnam H, Tran de Fremicourt K, Conversano A, Rimareix F, Simon M, Michiels S, Kolb F. Robotic prophylactic nipple-sparing mastectomy with immediate prosthetic breast reconstruction: a prospective study. Ann Surg Oncol. 2018,25(9):2579–86. https://doi.org/10.1245/s10434-018- 6555- x. Epub 2018 Jun 29. PMID: 29959612.

23. Lai HW, Chen ST, Lin SL, Chen CJ, Lin YL, Pai SH, Chen DR, Kuo SJ. Robotic nipple-sparing mastectomy and immediate breast reconstruction with gel implant: technique, preliminary results and patient-reported cosmetic outcome. Ann Surg Oncol. 2019,26(1):42–52. https://doi.org/10.1245/s10434-018-6704- 2. Epub 2018 Aug 14. PMID: 30109537.

24. Park HS, Lee J, Lee DW, Song SY, Lew DH, Kim SI, Cho YU. Robot-assisted nipple-sparing mastectomy with immediate breast reconstruction: an initial experience. Sci Rep. 2019,9(1):15669. https://doi.org/10.1038/s41598-019- 51744- 2. Erratum in: Sci Rep. 2020,10(1):7602. PMID: 31666551; PMCID: PMC6821761.

25. Houvenaeghel G, Bannier M, Rua S, Barrou J, Heinemann M, Knight S, Lambaudie E, Cohen M. Robotic breast and reconstructive surgery: 100 procedures in 2-years for 80 patients. Surg Oncol. 2019,31:38–45. https://doi.org/10.1016/j.suronc.2019.09.005. Epub 2019 Sep 10. PMID: 31526915.

26. Lai HW, Lin SL, Chen ST, Lin YL, Chen DR, Pai SS, Kuo SJ. Robotic nipple sparing mastectomy and immediate breast reconstruction with robotic latissimus Dorsi flap harvest—technique and preliminary results. J Plast Reconstr Aesthet Surg. 2018,71(10):e59–61. https://doi.org/10.1016/j.bjps.2018.07.006. Epub 2018 Aug 2. PMID: 30122600.

27. Kuo WL, Huang JJ, Huang YT, Chueh LF, Lee JT, Tsai HP, Chen SC. Robot-assisted mastectomy followed by immediate autologous microsurgical free flap reconstruction: techniques and feasibility in three different breast cancer surgical scenarios. Clin Breast Cancer. 2020,20(1):e1–8. https://doi.org/10.1016/j.clbc.2019.06.018. Epub 2019 Sep 4. PMID: 31780382.

28. Lai HW, Chen ST, Tai CM, Lin SL, Lin YJ, Huang RH, Mok CW, Chen DR, Kuo SJ. Robotic- versus endoscopic-assisted nipple-sparing mastectomy with immediate prosthesis breast reconstruction in the management of breast cancer: a case-control comparison study with analysis of clinical outcomes, learning curve, patient-reported aesthetic results, and medical cost. Ann Surg Oncol. 2020,27(7):2255–68. https://doi.org/10.1245/s10434-020-08223-0. Epub 2020 Feb 3. PMID: 32016631.

29. Lai HW, Chen ST, Mok CW, Lin YJ, Wu HK, Lin SL, Chen DR, Kuo SJ. Robotic versus conventional nipple sparing mastectomy and immediate gel implant breast reconstruction in the management of breast cancer—a case control comparison study with analysis of clinical outcome, medical cost, and patient-reported cosmetic results. J Plast Reconstr Aesthet Surg. 2020,73(8):1514–25. https://doi.org/10.1016/j.bjps.2020.02.021. Epub 2020 Feb 18. PMID: 32238306.

30. Lai HW, Toesca A, Sarfati B, Park HS, Houvenaeghel G, Selber JC, Cheng FT, Kuo WL, Peradze N, Song SY, Mok CW. Consensus statement on robotic mastectomy-expert panel from international endoscopic and robotic breast surgery symposium (IERBS) 2019. Ann Surg. 2020,271(6):1005–12. https://doi.org/10.1097/SLA.0000000000003789. PMID: 31977514.

31. Jones G, Yoo A, King V, Jao B, Wang H, Rammos C, Elwood E. Prepectoral immediate direct-to-implant breast reconstruction with anterior AlloDerm coverage. Plast Reconstr Surg. 2017,140(6S Prepectoral Breast Reconstruction):31S–8S. https://doi.org/10.1097/PRS.0000000000004048. PMID: 29166345.

32. Casella D, Di Taranto G, Marcasciano M, Sordi S, Kothari A, Kovacs T, Lo Torto F, Cigna E, Calabrese C, Ribuffo D. Evaluation of prepectoral implant placement and complete coverage with TiLoop bra mesh for breast reconstruction: a prospective study on long-term and patient-reported BREAST-Q outcomes. Plast Reconstr Surg. 2019,143(1):1e–9e. https://doi.org/10.1097/PRS.0000000000005078. PMID: 30303929.

33. Rathat G, Herlin C, Bonnel C, Captier G, Duraes M. Endoscopic nipple-sparing mastectomy with immediate prepectoral implant-based reconstruction: a case report. Am J Case Rep. 2019,20:1812–6. https://doi.org/10.12659/AJCR.919669. PMID: 31801936; PMCID: PMC6913238.

34. Parcells A, Spiro S. Exploration of robotic direct to implant breast reconstruction. Plast Reconstr Surg Glob Open. 2020,8(1):e2619. https://doi.org/10.1097/GOX.0000000000002619. PMID: 32095418; PMCID: PMC7015590.

24 胸肌前乳房重建：功能优势与成本－效益分析

编者：L. Cattelani, S. Polotto

译者：唐　军

24.1 胸肌前ＡＤＭ辅助乳房重建的功能评估

24.1.1 引言

当前，乳房重建已成为乳腺癌综合治疗的重要组成部分[1]。接受该手术的多为年龄较轻、预后良好的患者，对术后美学效果及功能恢复有较高期望。提升患者生活质量（QoL）应作为国家卫生体系的核心目标，也要求通过科技进步持续改善重建手术的近期与远期疗效。鉴于术后上肢功能障碍可引发慢性疼痛，导致患者生活质量显著下降，必须对各种术中重建技术的功能影响进行系统化评估[2]。

上肢功能评估体系包含客观检测与主观评价两个方面。客观评估通过标准化检测方法精确量化肌肉功能参数，而主观评价则侧重于患者自身感知与体验的采集。

24.1.2 乳房重建发展背景

自20世纪60年代首次开展乳房重建手术以来，为确保假体获得充分覆盖，开始采用胸肌后置入技术。然而，在紧密附着于胸壁的肌肉（胸大肌、前锯肌）下方人为创建置入空间需要部分松解肌肉，从而导致肌肉功能受损。

单纯胸肌后置入技术存在明显不足（如下极扩张受限、乳房下垂形态欠佳、难以置入300mL以上的假体等），由此又发展了双平面法，但该术式同样会导致明显的肌肉功能损失——需完全松解胸大肌下段起点以覆盖假体上极，而假体下极则置于皮下。

21世纪初，脱细胞真皮基质（acellular dermal matrices, ADMs）开始用于假体外下象限的覆盖，但直到近年，肌肉的有限损毁仍被认为是假体乳房重建的必要代价。

随着 ADMs 前覆盖及全包裹技术的应用，胸肌前乳房重建（prepectoral breast reconstruction, PPBR）应运而生。该技术

L. Cattelani (✉) · S. Polotto
Department of Breast Surgery, University Hospital of Parma, Parma, Italy

© The Author(s), under exclusive license to Springer Nature Switzerland AG 2023
R. Vidya, H. Becker (eds.), *Prepectoral Breast Reconstruction*,
https://doi.org/10.1007/978-3-031-15590-1_24

于原解剖位置重建乳房，假体位于胸肌前方，完全避免肌组织损伤（图24.1）。

显微外科技术［尤其腹壁下动脉穿支皮瓣（DIEP）重建术］是另一种理想重建方式，腹部组织在质与量上均属最佳选择。需要注意的是，并非所有患者都适用此类手术，并且游离皮瓣手术对术者的显微经验要求较高。

对于特定患者，扩大背阔肌肌皮瓣（LD皮瓣）或联合自体脂肪移植仍可作为即刻自体组织乳房重建的适宜选择[3,4]。

24.1.3 胸壁区域功能解剖学要点

胸大肌（pectoralis major, PM）具有维持肩关节稳定性的重要作用，主要负责肱骨内收、内旋及前屈运动。当手臂过度屈曲时，可使肱骨伸展；在肢体固定状态下，可通过收缩辅助躯体上提（如攀爬动作），并参与吸气运动。在止点处离断胸大肌会导致肩关节稳定性及上肢力量显著受损[5]。

前锯肌主要功能为使肩胛骨外展与外旋（上肢前举运动的关键），同时具有稳定肩胛骨对抗胸壁的作用，属辅助吸气肌。

背阔肌（latissimus dorsi, LD）主要参与肩关节内旋、上肢内收及后伸运动，可辅助举臂状态下的肢体下压动作，并在上肢活动中维持肩胛骨与胸壁贴合。双臂高举固定时，可产生躯干上提的攀爬功能，是划船、游泳等运动的重要动力肌。

24.1.4 上肢功能主观评估工具

主观量表是评估重建术后上肢功能受损的重要工具。尽管这类评估对某些功能障碍的检测精度不及客观测试，但能有效反映手术对患者日常生活的影响。

BREAST-Q量表（Memorial Sloan Kettering癌症中心与British Columbia大学联合研发）是目前应用最广泛的乳房重建术后生活质量（QoL）评估工具，其"胸区生理功能"模块（用于胸肌后/胸肌前重建评估）与"背部及肩部生理功能"模块（用于背阔肌皮瓣重建评估）对术后功能评价具有特殊价值。

其他常用评估工具包括：
- 上肢功能障碍问卷（Disabilities of the Arm, Shoulder, and Hand, DASH）及其简明版（quickDASH）。

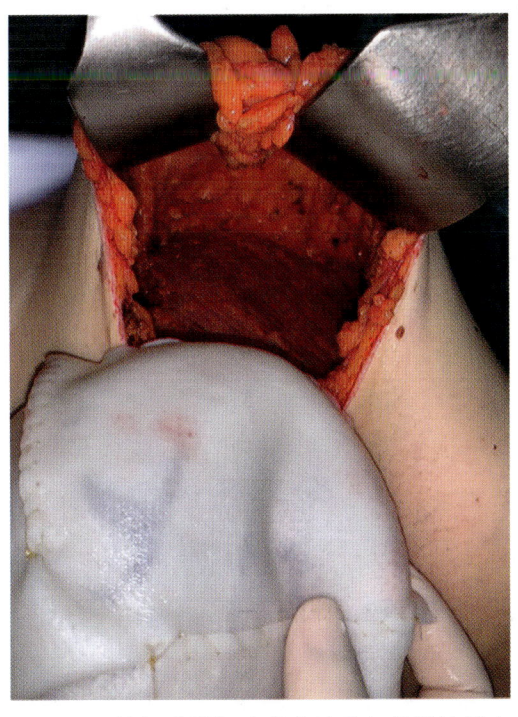

图24.1 前间隙脱细胞真皮基质包裹假体置入（胸大肌筋膜平面完整）。ADM，脱细胞真皮基质；PM，胸大肌

- 肩部疼痛与残障指数量表（Shoulder Pain and Disability Index, SPADI）。
- 美国肩肘外科医师协会标准化肩关节评估表（ASES）。
- 西安大略肩关节不稳定性指数（Western Ontario Shoulder Instability Index, WOSI）。
- 徒手肌力测试（Manual Muscle Test, MMT）。

24.1.5 上肢功能评估的客观验证测试

客观测试提供的原始数据可用于准确评估术后上肢功能（ULF）及其在随访期间的变化趋势。

- 等速测试（如等速测力法）被视为评估关节运动相关肌群力量与耐力的金标准[6]。最大自主等长收缩（MVIC）是通过应变计张力测定仪测量肌力的标准化简易测试。最大等速峰值力矩（MIPT）用于评估肩关节内外旋功能。等速肌力测试（IMPT）则提供肌力及功能信息。
- 肩关节被动与主动活动度（ROM）可通过量角器或数字倾斜仪客观测量。
- 单次最大重复负荷测试（1RM）旨在评估最大肌力。
- 最大自主收缩测试（MVC）。
- 表面或肌电图（EMG）。
- Constant-Murley 评分（CS）。

24.1.6 乳房切除与重建的功能影响

在评估乳房重建术的功能影响前，需考虑乳房切除相关并发症，因两类手术存在必然联系。20%~65% 的肿瘤性乳房切除术后患者会出现不同形式的持续性术后疼痛，统称为乳房切除术后疼痛综合征[7]。此类手术的常见症状包括胸大肌紧张、肌筋膜疼痛综合征、肩袖病变及粘连性关节囊炎。值得注意的是，长期随访发现很多患者持续存在上肢功能减退（ULF），提示术后开展康复治疗对改善患者生活质量至关重要[8]。

虽然前哨淋巴结活检（SLNB）很少引发长期功能障碍，但腋窝淋巴结清扫（ALND）术后出现上肢功能减退的概率较高。数据显示，接受 ALND 的患者在术后 6~12 个月（POM）存在明显的抬高与内收障碍，术后 2 个月仍存在肩关节外展与屈曲活动受限，约 30% 患者主诉上肢功能恶化[9-11]。有学者报告 44.8% 的乳房切除联合 ALND 患者（背阔肌 25.9%、前锯肌 24.0%，胸大肌 20.7%，冈下肌 19.0%，斜方肌 13.8%）出现肌筋膜疼痛综合征，证实触发点激活主要源于术中对肌群的操作，亦可累及未手术区域[7]。

胸肌后乳房重建术［包括直接假体置入术（DTI）与两阶段组织扩张器/假体置入术（TE/I）］均会对胸壁肌群（主要为胸大肌、前锯肌，偶累及腹直肌上部）造成损伤，导致明显的功能减退及肩关节稳定性受损。

Leonardis 等的研究表明，两阶段胸肌后 TE/I 重建术可能破坏肩关节功能结构，导致上肢力量及稳定性下降。肩关节失稳可严重影响日常生活活动能力，已成为患者主要困扰[12]。此外，研究亦显示，术后即使完整保留的胸大肌锁骨部功能也明显受损，代偿机制可能无法有效恢复上肢功能，部分患者甚至遗留永久性功能障碍[13]。

在 Leonardis 的后续研究中，作者比较了胸肌后与背阔肌皮瓣（LD 皮瓣）重建术，提出肩关节功能的保留应作为重建术式选择的核心考量因素。事实上，胸大肌（PM）与背阔肌（LD）是维持肩关节稳定性的主要肌肉，同时受损后难以通过代偿机制恢复功能[14]。

Kim 等研究发现，乳房切除胸肌后假体置入重建会显著影响肩关节活动度（ROM），肩关节屈曲与外展受限程度大于旋转，术后早期康复训练可能实现短期活动度完全恢复[10]。值得注意的是，术后 3 个月时三种重建方式（TE/I、LD 皮瓣、游离 TRAM 皮瓣）的上肢功能无显著差异，提示不同类型的重建均会导致大致同等程度的功能障碍；然而至术后 6 个月时，LD 皮瓣组患者有更明显的手臂内收与内旋功能障碍[15]。

De Haan 等通过研究进一步证实，胸肌后重建侧扭矩强度存在客观性显著下降[5]。

在术后早期，肌纤维被下方的假体或扩张器牵拉延长，导致患者常主诉乳房区域急性紧张感，部分可进展为慢性不适[13]。

胸大肌与皮下组织的直接接触会形成固定粘连，并且会因胸大肌运动加剧，最终引发动态畸形（animation deformity）。此外，少数患者因术中胸内、外侧神经损伤导致顽固性胸大肌不自主痉挛，此类损伤一旦形成极易慢性化。部分病例即使将假体转移至胸肌前仍无法缓解症状，需行胸大肌去神经化甚至肱骨附着点离断术[16]。

面对上述致残性术后并发症，部分患者最终选择取出假体或要求改行完全自体组织重建，需接受高难度修复手术。近年来，越来越多外科医生选择将存在问题的胸肌后假体重置于胸肌前，实现功能与美观的协同改善（图 24.2，图 24.3）。

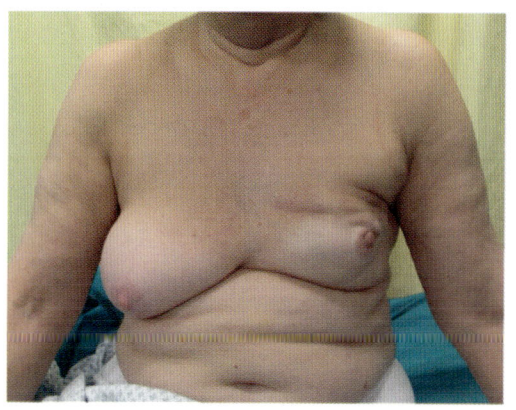

图 24.2　左胸肌后永久假体重建术后并发痛性动态畸形及包膜挛缩

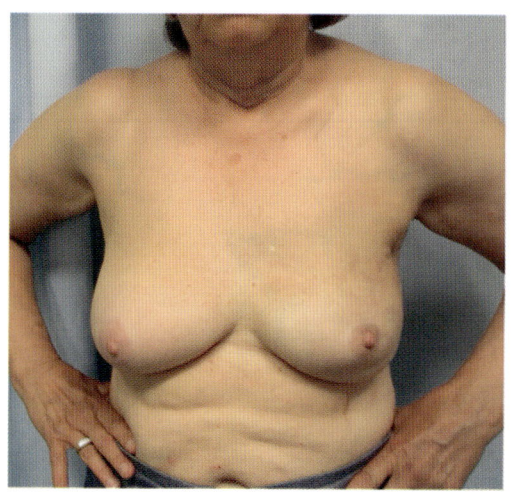

图 24.3　假体前间隙复位后美学与功能缺陷完全矫正

肌群活性下降也可通过仪器评估。超声检查可显示胸肌后相关肌群的纤维化改变与体积减小（厚度减少约50%），多普勒探头可检测肌群灌注降低[17]。

表24.1列出了胸肌后重建术的常见并发症，令人惊讶的是，患者通常将其视为正常现象而鲜少因此就诊。如后续章节所述，多数症状可通过将假体改置于胸肌前获得解决，或可经初始选择胸肌前术式直接规避。

Lee等对不同LD皮瓣乳房重建术后功能障碍进行系统综述，指出约41%患者主诉主观性上肢功能障碍。DASH量表评估显示日常生活与职业活动轻度受损，但运动及艺术相关活动障碍显著。尽管部分研究提示术后早期存在肩关节活动度与肌力明显受限，但90%~95%患者在术后1年肩关节功能可基本恢复至基线水平[3, 18, 19]。

DIEP皮瓣重建术可能造成供区功能损伤，表现为躯干屈伸轻度受限（部分病例不可逆）。Alba等研究发现，自体组织重建术后上肢疼痛程度显著高于胸肌后假体重建。此外，DIEP皮瓣也会影响上肢功能，表现为肩关节活动度下降约28.6%，徒手肌力检查结果与之相符[22]。

24.1.7 主动康复理疗策略

鉴于乳房手术会引发持续性上肢功能障碍及其对患者生活质量的影响，积极开展术后康复治疗以预防与减轻此类不良后果具有重要临床意义[23]。

术后早期肩关节活动应尽早实施：未行重建术者建议术后1周内开始，接受重建术者可于术后2周内启动。长期制动易导致肩关节功能障碍，而早期活动可显著改善术后1个月的肩关节外展与屈曲活动度[10]。

Phillips等研究强调，早期系统性康复计划不仅能有效改善患者躯体健康状态，减少误工问题，并且具有良好的成本效益[24]。

24.1.8 胸肌前乳房重建的功能优势

目前，关于胸肌前乳房重建（PPBR）功能结局的文献有限，但已有学者客观评价了其功能优势。

Schaeffer等比较了两阶段PPBR与即刻脱细胞真皮基质（ADM）辅助胸肌后假体置入术，以恢复术前肩关节活动度所需天数为指标。结果显示，PPBR组术后疼痛评分显著降低，阿片类药物需求减少，

表24.1 肌下乳房重建术常见并发症

手术耗时延长
恢复周期延长
术后疼痛加重且阿片类药物需求增加
治疗成本上升
胸大肌紧张
肌筋膜疼痛综合征
肩袖病变
粘连性关节囊炎
肩关节活动度受限
上肢力量减退
肩关节失稳
顽固性肌痉挛
动态畸形（animation deformity）
肌群萎缩/纤维化伴肌力下降
上肢功能客观性永久损伤
患者主观长期不适
美学效果欠佳

并且完全恢复主动肩关节活动时间较胸肌后组缩短50%（11.8天 : 24.2天）[25]。

Leonardis等证实，胸肌后重建技术导致肩功能损伤后，条件允许时建议优选PPBR以避免胸大肌离断导致上肢功能障碍[14]。Patel等研究发现，胸肌后重建术后胸大肌肌力客观下降约20%，QuickDASH与BREAST-Q量表提示上肢功能减退，其中躯体健康-胸部维度评分显著降低。尽管多数患者客观功能可恢复至基线，但主观评价与之不符，故推荐采用PPBR以减少胸肌后术式功能负担[26]。

2018年的一项前瞻性研究对胸肌后与胸肌前重建的功能结局进行了比较[27]，如表24.2所示，胸肌后组术后1周停用镇痛药比例仅为26.7%，而PPBR组达76.9%。

近期研究纳入乳房切除后接受辅助放疗（RT）的PPBR患者，发现BREAST-Q躯体健康-胸部维度评分在放疗组（92.9%）与非放疗组（94.0%）间无显著差异（$P<0.001$）[14, 28]。

24.2 胸肌前ADM辅助乳房重建的经济学评价

24.2.1 概述

多因素推动了乳房切除术在局部治疗与乳腺癌风险控制中的应用增加。伴随保乳技术的普及，即刻确定性乳房重建（BR）手术比例增高。欧洲乳腺诊疗质控标准建议70岁以下患者即刻重建率应>70%，但实际达标机构有限（表24.3）。

造成这一结果的原因极其复杂，涉及公共卫生体系内多种激励标准的差异。令人遗憾的是，在乳腺专科中心的质量评价指标中，尚未建立对手术美学与功能结果的评估体系。

尽管本研究无意深入剖析影响重建术式选择的所有变量，但仍要强调部分关键因素，以引导乳腺外科医师建立现代决策理念：在术式选择过程中主动规避因片面经济评估导致的认知偏差，而非被动接受其引发的矛盾性决策误区。

24.2.2 乳房重建率不高的原因

24.2.2.1 重建术式的可及性

延迟重建多采用自体游离皮瓣显微血管吻合技术，与假体重建相比，具有手术时间长、恢复周期久的特点。此类技术需在专科医疗中心通过大量病例实践方可掌握与维持。因此，此类中心必然无法广泛分布，导致复杂自体重建的候诊时间常以年计，成为患者选择重建术的重要阻碍因素。此外，远离重建中心的地理因素也被证实会降低患者意愿[29, 30]。

现有成本-效用分析多基于回顾性方法，并且仅采用患者主观乳房满意度问卷，未能充分体现胸肌前术式与其他方法相比的综合优势[31]。

事实上，尽管重建率正逐步提升，但其可及性仍存在显著的地域差异。高龄、低社会经济水平、低手术量机构是重建率低的独立预测因素。整形外科医师的密度差异亦可部分解释术式选择的地域特征[34]。

表 24.2 功能与满意度评分结果（BPI 简明疼痛量表，CM Constant-Murley 评分）

	第 1 组 (PPBR)				第 2 组（胸肌后）				P 值
	平均	置信区间	中值	方差	平均	置信区间	中值	方差	
首次手术后的对称性（单侧）	81.25%				10.81%				<0.001
手术时长（单侧）（分钟）	165			56.27	168.22			66.33	0.928
第 1 天 BPI	17.56	12.53–22.60	16.00	15.52	44.11	39.36–48.87	45.00	15.83	<0.001
第 7 天 BPI	8.23	3.24–13.22	1.00	15.39	21.96	16.37–27.54	20.00	18.59	<0.001
第 7 天 CM	65.67	62.65–68.69	69.00	9.31	52.36	48.68–56.03	53.00	12.23	<0.001
第 1 天 CM	71.62	68.74–74.49	75.00	8.87	60.36	57.19–63.52	62.00	10.54	<0.001
Dash	9.92	4.13–15.72	00.00.00	17.87	29.18	24.10–34.26	29.00	16.91	<0.001
Breast Q	92.21	89.28–95.13	94.00	9.03	76.07	71.70–80.44	79.00	14.55	<0.001
回归日常工作（天）	34.56	27.76–41.37	30.00	21.00	57.31	45.96–68.66	45.00	37.77	<0.001
	对乙酰氨基酚	酮洛芬	阿片类	无	对乙酰氨基酚	酮洛芬	阿片类	无	P 值
第 1 天镇痛药消耗	30.8%	61.5%	7.7%	0%	8.9%	66.7%	24.4%	0%	0.012
第 7 天镇痛药消耗	12.8%	10.3%	0%	76.9%	48.9%	24.4%	0%	26.7%	<0.001

表 24.3　部分国家乳房切除术后乳房重建的近似百分比

国家	重建比例	发表时间
澳大利亚	18%	2014
法国	27.4%	2012
英国	21.5%	2017
美国	43.3%	2014
加拿大	16%	2012
印度	55%	2017
瑞典	9.3%	2013
丹麦	14%	2010

即刻重建虽为理想选择，但实施面临诸多挑战：乳腺外科与整形外科的跨科协作复杂，乳房切除术后皮瓣质量评估存在不确定性，手术时长规划欠佳，术后监护责任划分模糊等问题频现。建议更多专科医师转型为肿瘤整形外科复合型人才，以提升即刻重建的可实施性。

通过严格患者筛选，假体直接置入术（尤其胸肌前术式）易掌握、便于推广，可使 70% 以上病例免于复杂手术或对侧整形[27]。ADM 辅助胸肌前重建术正引领乳房重建领域的革新，其术后并发症发生率仅为 6.4%[28]。

24.2.2.2　乳房重建术的接受度

多国乳房重建率低可能与患者对术式的接受度不足有关。研究显示，在充分知情的情况下，超过 80% 的乳房切除术后患者会考虑重建[33]。而在实际临床工作中，部分医师未向患者说明重建选项或仅将其作为备选方案；少数医师向患者阐释乳房切除重建是乳腺癌常规术式，是非保乳治疗的替代选择。显然，唯有对重建术式满怀热忱的外科医师方能有效说服患者，使其做出正确决策。

患者对延迟重建的顾虑主要源于二次手术需承担正常生活能力再度中断的风险及其他并发症（如 7% 输血风险）。尤其是 60 岁以上患者，常因担忧该选择被视为"出于女性虚荣心的显性诉求"而拒绝延迟重建，认为额外重建手术与单纯外观改善效益不匹配[33]。

值得注意的是，重建术的满意度感知无年龄差异性[35, 36]（图 24.4，图 24.5）。因此，乳腺外科与整形外科医师在患者接受度方面起着关键作用，需根据个体情况推荐最适宜的重建方案。

若能在切除乳房的同时完成重建且不增加制动时间、疼痛或瘢痕负担，将显著提升患者接受度。此外，一步法重建技术的推广有助于强化"重建是肿瘤治疗必要组成部分"的理念。

24.2.3　经济学评价基础

有限的公共资源要求外科医师引入新技术时需要进行成本评估，此类评价现已

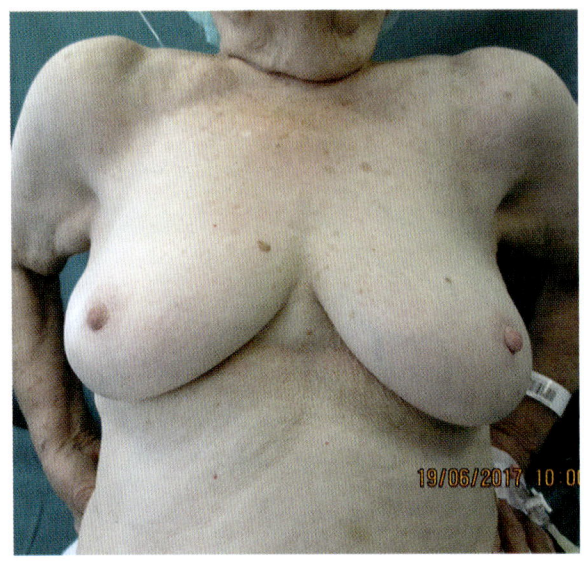 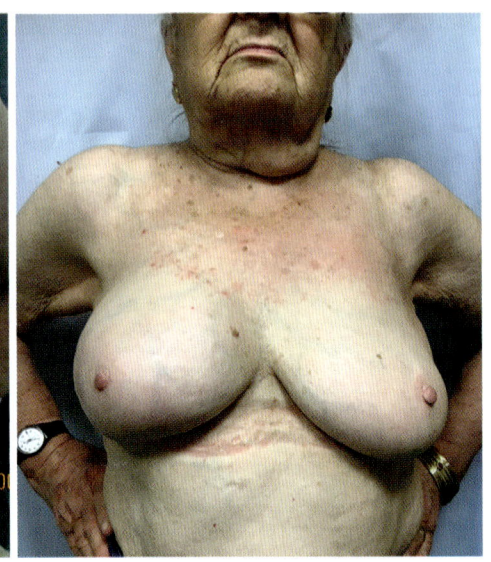

图 24.4 与图 24.5　82 岁患者强烈要求乳房重建：右侧脱细胞真皮基质胸肌前重建术前（图 24.4）与术后 6 个月（图 24.5）。虽存在轻微不对称，患者对重建乳房满意度高。PPBR，前间隙乳房重建术；DTI，直接假体置入；ADM，脱细胞真皮基质

普遍应用。多数情况下，单纯评估院内成本易陷入复杂领域。当前成本评价体系往往忽视医疗价值，单一成本控制策略的效果有时甚至适得其反。

事实上，尽管每家医院都高度关注自身预算，但特定干预措施引发的躯体与心理后遗症，最终仍将由社会医疗资源承担。必须明确，国家公共卫生系统的核心使命不仅是控制成本，更是通过应对重大疾病促进社会福祉。现行医疗绩效指标多聚焦投入与产出，却忽视了一系列患者关注的结局指标，包括疼痛、功能状态、生存质量（QoL）及就医体验等。评估乳房重建时，不宜仅参照医保报销额度（多数国家报销比例与真实成本不匹配）。此外，两阶段手术因可获得两次独立报销，可能导致医院不合理的财务偏好。

因此，正确的评价体系应基于成本 - 价值比来构建。新术式在直接成本上常高于传统方法，现有成本 - 效果分析方法虽见诸文献，但在量化院外效用方面仍存不足。尽管实施困难，但需重点分析医疗领域外的干预后果（如经济生产力、病假津贴、社会服务、康复支出）[37]。

从患者与支付方视角来看，不同重建方式的比较需纵向分析创新技术的所有优劣势，并对完整治疗周期涉及的服务与活动进行量化，从而建立更精准的价值评估模型[38]。下文基于我院胸肌前 / 后假体重建的评估经验，结合近期自体重建文献数据[39-44]，对各结局指标进行量化分析。

24.2.3.1　手术时间

乳房切除术联合自体游离皮瓣重建术耗时 > 360min；胸肌后两阶段组织扩张器 / 假体置入（TE/I）重建术总时长 ≥ 210min，胸肌后直接假体置入术需要约

150min；胸肌前重建术（PPBR）因可于乳房切除及腋窝切口缝合同期完成 ADM 包裹假体操作，并且无须制备肌袋，总时长仅约 90min。术式革新节约了手术室资源（每小时成本 823 欧元）及患者麻醉药物用量。

24.2.3.2　住院时长

在住院时间方面，自体游离皮瓣重建平均 3.9~4.8 天，胸肌后假体重建约为 2.1 天，而胸肌前一步法重建住院不足 24 小时。以每日住院成本 400 欧元计算，胸肌前术式较胸肌后术式与自体组织重建分别节省 1 天与 3.5 天的住院费用。

24.2.3.3　疼痛与镇痛需求

胸肌前重建术疼痛轻微，患者术后仅需口服对乙酰氨基酚，1 周内无需强效镇痛药，支持其"日间手术"模式。与其他术式相比，本方法无须使用麻醉性镇痛药，既避免了药物的不良反应，也规避了近年备受关注的术后吗啡类衍生物依赖风险。研究表明，胸肌前术式镇痛药物成本较胸肌后术式降低 60%。复杂重建术引发的高强度疼痛相关不适，可显著影响患者心理体验与恢复周期，应作为价值评估的重要负面因素[45]。

24.2.3.4　躯体与功能完整性

目前，在疗效等同的前提下，维持机体结构完整性已上升为首要考量，其重要性甚至可比拟生存获益。无论对于职业或日常生活，保留患者动态生活方式需高度关注各类治疗（尤其手术干预）的远期影响。与胸肌后重建术相比，胸肌前重建术可在保全肌群的前提下实现乳房重建，从而完全保留上肢功能。

自体组织重建术可能引发供区显著改变，常见问题包括额外瘢痕、腹壁薄弱化风险，甚至原发疾病区域外的毁损性并发症。因手术干预引发的新发健康问题会严重削弱治疗整体价值，一旦出现此类损害，所有结局指标需重新评估。最大限度减少此类缺陷是重建术创新的核心目标。胸肌前重建术可有效规避治疗相关附加负担，同时保留机体结构为未来可能的重建术式选择留有余地。或许应摒弃"以功能残缺换取疾病治愈"的传统思维模式。

24.2.3.5　恢复正常活动时间

重建术后全面恢复日常活动所需时间是患者关注的核心结局指标，亦是术式价值评估的重要维度。肌群保全型重建术允许早期上肢活动，基本无需康复理疗（使用率趋近于零）；胸肌后假体重建后需要理疗干预的概率为 50%，自体组织重建术为 25%。每周期理疗费用（含理疗评估）约 700 欧元。

关于术后恢复期，胸肌前一步法重建术平均为 30 天，胸肌后直接假体置入术为 55 天，两阶段 TE/I 重建术因二次手术需要额外增加 25 天，自体组织重建术则为 65 天。误工日均成本估算为 62.5 欧元。

由此可见，胸肌前直接假体重建术通过减少误工时间（无需理疗）、降低门诊复诊频次（每次 45 欧元），较其他术式会进一步节省社会经济成本。

24.2.3.6 重建乳房的稳定性与修复手术需求

评估不同乳房重建术式时,因远期功能或美学改变需要二次干预的可能性是核心结局指标,涉及乳房形态早期稳定性与长期可接受性。

传统观点认为,自体组织重建术在长期柔软度与形态自然性方面显著优于胸肌后假体重建,后者常伴有较高比例的不良形态改变,如严重动态畸形(30%)、III/IV级Baker包膜挛缩、假体上内侧移位、躯干上部慢性疼痛等,非计划性翻修率近30%[46]。单次翻修术花费约3 400欧元。自体组织重建术(放疗除外)总体稳定性较高,但40%以上病例需皮瓣修整以优化形态。

我院对480例胸肌前一步法重建乳房患者随访5年发现,非计划性手术翻修率仅3.3%(主要与放疗后不良改变相关)。未放疗患者未发现包膜挛缩、动态畸形或假体移位,乳房初始柔软度与自然形态基本保持稳定(图24.6,图24.7)。

因假体迟发性感染/外露或皮肤坏死而需要取出假体者共4例,因假体濒临外露或放疗后包膜挛缩行修复术3例,进行性加重的不可接受性下垂矫正2例,7例通过脂肪移植术改善皱褶。

24.2.3.7 美学效果与患者满意度

采用标准化量表工具通过患者问卷评估患者美学满意度及重建相关生活质量。一项前瞻性研究应用BREAST-Q量表(Memorial Sloan Kettering癌症中心与British Columbia大学,2006年),对ADM辅助胸肌前一步法重建术(PPBR)与胸肌后直接假体置入(DTI)或两阶段组织扩张器/假体(TE/I)重建进行了比较,结果如表24.4所示。PPBR组各项评分均显著更优($P<0.001$)。值得注意的是,

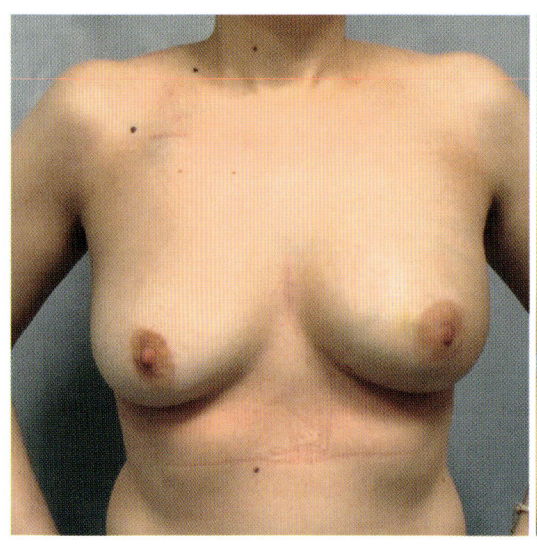
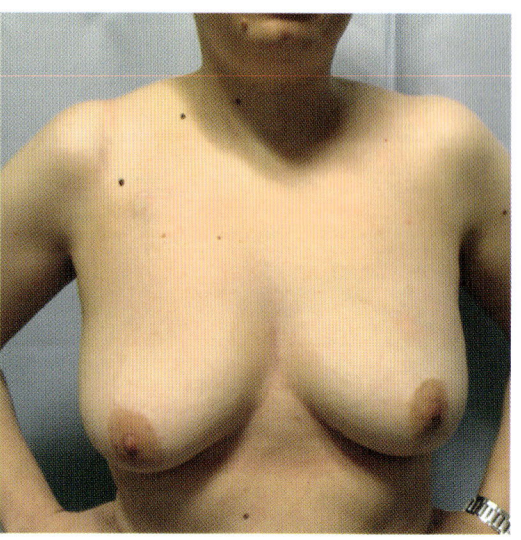

图24.6与图24.7 51岁患者左侧脱细胞真皮基质直接假体胸肌前重建术后27天(图24.6)与术后3年(图24.7)。乳房柔韧性及形态随时间保持完美稳定。PPBR,前间隙乳房重建术;DTI,直接假体置入;ADM,脱细胞真皮基质

表 24.4　BREAST-Q™ 评分结果：分值越高代表结局越好

BREAST-Q™ 重建模块术后（平均分数 ± 标准差）	PPBR（n=39）	胸肌后（n=45）	P 值
乳房满意度	90.1 ± 4.5	73.5 ± 9.7	<0.001
心理社会健康	94.3 ± 2.7	79.4 ± 8.4	<0.001
躯体健康 – 胸部维度	95.1 ± 4.7	68.1 ± 7.5	<0.001
性健康	9.7 ± 14.9	64.9 ± 18.7	<0.001
假体满意度	7.1 ± 0.7	3.4 ± 1.5	<0.001

PPBR，胸肌前乳房重建；*BR*，乳房重建

在单侧乳房切除术病例中，胸肌前组对称满意度达 81.25%，显著高于胸肌后组的 10.81%（$P<0.001$）[27]。

24.2.4　院内成本

各项术式院内成本汇总见表 24.5。

24.2.5　结局指标的货币化评估

各结局指标的货币化评估结果见表 24.6。

结合表 24.5 与表 24.6 的数据，可对各术式全周期经济结果进行评估（表 24.7）。

需要指出的是，胸肌前一步法 PPBR 在躯体完整性维护、疼痛控制及美学满意度等维度的优势虽难以货币化衡量，但显著提升了术式的综合价值与临床可接受性。

24.3　小结

现有证据表明，在功能预后方面，胸肌前假体乳房重建术（PPBR）显著优于其他假体置入式重建手术。因此，胸肌保留技术应作为乳房切除术后重建计划的首选考量。

该技术与肿瘤整形团队的诊疗路径的完美整合，不仅能最大限度规避传统术式对患者功能状态的永久性损伤，更为乳腺癌最佳保守治疗路径赋予独特价值。

推荐对各类乳房重建术的功能预后进行系统评估，以持续优化手术方案。重建策略的微创性、时效性与稳定性应作为决策分析的核心要素，此举亦是社会核心价值与预期优先级的医学映现。

综合成本–效益分析，胸肌前即刻乳房重建虽涉及脱细胞真皮基质的额外支出，仍应被视为优于传统干预的优选方案，同时其对伦理方面的可及性与接受度的提升贡献显著。未来，乳房重建外科医师须充分权衡多方利益，致力于制订最优个体化治疗方案。

24.4　要点与临床建议

- 乳房切除术后生活质量与上肢功能恢复

表24.5 各术式规划重建周期内医疗成本（单位：欧元，2018财政年度）

	第一次门诊就诊+术前检查	手术室+工作人员（823欧元/小时）	置入材料	住院费用（400欧元/天）	门诊就诊/药物（每次45欧元）	总计
单步PPBR+ADM（完全覆盖）	97.5	1 234	（假体550+ADM3 000）3 550	400	135	5 416
胸肌后DTI（无ADM）	97.5	2 057	550	840	135	3 679
两步胸肌后TE/I（无ADM）	（97.5×2）195	（2 057+1 234）3 291	（扩张器550+假体550）1 100	（第1步840+第2步600）1 440	（第1步360+第2步135）495	6 521
自体游离皮瓣	300	4 938	0	1 740	225	7 203

PPBR，胸肌前乳房重建；*ADM*，脱细胞真皮基质；*DTI*，直接置入；*TE/I*，组织扩张器/内置物

表24.6 院外非计划性（早期与晚期）手术翻修联合对称化手术费用（欧元计价，2018财年）

	因完成重建手术而缺勤的天数（62 欧元/天）	物理治疗（700 欧元/每个周期）	早期再手术并发症（平均费用 2 170 欧元）	对称化 [单侧乳房切除术后]（平均费用 2 845 欧元）	后期修正/重塑手术（平均费用 3 482 欧元）	总计
单步 PPBR+ADM（完全包囊）	1 875	概率 0%，0	概率 3.2%，68.4	概率 18.7%，532	概率 3.3%（包括脂肪塑形），114.9	2 590
胸肌后 DTI（无 ADM）	3 457	概率 50%，350	概率 17.1%[47]，371	概率 89.2%，2 537	概率 30%，1 044	7 759
丙步胸肌后 TE/I（无 ADM）	5 312	概率 50%，350	概率 11.4%，247.4	概率 89.2%，2 537	概率 30%，1 044	9 517
自体游离皮瓣	4 062	概率 25%，175	概率 5.8%[48]，125.9	概率 39%，1 109	概率 17%，592	6 064

PPBR，胸肌前乳房重建；ADM，脱细胞真皮基质；DTI，直接置入；TE/I，组织扩张器/内置物

表 24.7 不同重建术式总成本（含院内支出、院外费用及社会保障成本，随访 ≥4 年）

单步 PPBR+ADM（完全包裹）	8006 欧元
胸肌后 DTI（无 ADM）	11,438 欧元
两步胸肌后 TE/I（无 ADM）	16,038 欧元
自体游离皮瓣	13,267 欧元

PPBR，胸肌前乳房重建；*ADM*，脱细胞真皮基质；*DTI*，直接置入；*TE/I*，组织扩张器 / 内置物

直接相关。
- 肿瘤外科医师应通过主客观量表对重建术的功能影响进行系统评估。
- 胸肌前重建可保留肩关节稳定性，减轻术后疼痛，加速社会功能回归。
- 参照欧洲标准，70 岁以下患者即刻重建率应＞ 70%。
- 经济学评估须纳入直接医疗成本、远期翻修成本及躯体完整性维护效益。
- 长期随访证实，胸肌前重建术预后稳定，对多数病例推荐作为首选方案。

参考文献

1. Albornoz CR, Bach PB, Mehrara BJ, et al. A paradigm shift in U.S. Breast reconstruction: increasing implant rates. Plast Reconstr Surg. 2013,131(1):15–23.
2. Ness KK, Wall MM, Oakes JM, et al. Physical performance limitations and participation restrictions among cancer survivors: a population-based study. Ann Epidemiol. 2006,16:197–205.
3. Cattelani L, Spotti A, Pedrazzi G, et al. Latissimus dorsi myocutaneous flap in immediate reconstructtion after salvage mastectomy post-lumpectomy and radiation therapy. Plast Reconstr Surg Glob Open. 2019,7(7):e2296.
4. Sood R, Easow JM, Konopka G, et al. Latissimus dorsi flap in breast reconstruction: recent innovations in the workhorse flap. Cancer Control. 2018,25(1):1073274817744638.
5. de Haan A, Toor A, Hage JJ, et al. Function of the pectoralis major muscle after combined skin-sparing mastectomy and immediate reconstruction by subpectoral implantation of a prosthesis. Ann Plast Surg. 2007,59(6):605–10.
6. Meldrum D, Cahalane E, Conroy R, et al. Maximum voluntary isometric contraction: reference values and clinical application [published correction appears in Amyotroph Lateral Scler. 2008,9(1):63]. Amyotroph Lateral Scler. 2007,8(1):47–55.
7. Torres Lacomba M, Mayoral del Moral O, Coperias Zazo JL, et al. Incidence of myofascial pain syndrome in breast cancer surgery: a prospective study. Clin J Pain. 2010,26(4):320–5.
8. Hayes SC, Rye S, Battistutta D, et al. Upper-body morbidity following breast cancer treatment is common, may persist longer-term and adversely influences quality of life. Health Qual Life Outcomes. 2010,8:92.
9. Helms G, Kühn T, Moser L, et al. Shoulder-arm morbidity in patients with sentinel node biopsy and complete axillary dissection—data from a prospective randomised trial. Eur J Surg Oncol. 2009,35(7):696–701.
10. Kim KH, Yeo SM, Cheong IY, et al. Early rehabilitation after total mastectomy and immediate reconstruction with tissue expander insertion in breast cancer patients: a retrospective case-control study. J Breast Cancer. 2019,22(3):472–83.
11. Sagen A, Kaaresen R, Sandvik L, et al. Upper limb physical function and adverse effects after

breast cancer surgery: a prospective 2.5-year follow-up study and preoperative measures. Arch Phys Med Rehabil. 2014,95(5):875–81.
12. Rancourt D, Hogan N. Stability in force-production tasks. J Mot Behav. 2001,33(2):193–204.
13. Leonardis JM, Lyons DA, Giladi AM, et al. Functional integrity of the shoulder joint and pectoralis major following subpectoral implant breast reconstruction. J Orthop Res. 2019,37(7):1610–9.
14. Leonardis JM, Diefenbach BJ, Lyons DA, et al. The influence of reconstruction choice and inclusion of radiation therapy on functional shoulder biomechanics in women undergoing mastectomy for breast cancer. Breast Cancer Res Treat. 2019,173(2):447–53.
15. Myung Y, Choi B, Kwon H, et al. Quantitative analysis of shoulder function and strength after breast reconstruction: a retrospective cohort study. Medicine (Baltimore). 2018,97(24):e10979.
16. Govshievich A, Kirkham K, Brull R, et al. Novel approach to intractable pectoralis major muscle spasms following submuscular expander-implant breast reconstruction. Plast Surg Case Studies. 2015,1(3):68–70.
17. Roxo AC, Nahas FX, Pinheiro Rodrigues NC, et al. Functional and volumetric analysis of the pectoralis major muscle after submuscular breast augmentation. Aesthet Surg J. 2017,37(6):654–61.
18. Lee KT, Mun GH. A systematic review of functional donor-site morbidity after Latissimus dorsi muscle transfer. Plast Reconstr Surg. 2014,134(2):303–14.
19. de Oliveira RR, do Nascimento SL, Derchain SF, et al. Immediate breast reconstruction with a Latissimus dorsi flap has no detrimental effects on shoulder motion or postsurgical complications up to 1 year after surgery. Plast Reconstr Surg. 2013,131(5):673e–80e.
20. Atisha D, Alderman AK. A systematic review of abdominal wall function following abdominal flaps for postmastectomy breast reconstruction. Ann Plast Surg. 2009,63(2):222–30.
21. Lee KT, Park JW, Mun GH. Impact of rectus muscle injury during perforator dissection on functional donor morbidity after deep inferior epigastric perforator flap breast reconstruction. Plast Reconstr Surg Glob Open. 2019,7(10):e2484.
22. Alba B, Schultz B, Qin LA, et al. Postoperative upper extremity function in implant and autologous breast reconstruction. J Reconstr Microsurg. 2020,36(2):151–6. https://doi.org/10.1055/s-0039- 1698439.
23. Ballal H, Hunt C, Bharat C, et al. Arm morbidity of axillary dissection with sentinel node biopsy versus delayed axillary dissection. ANZ J Surg. 2018,88(9):917–21.
24. Phillips CJ, Phillips R, Main CJ, et al. The cost effectiveness of NHS physiotherapy support for occupational health (OH) services. BMC Musculoskelet Disord. 2012,13:29.
25. Schaeffer CV, Dassoulas KR, Thuman J, et al. Early functional outcomes after prepectoral breast reconstruction: a case-matched cohort study. Ann Plast Surg. 2019,82(6S Suppl 5):S399–403.
26. Patel AU, Day SJ, Pencek M, et al. Functional return after implant-based breast reconstruction: a prospective study of objective and patient-reported outcomes. J Plast Reconstr Aesthet Surg. 2020,73(5):850–5.
27. Cattelani L, Polotto S, Arcuri MF, et al. One-step prepectoral breast reconstruction with dermal matrix-covered implant compared to submuscular implantation: functional and cost evaluation. Clin Breast Cancer. 2018,18(4):e703–11.
28. Polotto S, Bergamini ML, Pedrazzi G, et al. One-step prepectoral breast reconstruction with porcine dermal matrix-covered implant: a protective technique improving the outcome in post-mastectomy radiation therapy setting. Gland Surg. 2020,9(2):219–28.
29. Albornoz CR, Cohen WA, Razdan SN, et al. The

29. impact of travel distance on breast reconstruction in the United States. Plast Reconstr Surg. 2016,137(1):12–8.
30. Roughton MC, Di Egidio P, Zhou L, et al. Distance to a plastic surgeon and type of insurance plan are independently predictive of postmastectomy breast reconstruction. Plast Reconstr Surg. 2016,138(2):203e–11e.
31. Cattelani L, Polotto S. The economics of prepectoral breast reconstruction. Plast Reconstr Surg. 2018,142(3):415e–7e.
32. Ilonzo N, Tsang A, Tsantes S, et al. Breast reconstruction after mastectomy: a ten-year analysis of trends and immediate postoperative outcomes. Breast. 2017,32:7–12.
33. Retrouvey H, Zhong T, Gagliardi AR, et al. How patient acceptability affects access to breast reconstruction: a qualitative study. BMJ Open. 2019,9(9):e029048.
34. Régis C, Le J, Chauvet MP, et al. Variations in the breast reconstruction rate in France: a nationwide study of 19,466 patients based on the French medico-administrative database. Breast. 2018,42:74–80.
35. Sisco M, Johnson DB, Wang C, et al. The quality-of-life benefits of breast reconstruction do not diminish with age. J Surg Oncol. 2015,111(6):663–8.
36. Johnson DB, Lapin B, Wang C, et al. Advanced age does not worsen recovery or long-term morbidity after postmastectomy breast reconstruction. Ann Plast Surg. 2016,76(2):164–9.
37. Porter ME. What is value in health care? N Engl J Med. 2010,363(26):2477–81.
38. Glasberg SB. The economics of prepectoral breast reconstruction. Plast Reconstr Surg. 2017,140(6S Prepectoral Breast Reconstruction):49S–52S.
39. Momeni A, Ramesh NK, Wan D, et al. Postoperative analgesia after microsurgical breast reconstruction using liposomal bupivacaine (Exparel). Breast J. 2019,25(5):903–7.
40. Thacoor A, van den Bosch P, Akhavani MA. Surgical management of cosmetic surgery tourism-related complications: current trends and cost analysis study of the financial impact on the UK National Health Service (NHS). Aesthet Surg J. 2019,39(7):786–91.
41. Nguyen PD, Herrera FA, Roostaeian J, et al. Career satisfaction and burnout in the reconstructive microsurgeon in the United States. Microsurgery. 2015,35(1):1–5.
42. Highton L, Johnson R, Kirwan C, et al. Prepectoral implant-based breast reconstruction. Plast Reconstr Surg Glob Open. 2017,5(9):e1488.
43. Frey JD, Salibian AA, Karp NS, et al. Examining length of hospital stay after microsurgical breast reconstruction: evaluation in a case-control study. Plast Reconstr Surg Glob Open. 2017,5(12):e1588.
44. Liu C, Momeni A, Zhuang Y, et al. Outcome analysis of expander/implant versus microsurgical abdominal flap breast reconstruction: a critical study of 254 cases. Ann Surg Oncol. 2014,21(6):2074–82.
45. Roth RS, Qi J, Hamill JB, et al. Is chronic postsurgical pain surgery-induced? A study of persistent postoperative pain following breast reconstruction. Breast. 2018,37:119–25.
46. Becker H, Fregosi N. The impact of animation deformity on quality of life in post-mastectomy reconstruction patients. Aesthet Surg J. 2017,37(5):531–6.
47. Bennett KG, Qi J, Kim HM, et al. Comparison of 2-year complication rates among common techniques for postmastectomy breast reconstruction. JAMA Surg. 2018,153(10):901–8.
48. Fischer JP, Nelson JA, Au A, et al. Complications and morbidity following breast reconstruction—a review of 16,063 cases from the 2005–2010 NSQIP datasets. J Plast Surg Hand Surg. 2014,48(2):104–14.

25 生物合成支架在胸肌前重建中的应用

编者：Hilton Becker
译者：赵海东

25.1 概述

近年来，胸肌剥离术式应用频率显著降低。该术式存在诸多弊端，包括延长手术时间、加重创伤、破坏组织解剖层次、加重术后疼痛、延长恢复周期，并可能引发动态畸形、慢性不适、疼痛及肩关节功能障碍等[1~3]。其主要优势在于能为假体（尤其上极区域）提供充分覆盖。为弥补覆盖不足，生物基质材料、合成补片及脂肪移植技术的应用已取得阶段性成功。目前，基质材料联合组织扩张器在假体即刻乳房重建中的应用日趋普遍[4]。2003年首次报道了补片应用于乳房修复术[5]，2005年拓展至乳房重建领域[6]。

生物基质虽可提供额外支撑，但存在成本高昂、整合失败及感染等不足。由可吸收或不可吸收纤维编织的合成补片（作为内置支撑结构）的应用亦取得一定的效果[7,8]。不可吸收补片质地过硬，而可吸收补片过薄并且最终会降解，因此采用多层长效可吸收补片可获得更优效果。若皮瓣厚度足以容纳移植物，则脂肪移植可产生显著获益。补片与皮瓣形成的"夹层效应"可促进移植脂肪存活，多层补片叠加更能有效增厚皮瓣（图25.1）。

为优化DuraSorb（长效可吸收补片）的功能特性，研究团队首先尝试将其浸于富血小板血浆（platelet-rich plasma, PRP）中，但发现该材料对PRP的吸附能力欠佳（图25.2）。继而通过构建三维立体补片

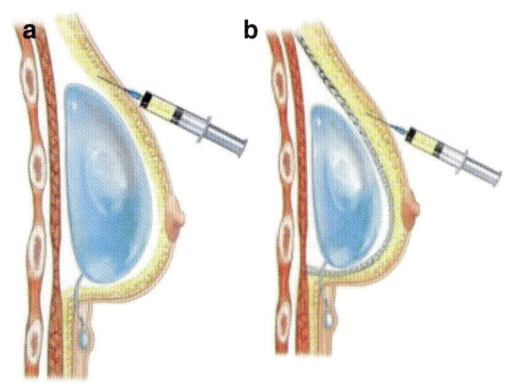

图25.1 （a）皮瓣内脂肪注射受限；（b）补片衬垫形成夹层结构实现大容量脂肪填充

H. Becker (✉)
Department of Surgery, Charles E. Schmidt College of Medicine, Boca Raton, FL, USA
Florida Atlantic University, Boca Raton, FL, USA
e-mail: Hilton@beckermd.com

并涂覆脂肪组织，开发了新型复合支架：当 PRP 作用于该结构时，可形成具有生物活性的合成支架。该支架具备渐进性软化特性（术后 3 个月硬度下降 42%±6%），并能有效固持脂肪移植物（6 个月存活率提升至 78%±9%），如图 25.3 所示。此项技术将 PRP 与脂肪强化的合成补片结合，显著促进了胸肌前重建术后的创面愈合与美学效果的优化。

25.2 手术步骤

术前须与患者签署详细知情同意书，充分说明手术方案、替代治疗方式、潜

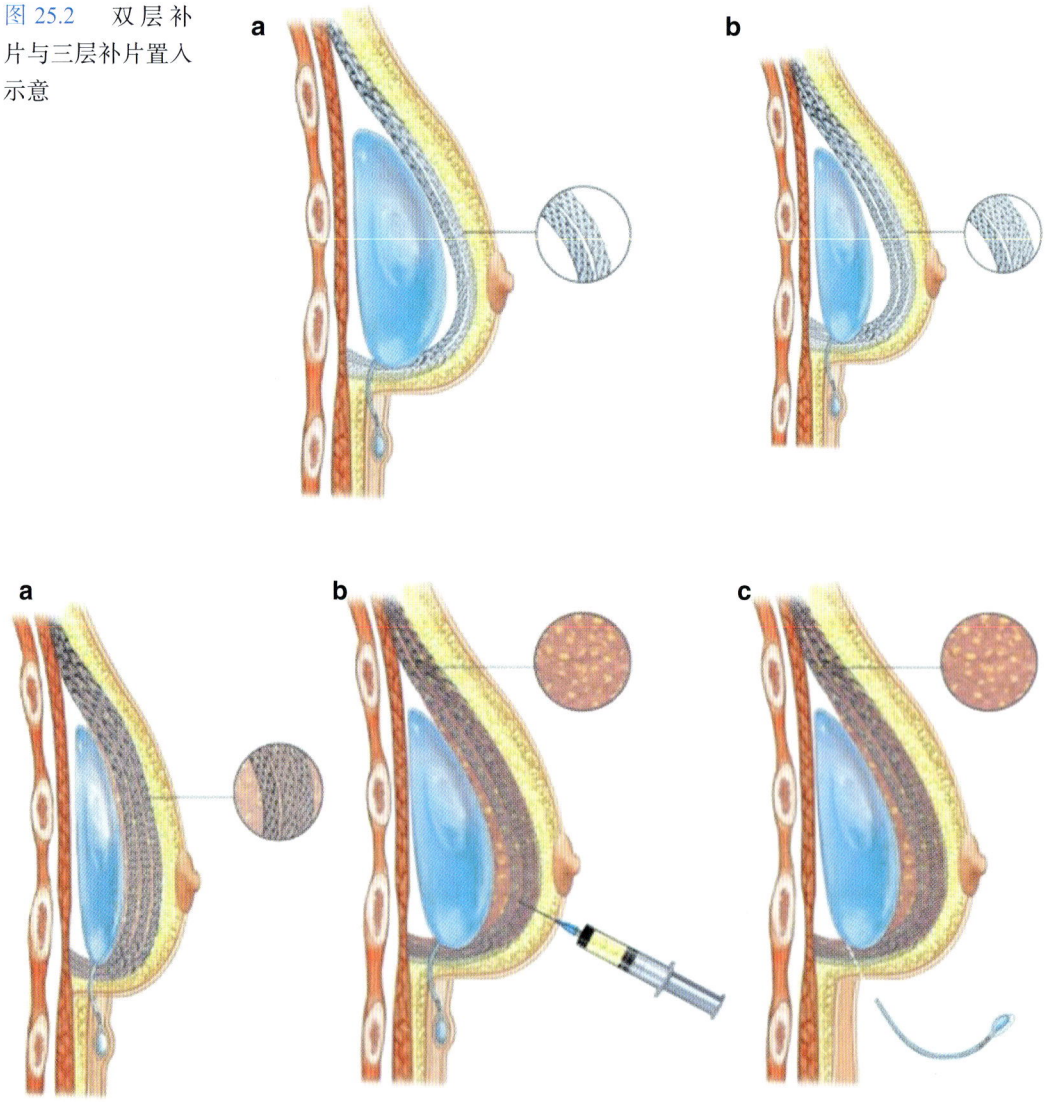

图 25.2 双层补片与三层补片置入示意

图 25.3 （a）用生物补片（复合富血小板血浆与脂肪）覆盖假体上方；（b）2~3 个月后在补片内注射脂肪；（c）注射端口移除后视图

25 生物合成支架在胸肌前重建中的应用

在获益及风险。生物合成支架采用多层 DuraSorb（聚二氧环己酮）或 Galafex（聚-4-羟基丁酸酯网状材料）构建。

供区局部注射稀释罗哌卡因与肾上腺素混合液后，用 4mm 或 5mm 切割套管获取脂肪移植物以最大化基质血管成分（SVF）含量[9]。脂肪经冲洗过滤去除油性成分后，平铺于网状材料或置入网状袋内。随后将富血小板血浆（PRP）与钙剂、凝血酶复合物补充至脂肪-网状材料复合体[10-12]。亦可折叠 6cm×6cm 网格材料，采用聚二氧环己酮（PDS）缝线构建锥状结构（图 25.4，图 25.5），适用于修复组织缺损（如保乳术后即刻修复或小体积假体置换重建术）。

闭合负压引流管经长皮下隧道置入后缝合固定。深部组织用 3-0 薇乔线分层间断缝合，皮肤用 4-0 单乔线（Ethicon）双层缝合。术区以弹力胶布塑形固定。

胸肌前即刻乳房重建标准术式采用可调节假体。假体置入时应适量充气以避免皮瓣血运障碍[13]。假体表面覆盖生物补片，

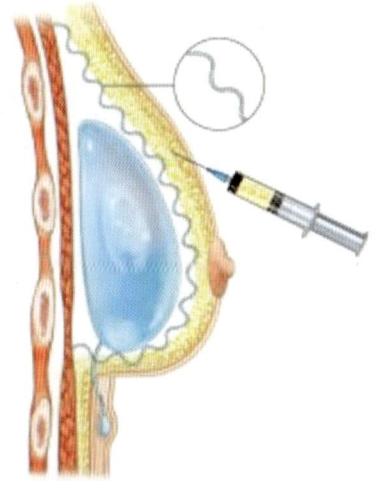
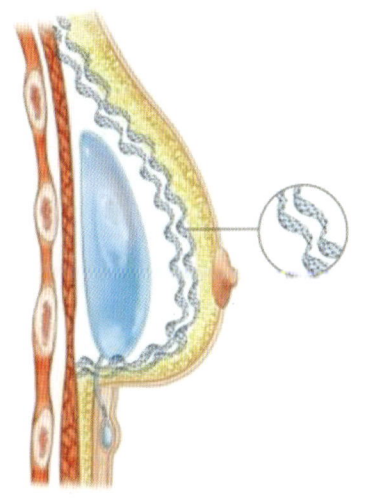
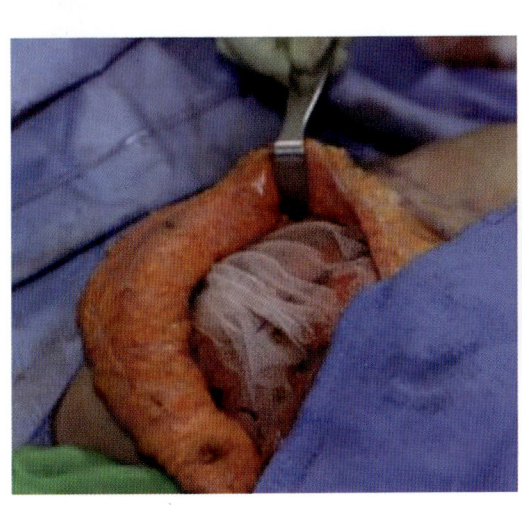

图 25.4 波纹状补片

该补片具有一定容积支撑功能。后续可通过向假体注水逐步扩容，待达到预期体积后移除注水阀，保留具有良好软组织覆盖的小体积永久假体。若术后自体脂肪移植量充足，可完全移除假体实现全自体组织重建。术后应配合外源性容积扩张装置维持支架形态，促进组织长入。最早于术后2个月可进行二次脂肪移植。

在经严格筛选的病例中，可采用多层生物补片替代假体行乳房重建，通过多层补片叠加塑形，可构建个性化乳房轮廓。初次手术1~2个月后可行二次脂肪移植（图25.6~25.10）。

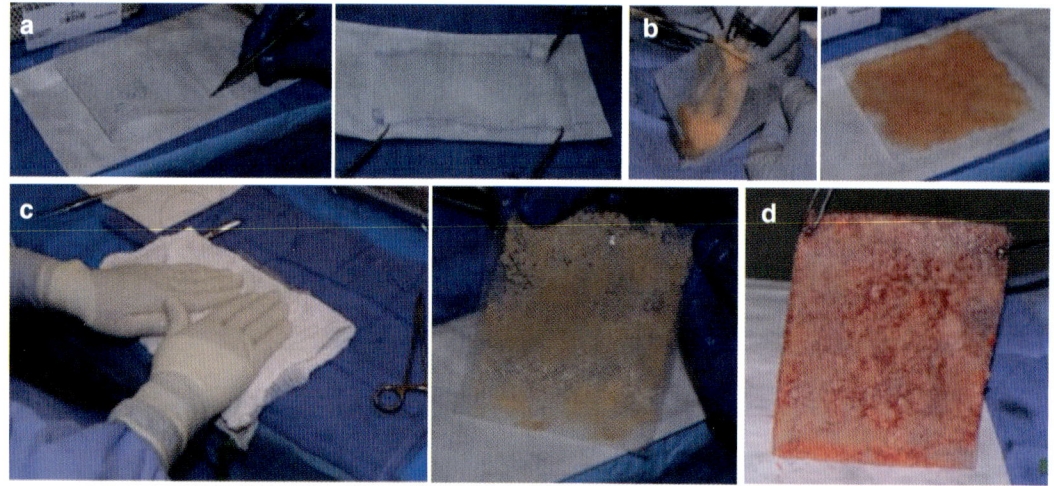

图 25.5　生物补片制备流程：（a）双层补片缝合形成袋状；（b）脂肪浸渍补片；（c）轻拍晾除游离油滴；（d）添加富血小板血浆

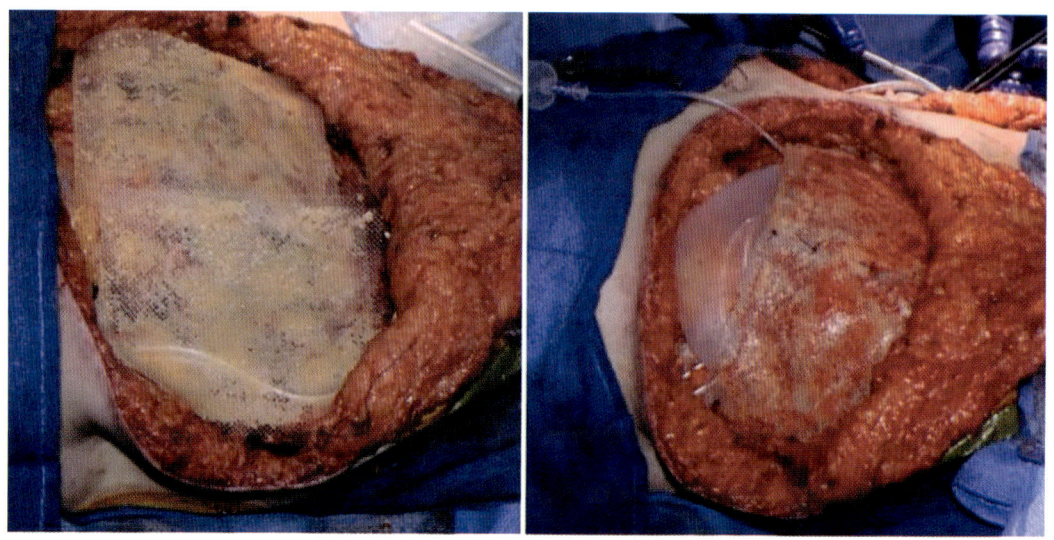

图 25.6　闭合前置入负载 PRP 脂肪的补片

25 生物合成支架在胸肌前重建中的应用

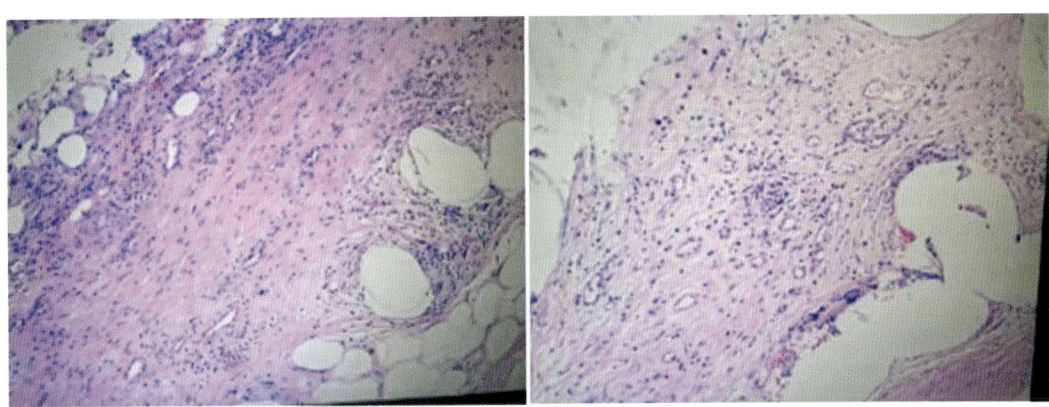

图 25.7 术后 6 周组织学切片：可见新生血管、胶原沉积及脂肪细胞存活

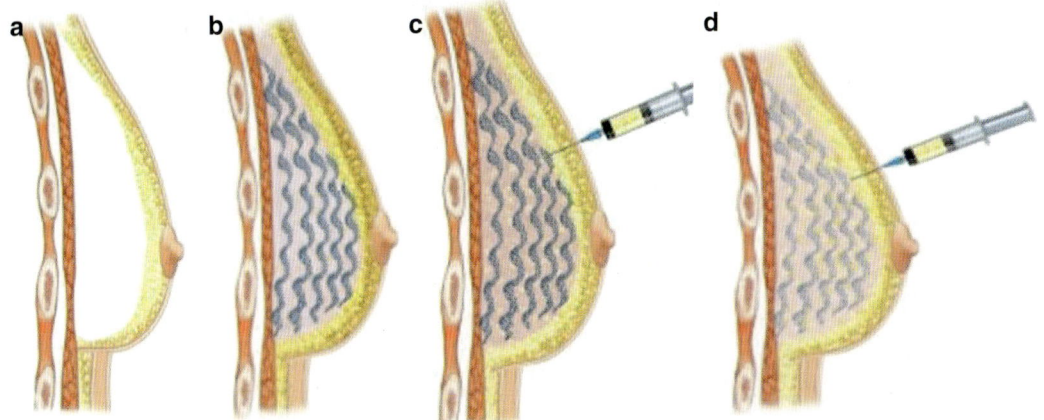

图 25.8 增量容积生物支架构建步骤：（a）乳房切除术后创面；（b）置入生物支架；（c）初次脂肪移植；（d）二次脂肪移植后补片逐步降解

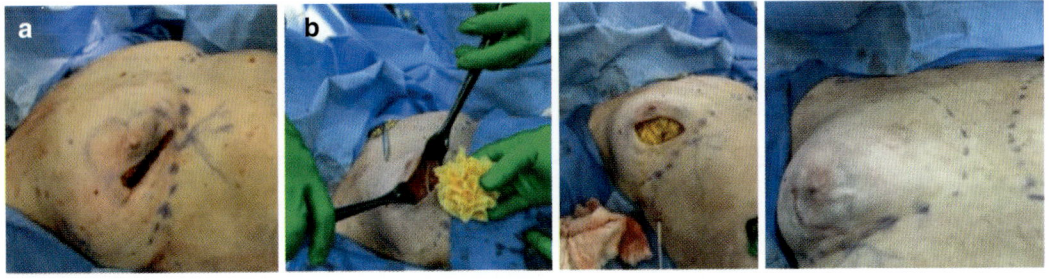

图 25.9 保乳术后应用：（a）肿块切除术后；（b）制备并置入生物补片

25.2.1 结果

本中心 1 年内完成生物补片乳房重建 30 余例，包括：

1. 保乳术后缺损修复（女性，9 例）。

2. 胸肌前可调节盐水假体即刻乳房重建（图 25.3）。

3. 无假体即刻乳房重建（图 25.11）。

297

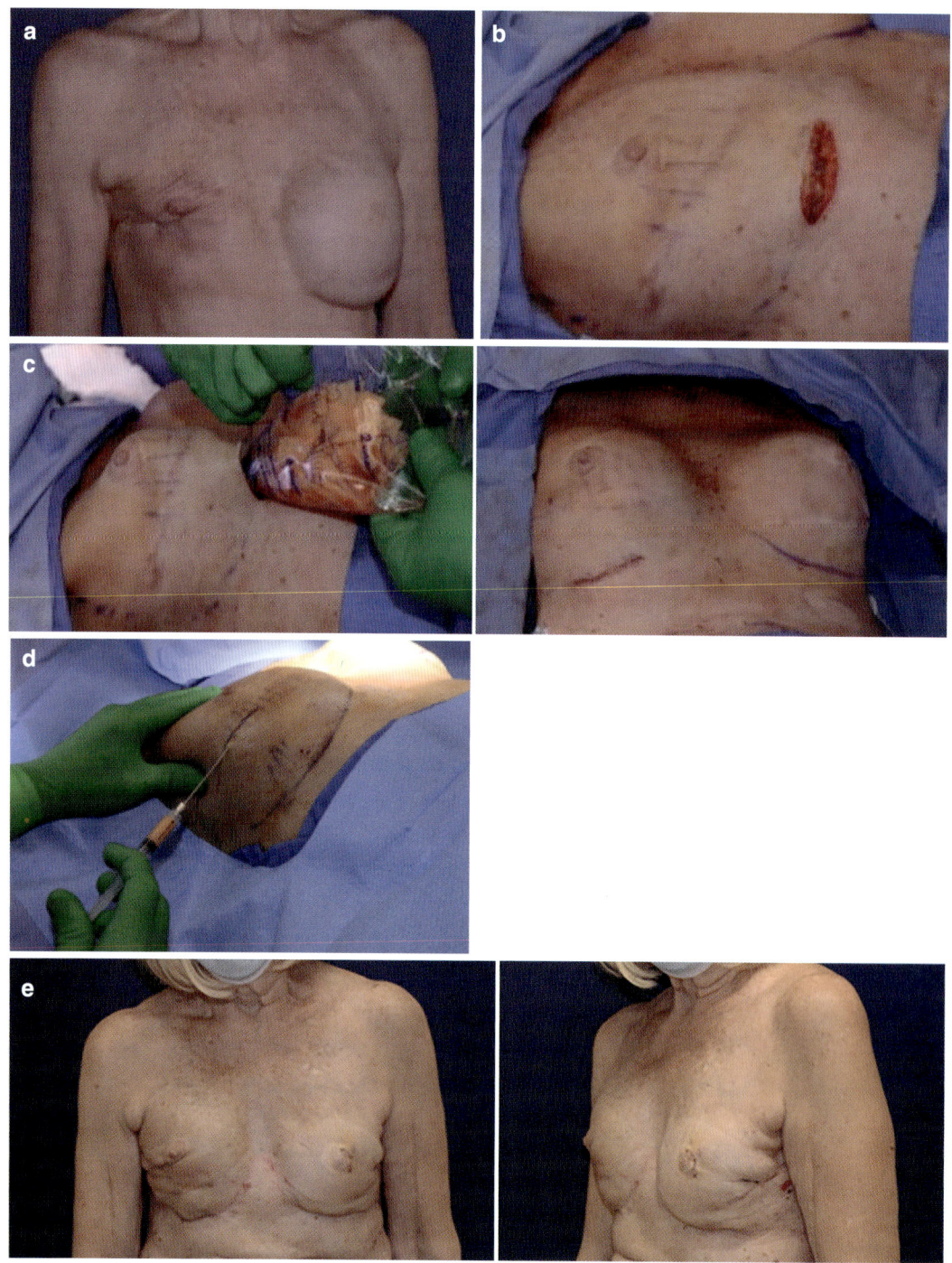

图 25.10　延期重建：（a）乳房切除术后右侧扩张器丢失（放疗后）；（b）囊腔制备；（c）Keller 漏斗辅助置入生物补片；（d）术后 2 个月补片内脂肪注射；（e）最终效果

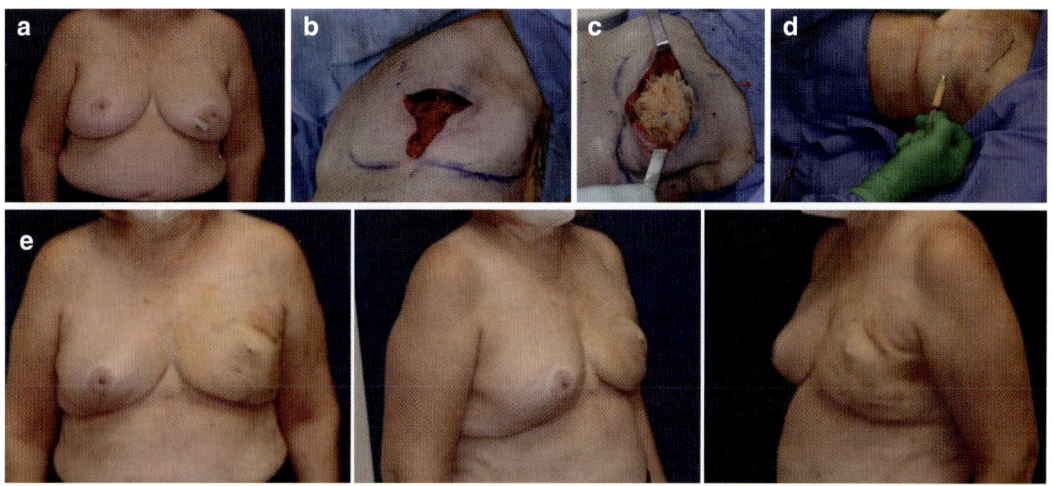

图 25.11　即刻重建：（a）左乳癌术前；（b）左乳切除术后；（c）生物补片置入；（d）术后 6 周脂肪移植；（e）术后 2 个月效果

4. 乳房修复性重建（图 25.10）。

随访显示支架结构维持良好，仅 1 例接受放疗患者发生感染。目前持续通过定期随访评估患者满意度、并发症发生率及美学效果（标准化摄影记录）。

25.3　讨论

本技术源于团队前期肌腱愈合研究。传统观点认为肌腱缺乏内在修复能力[14]。本团队通过组织培养实验发现，经钻孔处理的肌腱缺损区仅边缘产生薄层成纤维细胞；若向缺损区注入富血小板血浆（PRP），则成纤维细胞会迅速向 PRP 基质迁移并分泌胶原；施加张力后，细胞活性增强且沿应力方向有序排列[15]。据此推测，生物合成支架在体内可能呈现类似的再生行为。

PRP 的应用可促进组织整合并加速创面愈合，核心机制是通过局部高浓度生长因子释放来实现生物学调控，这一特性使其成为外科领域重要的生物增效手段。

再生组织工程学在外科领域的应用日益广泛。Rehnke 等[16]曾报道利用三维支架结构实现乳房重建。

本技术通过将富含基质血管成分（SVF）及富血小板血浆（PRP）的三维支架置入网状间隙，可诱导周围组织与脂肪长入支架内部，形成具有再生潜力的自体组织，为后续脂肪移植创造理想微环境。既往研究虽报道过脂肪涂布补片技术成功用于乳房重建，但若脂肪未直接接触血供（尤其当补片间隙较大时），其存活率显著受限。因此，本团队创新性采用 SVF 包被海绵状补片——该结构富含胶原及活性细胞成分，可依赖组织液存活，其内部 PRP 填充的网状空间则为细胞长入提供理想基质（图 25.7）。

25.4 小结

应用生物合成材料补片实施胸肌前重建术，是改善乳房切除术后皮瓣状态（尤其是代偿胸肌缺损的上极区域）的理想选择。

该材料补片不仅可用于修复肿瘤切除形成的组织缺损，亦可在不依赖皮瓣或假体的情况下实现乳房重建。

对于已构建的支架结构，可通过Ⅱ期脂肪移植手术实现进一步扩容。

参考文献

1. Becker H, Fregosi N. The impact of animation deformity on quality of life in post-mastectomy reconstruction patients. Aesthet Surg J. 2017,37（5）:531–536. https://doi.org/10.1093/asj/sjw264. PMID: 28158447.
2. Gabriel A, Sigalove S, Sigalove NM, Storm-Dickerson TL, Rice J, Pope N, Maxwell GP. Prepectoral revision breast reconstruction for treatment of implant-associated animation deformity: a review of 102 reconstructions. Aesthet Surg J. 2018,38（5）:519–526. https://doi.org/10.1093/asj/sjx261. PMID: 29365064.
3. Campbell CA, Losken A. Understanding the evidence and improving outcomes with implant-based prepectoral breast reconstruction. Plast Reconstr Surg. 2021,148（3）:437e–450e. https://doi.org/10.1097/PRS.0000000000008229. PMID: 34432700.
4. Hallberg H, Rafnsdottir S, Selvaggi G, et al. Benefits and risks with acellular dermal matrix（ADM）and mesh support in immediate breast reconstruction: a systematic review and meta-analysis. J Plast Surg Hand Surg. 2018,52（3）:130–147. https://doi.org/10.1080/2000656x.2017.1419141.
5. Duncan D. Correction of implant rippling using allograft dermis. Aesthet Surg J. 2001,21（1）:81–84. https://doi.org/10.1067/maj.2001.113438.
6. Spear SL, Parikh PM, Reisin E, Menon NG. Acellular dermis-assisted breast reconstruction. Aesthet Plast Surg. 2008,32（3）:418–425. https://doi.org/10.1007/s00266–008–9128–8.
7. Becker H, Lind JG II. The use of synthetic mesh in reconstructive, revision, and cosmetic breast surgery. Aesthet Plast Surg. 2013,44（4）:1120–1127. https://doi.org/10.1007/s00266–020–01822-y.
8. Logan Ellis H, Asaolu O, Nebo V, Kasem A. Biological and synthetic mesh use in breast reconstructive surgery: a literature review. World J Surg Oncol. 2016,14（1）:121. https://doi.org/10.1186/s12957–016–0874–9.
9. Becker H, Vazquez OA, Rosen T. Cannula size effect on stromal vascular fraction content of fat grafts. Plast Reconstr Surg Glob Open. 2021,9（3）:e3471. https://doi.org/10.1097/GOX.0000000000003471. PMID: 33907655; PMCID: PMC8062151.
10. Gabling VLW, Açil Y, Springer IN, Hubert N, Wiltfang J. Platelet-rich plasma and platelet-rich fibrin in 13 human cell culture. Oral Surg Oral Med Oral Pathol Oral Radiol Endod. 2009,108（1）:48–55. https://doi.org/10.1016/j.tripleo.2009.02.007.
11. Gentile P, Calabrese C, De Angelis B, et al. Impact of the different preparation methods to obtain autologous non-activated platelet-rich plasma（A-PRP）and activated platelet-rich plasma（AA-PRP）in plastic surgery: wound healing and hair regrowth evaluation. Int J Mol Sci. 2020,21（2）:431. https://doi.org/10.3390/ijms21020431.
12. De Angelis B, D'Autilio MF, Orlandi F, et al. Wound healing: in vitro and in vivo evaluation of a biofunctionalized scaffold based on hyaluronic acid and platelet-rich plasma in chronic ulcers. J Clin Med. 2019,8（9）:1486. https://

doi.org/10.3390/jcm8091486.

13. Becker H, Mathew PJ. Immediate prepectoral breast reconstruction in suboptimal patients using an air-filled spacer. Plast Reconstr Surg Glob Open. 2019,7（10）:e2470. https://doi.org/10.1097/GOX.0000000000002470. PMID: 31772895; PMCID: PMC6846304.

14. Becker H, Graham MF, Cohen IK, Diegelmann RF. Intrinsic tendon cell proliferation in tissue culture. J Hand Surg Am. 1981,6（6）:616–619. https://doi.org/10.1016/s0363-5023（81）80146-3. PMID: 7310091.

15. Graham MF, Becker H, Cohen IK, Merritt W, Diegelmann RF. Intrinsic tendon fibrosis: documentation by in vitro studies. J Orthop Res. 1984,1（3）:251–256. https://doi.org/10.1002/jor.1100010304. PMID: 6481508.

16. Rehnke RD, Schusterman MA II, Clarke JM. Breast reconstruction using a three-dimensional absorbable mesh scaffold and autologous fat grafting: a composite strategy based on tissue-engineering principles. Plast Reconstr Surg. 2020,146（4）:409e–413e.